D0730892

Author **James E. Marti** is Executive Director of the Holistic Medical Research Foundation in San Anselmo, California, and has acted as a consultant to Fortune 500 companies in the U.S. and Europe. He served as coordinator of the Nonviolence Studies Program at Syracuse University, the first program of its kind in the U.S. to offer yoga, meditation, and stress reduction for academic credit. He subsequently founded the National Academy of Peace Committee, which successfully lobbied Congress to create the U.S. Peace Institute in 1976. His books include *The World Model* and the *New Book of World Rankings*.

Foreword writer and leading natural medicine authority **Michael T. Murray** maintains a private medical practice and serves on the faculty and the board of trustees at Bastyr University in Seattle, Washington. He is the author of several books on natural medicine, including *The Healing Powers of Herbs*, *The Getting Well Naturally Series*, *The Healing Power of Foods*, and *Alternatives to Over-the-Counter and Prescription Drugs*.

Andrea Hine holds degrees in cultural anthropology and Oriental and African Studies. She was the editor of the *New Book of World Rankings* and is currently editor and copywriter for the award-winning *Small Business Success*, the official national publication of the U.S. Small Business Administration. She also writes a biweekly column on small business issues.

MEDICAL ADVISORY BOARD

THE
Alternative
HEALTH &
MEDICINE
ENCYCLOPEDIA

ALSO FROM VISIBLE INK PRESS

Zimmerman's Complete Guide to Nonprescription Drugs

AS SEEN ON "DONAHUE"

> "The most comprehensive guide to over-the-counter drugs we've seen. . . . A highly recommended household reference." —*Publisher's Weekly*

Seventy-five chapters packed with product information and ratings take the guesswork out of choosing alternative treatments. By identifying safe and effective active ingredients in major brands, you'll discover less costly generic replacements that offer the same results.

2nd Ed. • Edited by David R. Zimmerman • 6" x 9" Paperback • 1,184 pp. • ISBN 0-8103-9421-9

The Best Hospitals in America

REVISED AND EXPANDED FROM THE POPULAR 1987 EDITION.

This guide to 87 top-rated medical facilities in the U.S. and Canada is written from a patient's point of view, drawing valuable input from physicians and other medical personnel to help you make and evaluate healthcare choices.

2nd Ed. • Edited by John Wright and Linda Sunshine • 6"x 9" Paperback • 500 pages • ISBN: 0-8103-9887-7

THE

Alternative
HEALTH &
MEDICINE
ENCYCLOPEDIA

JAMES MARTI
with Andrea Hine

Foreword by
DR. MICHAEL T. MURRAY

VISIBLE
INK
PRESS

DETROIT • WASHINGTON, D.C. • LONDON

The Alternative Health & Medicine Encyclopedia

Published by **Visible Ink Press**™
a division of Gale Research Inc.
835 Penobscot Bldg.
645 Griswold St.
Detroit MI 48226-4094

VISIBLE INK PRESS™ is a trademark of Gale Research Inc.

The Library of Congress has cataloged the Gale Research Inc. edition as follows:

Marti, James.
    The alternative health & medicine encyclopedia / by James Marti.
        p.   cm.
    Includes bibliographical references and index.
    ISBN 0–8103–9580–0
    1. Holistic medicine.   I. Title.   II. Title: Alternative health and medicine encyclopedia.
    R733.M38   1995
    615.5´3´03—dc20   94–34460
                                                                                    CIP

ISBN 0-8103-8303-9

Product Design Manager: Cynthia Baldwin
Cover and Page Design: Pamela A. E. Galbreath

Visible Ink Press books are available at special discounts for bulk purchases, for sales promotions, fund-raising, or educational purposes. Special editions can be created to specifications. For more information, contact: Special Markets Manager, Visible Ink Press, 835 Penobscot Bldg., 645 Griswold St., Detroit MI 48226.

CONTENTS

Chapter 1:
WHAT IS ALTERNATIVE MEDICINE?
Acupuncture and Acupressure • Ayurvedic Medicine •
Biofeedback • Botanical Medicine • Chiropractic Medicine •
Exercise • Homeopathy • Hypnosis • Meditation • Transcendental
Meditation • Naturopathic Medicine • Nutrition • Osteopathic
Medicine • Visualization Therapies • Yoga • Hydrotherapy •
Massage • Music Therapy • Alexander Technique • Aston
Patterning • Feldenkrais Method • Hellerwork • Kinesiology •
Rolfing • Choosing Alternative Care

Chapter 2:
NATURAL NUTRITION
Required Nutrients • Calories • Carbohydrates • Cholesterol •
Fiber • Lipids • Proteins • Recommended Dietary Allowance •
Nutrition for Children • Nutrition for the Elderly • Overweight
Americans • Weight-Loss Programs • Obesity • Anorexia
Nervosa • Bulimia

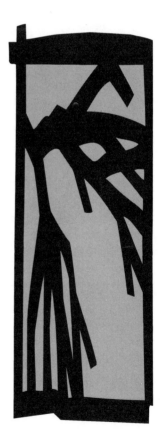

A paradigm is defined as a model used to explain events. As our understanding of the environment and the human body evolves, new paradigms emerge, including a new one for medicine. While the old medical paradigm viewed the body basically as a machine, the new paradigm focuses on the interconnectedness of body, mind, emotions, social factors, and the environment in determining health status. Rather than relying on drugs and surgery, the new model utilizes natural, noninvasive techniques to promote health and healing. Many of these healing techniques are now labeled as "alternative."

The Alternative Health & Medicine Encyclopedia provides information on some of the major components of this new medical paradigm. As this book details, alternative medicine emphasizes achieving health, not just eliminating disease; treatments that address underlying causes rather than just symptoms; and an integrated approach that treats the whole patient as opposed to specialization. The alternative therapies covered in this volume stress the role of diet, lifestyle, and preventative measures, a distinct contrast to conventional medicine's use of high technology. An additional difference of the new model is the importance of empathy and caring on the part of the physician. The alternative medicine practitioner is looked upon as a partner in the healing process–someone who informs, counsels, and assists the patient in making health-care choices.

An interesting aspect of the emerging medical paradigm is that it draws from the healing wisdom of many lands and cultures, including India (Ayurvedic), China (Taoist), and Greece (Hippocratic). Based on these traditions, four time-tested medical principles are being incorporated into modern medicine. I believe these four principles define the philosophy and foundation of natural medicine whether they are utilized by a naturopath (N.D.), medical doctor (M.D.), osteopath (D.O.), chiropractor (D.C.), or other health practitioner. These principles will assuredly continue to stand the tests of time.

Principle 1. The Healing Power of Nature. The human body has considerable power to heal itself. The role of the physician is to facilitate and enhance this process. Increasing evidence supports the contention that the healing process is best enhanced with the aid of natural, nontoxic therapies. The tremendous healing power of the mind is of particular interest.

Principle 2. First Do No Harm. As Hippocrates said, "Above all else, do no harm." In our current medical system, potential harm lies not only in drugs and surgical operations, but also in the inappropriate application of medications and procedures.

Principle 3. Identify and Treat the Cause. Of vital importance is the treatment of the underlying causes of a disease rather than simply suppressing the symptoms. Evidence is accumulating that many drug treatments are effective only in suppressing the symptoms, while many natural treatments actually address the cause.

Principle 4. The Physician as Teacher. The primary meaning of the word "doctor" is teacher. The physician's role is to teach the patient about achieving health and avoiding disease. As Thomas Edison once said, "The doctor of the future will give no medicine, but will interest his patient in the care of the human frame, in diet, and in the cause and prevention of disease."

The conventional medical doctor simply does not have time to teach. The typical first office visit lasts less than seven minutes, which usually provides only enough time for a doctor to make a quick diagnosis and write a prescription. In contrast, a typical first office visit with an alternative health-care practitioner is much more in-depth and may last an hour or longer. But making a careful assessment of a patient's health status and diagnosing disease is only one part of the healing process. Since alternative health-care providers consider teaching to be one of their primary goals, the time devoted to discussing and explaining principles of health is one of the aspects that sets them apart from conventional medical doctors.

Alternative medicine is a term I believe will be short-lived because what is now considered "alternative" will soon become part of the conventional medical approach. The nineteenth-century German philosopher Arthur Schopenhauer stated that all truth goes through three steps: First, it is ridiculed. Second, it is violently opposed. Finally, it is accepted as self-evident. At one time, alternative therapies were violently opposed by conventional medical groups, although numerous medical organizations that in the past had spoken out strongly against alternative medicine now endorse many aspects of it. For example, since the early 1900s, naturopathic physicians have extolled the value of eating more high-fiber foods; reducing the intake of refined sugars, fats, and cholesterol; and increasing the intake of dietary antioxidants. These same recommendations are now endorsed by the U.S. National Academy of Sciences, American Cancer Society, American Heart Association, and the American Diabetic Association. Another example is that at one time acupuncture was viewed as total quackery by the medical establishment. Now it is becoming much more widely accepted and is even taught at several medical schools across the United States.

The growing adoption of the principles and healing techniques of alternative medical practitioners by conventional medicine illustrates the paradigm shift occurring in medicine. Treatments once scoffed at are now becoming generally accepted as effective. In fact, in many instances clinical research is demonstrating that natural alternatives offer significant benefits over conventional medical treatments. In the future many of the concepts, philosophies, and techniques now considered alternative will be incorporated into conventional medical practice. How soon this shift occurs will depend upon how effectively the alternative medical community can get the information to consumers. *The Alternative Health & Medicine Encyclopedia* is a powerful step in the right direction.

Michael T. Murray, N.D.

Michael T. Murray is widely regarded as one of the world's leading authorities on natural medicine. In addition to maintaining a private medical practice, he serves on the faculty and the board of trustees at Bastyr University in Seattle, Washington. He is the coauthor of A Textbook of Natural Medicine, *the definitive textbook on naturopathic medicine for physicians,* The Encyclopedia of Natural Medicine, *and* Botanical Influences on Illness. *He has also written* The Healing Powers of Herbs, The Getting Well Naturally Series, The Healing Power of Foods, *and* Natural Alternatives to Over-the-Counter and Prescription Drugs.

PREFACE

In 1990, my mother developed breast cancer at the age of 78. A tennis instructor for four hours each day, she was told she would have to completely discontinue her physical activity and undergo radiation therapy. At the time, I was the executive director of the San Francisco Medical Research Foundation, one of the first American holistic medical foundations researching orthomolecular, nutritional, and psychoimmunological therapies for chronic degenerative diseases. I was familiar with Dr. Bernie Siegel's pioneering work with cancer patients, and advised my mother to visualize her radiation treatments as healing white light that would kill the cancer cells. I also sent her a daily supply of vitamin C crystals, chlorophyll, Green Magma (a green barley leaf from Sweden), and aloe vera juice to maintain the strength of her immune system. My mother took the botanical supplements each morning, underwent radiation treatments in her tennis togs, and afterward went out and played competitive senior tennis matches. Her cancer went into remission within three months.

My mother had been a competitive athlete for most of her life and, given her level of physical fitness, her recovery did not seem unusual to me. Recently, however, quite a number of remarkable cases of "spontaneous remission" cases involving ordinary people of different ages and levels of fitness have been documented. We now know from the studies of Dr. Siegel, Dr. Andrew T. Weil, Dr. David Spiegel, Dr. Dean Ornish, Dr. Deepak Chopra, and other leading alternative medical specialists that self-healing is a power that each of us possesses.

Alternative, or holistic, medicine is composed of many specialized therapies, each of which might be said to constitute a spoke on a wheel. Taken as a whole, they provide a comprehensive program for maintaining robust health and extending normal life span. Each of us inherits a set of biogenetic cards from our parents, which to some extent determines our ability to resist disease. Yet whatever advantages or limitations we inherit, we are all ultimately responsible for our own personal health. Consciously or unconsciously, we make choices every day regarding nutrition, exercise, vitamins and minerals, botanical supplements, stress reduction, avoiding toxins, and living harmoniously with the environment.

The Alternative Health & Medicine Encyclopedia presents the latest international medical data drawn from the disciplines of orthomolecular medicine, homeopathy, naturopathy, biochemistry, nutrition, psychoimmunology, chiropractic, bodywork, and Ayurvedic and Chinese medicine. Primary research was conducted at the UC Berkeley Medical Library and the Lane Medical Library at Stanford University. For international and foreign language journals, we relied on computerized Medline searches at the Marin General Hospital Library in Kentfield, California. Head librarian Kathy Resnick helped us comb through hundreds of foreign journal articles that had been translated and summarized in English. In some cases, the month, volume, number, or page numbers were not provided, especially for Chinese, Japanese, and Russian journals. Nevertheless, readers can still find the articles by author, title, and year in most medical libraries, or by Medline.

Our hope in writing this book is to clearly present the different specialized therapies that fall under the umbrella of alternative medicine. Which program or therapy will be right for you is a highly individual matter. The diversity of alternative medicine is its strength. There are many different paths to whole body health, although the goal of holistic practitioners is always the same: to empower the individual to achieve his or her personal best—the highest level of health possible. In one sense, alternative medicine is ultimately about attaining higher levels of consciousness and self-knowledge. We sincerely hope the information provided in this book empowers you to live a long, meaningful, and healthy life.

ACKNOWLEDGMENTS

A book of this scope is never the product of one individual's work. I have benefitted from a number of personal and professional acquaintances, without whose support this book would not have been possible. Foremost among these is Andrea Hine, my Stanford University colleague and co-author, with whom I have worked since 1989. This book is very much the product of her remarkable mind, careful research, and meticulous editing and writing.

This book afforded Ms. Hine and me the unique opportunity to collaborate with medical practitioners who are both competent and compassionate, and we wish to recognize the physicians and researchers who served on the *Encyclopedia*'s Medical Advisory Board. They are all prominent in their areas of specialty, and we thank them.

We are also indebted to several fine texts in medicine which were consulted in outlining this book. Specifically, we would like to acknowledge the *Encyclopedia of Natural Medicine,* by Michael Murray and Joseph Pizzorno, *Alternative Medicine: The Definitive Guide,* produced by the Burton Goldberg Group, *Prescriptions for Nutritional Healing,* by James Balch and Phyllis Balch, and *Health and Wellness: A Holistic Approach,* by Gordon Edlin and Eric Golanty.

Personally, I am especially grateful to Jane Hoehner, my editor at Gale Research, who shared the vision of this book and made it possible. She, along with Larry Baker, Diane Dupuis, Ellen Paré, and Dedria Bryfonski, believed in the importance of providing readers with holistic medical alternatives. Marlene Lasky and Maria L. Franklin of Gale's permissions staff worked tirelessly under a nearly impossible deadline. Lori Harper, my literary agent, is the best at what she does, combining integrity, intelligence, competence, and a wry sense of humor. I also am deeply indebted to Dr. Raphael Ornstein, founder of the San Francisco Medical Research Foundation, who has been my friend and colleague since 1980. Many of the discussions in this book are derived from our conversations over the years.

Most of all, I remain very grateful to the pioneers of alternative medicine. In the 1970s it was difficult for holistic practitioners to find a forum to present their life-enhancing views. In the last 25 years, the works of Dr. Herbert Benson, Dr. Joan Borysenko, Dr. Deepak Chopra, Dr. Dean Ornish, Dr. Raphael Ornstein, Dr. Kenneth Pelletier, Dr. Bernie

Siegel, and Dr. Andrew T. Weil have achieved international prominence. The popularity of their work is due, I believe, to vision and dedication. These practitioners, like holistic practitioners everywhere, believe passionately in the remarkable powers of the body to heal itself, in the higher powers of the mind, and in the idea that life is for all of us a journey toward higher consciousness. This book serves as a testament to their work.

INTRODUCTION

We live in extraordinary times and are witnessing an evolution of medical discoveries our ancestors would not have conceived possible. Virtually every day new breakthroughs are revealed, offering the promise that each of us may live longer, healthier lives free of medical complications. Many of these discoveries are being developed by medical practitioners and researchers in the alternative field—a wide variety of disciplines with a long history of success, and an increasingly broad number of adherents.

Dr. David Eisenberg of Harvard Medical School summarized a representative survey he conducted in a January 1993 article in the *New England Journal of Medicine,* which showed that more than 33 percent of American people preferred alternative medical treatments over conventional methods. The conditions for which most of those surveyed sought holistic medical care were cancer, arthritis, chronic back pain, AIDS, gastrointestinal problems, chronic renal failure, and eating disorders. Eisenberg's survey indicated that most Americans used alternative therapies in addition to conventional medical treatment or after conventional medical therapy had failed. To many Americans, alternative medicine was more accessible, more

humane, and more likely to treat the whole person rather than the symptoms only.

Partly as a response to the growing popularity of alternative medicine in the United States, President Clinton signed into law on June 14, 1993, the National Institutes of Health Revitalization Act, now known as Public Law 103-43. In the law, Congress permanently established the Office of Alternative Medicine (OAM) within the Office of the Director of National Institutes of Health. The purpose of OAM is "to facilitate the evaluation of alternative medical treatment modalities, including acupuncture and Oriental medicine, homeopathic medicine and physical manipulation therapies."

How to Use This Book

The Alternative Health & Medicine Encyclopedia is designed to acquaint readers of different ages, backgrounds, and interests with the major components of alternative medicine. As a medical system, alternative medicine is holistic—it views the mind and body as a living integrated system, and is based on the premise that the mind and body continually interact. For example, negative thoughts and emotions can adversely affect the body and lead to physiological disorders.

In turn, physiological imbalances can directly impact the mind and lead to psychological or emotional disorders.

Chapter 1 presents an overview of each specialty, from complete systems such as Ayurvedic medicine to very specialized bodywork therapies such as Aston Patterning. After reading Chapter 1, readers can turn directly to chapters that may be of particular interest to them. Beginning with Chapter 2, the specific components of alternative medicine are described in detail. The progression of the 19 chapters provides a comprehensive manual to maintaining vibrant health through nutrition, orthomolecular medicine, botanical medicine, detoxification, stress reduction, and psychoimmunological therapies such as positive thinking. Chapter 9 begins the discussion of alternative treatments for specific disorders. The index at the back of the book provides a quick reference to pages that discuss specific topics. There is a listing of resources included at the end of each chapter that cites references and additional books and articles on the topics discussed, as well as related organizations that can provide more information.

Chapter 1: What is Alternative Medicine?

The major components of modern alternative medicine detailed in Chapter 1 are based on holistic concepts of health that have been an integral aspect of the belief systems and healing practices of many cultures throughout history. Respect for and understanding of the unity of mind and body, for example, have always been basic precepts of the healing systems of Ayurvedic medicine, Chinese medicine, homeopathy, naturopathy, and chiropractic. In alternative medicine, health is defined as more than the absence of disease—it is the result of all our bodily systems being harmoniously in balance with each other and with the environment. In this state of equilibrium, our defense mechanisms and our immune system can efficiently respond to most of the hazards that life presents, whether these are pathogenic (disease-causing) organisms, toxic substances, or environmental or emotional stress factors.

Chapter 2: Natural Nutrition

Nutrition has always been one of the key components of alternative medicine because humans cannot live without nutrients. As Chapter 2 suggests, poor dietary habits comprise two separate problems: 1) many Americans overeat what they shouldn't eat—fats, oils, meats, and processed food, and 2) they often underconsume what they should eat—fresh, organically grown fruits and vegetables, whole grains, seeds, nuts, and fish.

Chapter 3: Vitamins

Chapter 3 summarizes a large body of research linking vitamin deficiencies to certain diseases—and describes how vitamin supplements have proven helpful in preventing them. All of the major vitamins are discussed, including the Recommended Dietary Allowances (RDA) for each and the foods in which they can be found.

Chapter 4: Minerals and Trace Elements

Minerals and trace elements are essential parts of enzymes that play an important role in many physiological processes. Most minerals and trace elements are available in foods, especially fresh fruits and vegetable. Chapter 4 discusses all of the important minerals and trace elements, the foods that contain them, daily recommended dosages, and how specific mineral deficiencies or excesses have been linked to chronic diseases.

Chapter 5: Botanical Medicines

More than 5,000 botanical plants have been extensively tested for medicinal uses. Chapter 5 analyzes more than 20 botanical medicines that have proven effective in clinical trials in treating common medical disorders, including botanicals that are widely used in the United States.

Chapter 6: Exercise

The human body stays healthy longer when it is regularly exercised—and most studies suggest that people should exercise at least three times a week for 20 minutes in order to prevent chronic degenerative disorders. Chapter 6 details 11 important medical benefits of exercise, surveys several important types of exercise, and provides physical activity guidelines for children, the elderly, and the disabled.

Chapter 7: Strengthening the Immune System

Every day people risk being exposed to more than 10,000 environmental toxins, many of which are poisonous. Many people suffer from chronic health problems simply because their bodies do not effectively eliminate toxins that can weaken the immune system. Chapter 7 discusses the most common (and often dangerous) toxins in the air, water, and foods, and suggests that one safe and effective method of eliminating toxic debris is through gentle detoxification programs which rejuvenate the immune system.

Chapter 8: Coping with Stress

The modern Western lifestyle is physically and emotionally stressful, and an estimated 70 to 80 percent of Americans who visit a physician suffer from stress-related disorders. Chapter 8 analyzes how the body responds to stress and provides alternative therapies for reducing stress and coping with its effects, including exercise, guided imagery, yoga, meditation, biofeedback, massage, group support, and nutritional, vitamin, and mineral therapies.

Chapter 9: Stress-Related Disorders

The direct relationship between stress and disease is now well known and widely accepted. Chapter 9 presents a variety of alternative therapies for preventing, treating, or reversing such stress-related disorders as headaches, hypertension, irritable bowel syndrome, ulcers, and atherosclerosis.

Chapter 10: Drug Abuse and Addiction

Many people take pharmaceutical drugs to relieve headaches, indigestion, tension, cramps, fatigue, or anxiety. In addition, an increasing number of people now take "recreational" or psychoactive drugs that stimulate pleasurable feelings and can alter thoughts, feelings, perceptions, or moods. An estimated 520,000 Americans die each year as a result of drug abuse, particularly cigarettes, alcohol, and hard drugs. Chapter 10 describes alternative treatments for drug dependencies and addiction that combine nutrition, exercise, vitamin and botanical supplements, and lifestyle changes.

Chapter 11: Mental Health Disorders

Everyone experiences emotionally stressful times and most people successfully develop ways to cope with these episodes. Some people, however, find it difficult to control their own thoughts, moods, fears, or emotional reactions to stressful life experiences. These individuals suffer from a variety of mental health disorders, including depression, panic disorders, or psychotic states such as schizophrenia. Chapter 11 suggests that alternative or holistic therapies such as nutrition, vitamins, minerals, amino acids, hormones, botanical medicines, exercise, and massage, when used in conjunction with psychotherapy, behavioral therapy, or psychoanalysis, can help treat many mental health disorders.

Chapter 12: Common Male Health Problems

The most common health problems in men involve disorders of the genitourinary system, which includes the bladder, urethra, prostate gland, penis, and testicles. Chapter 12 discusses alternative treatments for common health problems, such as low sexual energy, impotence, enlarged prostate (benign prostatic hypertrophy), and prostatitis.

Chapter 13: Common Female Health Problems

The average American woman can now expect to live a third of her life after menopause due to increased longevity rates. Approximately 40 million American women are now in or past menopause, and another 20 million will reach that stage of life in the next decade. Chapter 13 discusses new alternative therapies for preventing and treating common female health problems, including premenstrual syndrom (PMS), dysmenorrhea, vaginitis, and fibrocystic breast disease.

Chapter 14: Pregnancy, Childbirth, and Infant Care

Because the expectant mother and child are one biological organism until the moment of birth, whatever the woman puts into her body will most likely be passed on to her baby. Chapter 14 outlines a holistic approach to pregnancy, birthing, and infant care. It answers many of the common questions pregnant women ask about what foods and vitamin and mineral supplements they should consume, and the type and amount of exercise they should maintain.

Chapter 15: Dental Care

A comprehensive holistic approach to dental care is extremely important because the mouth is a primary site of many types of infection. As a result, dentists are often the first practitioners to diagnose cancers of the mouth, bulimia, diabetes, and other medical disorders. Chapter 15 presents guidelines for a thorough program of dental care and treating common dental disorders.

Chapter 16: Eye, Ear, Nose, and Throat Disorders

The eyes, ears, nose, and throat, along with the skin and mucous membranes, serve as the body's first line of defense against external toxins and infectious organisms. Chapter 16 focuses on alternative medical approaches to keeping these organs healthy and treating a wide variety of disorders that can affect them.

Chapter 17: Cancer

Currently, one out of every five Americans is likely to develop cancer during his or her lifetime, and in that group, one person in five is likely to die from it. It is estimated that 80 percent of all cancers could be prevented if people ate nutritious low-fat foods, did not smoke, and limited other unhealthy behaviors. Chapter 17 outlines several holistic options for treating cancer. Both alternative and conventional therapies, when given sufficient time to work, have helped people become healthier cancer patients— physically and emotionally. Alternative cancer therapies can in some cases help shift the balance toward improved outcomes.

Chapter 18: Heart Disorders

More Americans die each year from cardiovascular disease than from all other causes of death combined, including cancer, AIDS, infectious diseases, accidents, and homicides. Although heart disease causes nearly half of all deaths in the U.S., it is one of the most preventable chronic diseases. Eighty-five percent of all heart attacks, for example, are caused by atherosclerosis—the hardening of the coronary arteries that blocks blood flow to the heart. Chapter 18 outlines several holistic approaches to treating and reversing coronary artery disease.

Chapter 19: Aging

No matter how conscientious people are about diet, nutrition, exercise, vitamins, minerals, and botanical medicines, everyone ages. Although scientists have not been able to reverse the normal aging process, Chapter 19 outlines therapies that people can use to improve their strength, flexibility, and energy levels and subsequently protect themselves against age-related disorders such as Alzheimer's disease, senile dementia, and osteoporosis.

The Future of Alternative Medicine

In the next 50 years the rising cost of health care around the world and the public's demand for safer, less expensive medical therapies will produce new medical treatments that more fully integrate the mind and body. The conclusion brings together the members of the Medical Advisory Board established for *The Alternative Health & Medicine Encyclopedia,* who, in a roundtable format, discuss what alternative medicine will be like in the year 2050 and what new treatments might be available.

Interestingly, and not surprisingly, there was not complete consensus among the board members as to the future of alternative medicine, particularly in terms of the role technology will play. While they all agreed that people will be more interested in alternative medicine as a whole, some felt their own specialties, such as homeopathy, acupuncture, or chiropractic, would assume greater prominence. Several suggested that remarkable new therapies such as immunomodulating botanical or homeopathic remedies will emerge that slow the onset of the aging process. In the absence of consensus, the present disagreement as to what alternative medicine will produce in the future challenges proponents of each specialized area to further research their own disciplines as well as other fields of expertise. In the long run, this debate should result in new medical practices that will incorporate the proven and most helpful therapies from many different approaches.

One criticism shared by many people who find themselves dissatisfied with conventional medicine is that it tends to overlook innate emotional and psychological healing mechanisms. One reason that alternative, or holistic, medicine has become increasingly popular is because it puts the human touch into medical treatment. This approach is aptly summarized by Dr. Ed Weiss, acupuncturist and member of *The Alternative Health & Medicine Encyclopedia*'s Medical Advisory Board, who states: "I think it's being a human being, acting like a human being, being perceptive like a human being, and expressing love for your patient that leads to health. That's the most important thing holistic medicine should offer."

Chapter 1

WHAT IS ALTERNATIVE MEDICINE?

In the winter of 1988, San Francisco cardiologist Dean Ornish shocked the medical community when he proved that forty patients with advanced heart disease could actually shrink the fatty plaque deposits that were progressively blocking their coronary arteries. As the deposits were reduced, the patients' arteries began to open and oxygen was able to reach their hearts. As a result, most of the patients no longer suffered from chest pains or were no longer at risk of having another heart attack.

What was amazing about Ornish's clinical experiment was the therapy he used to make the plaque disappear. Ordinarily, Western heart specialists use surgery to reopen the clogged artery or bypass the artery altogether. Instead, Ornish used nature—the innate healing power of the body itself. Some of his patients "reversed" their disease with yoga, meditation, a low-cholesterol diet, exercise, and group therapy. After approximately one year of lifestyle changes, their clogged heart arteries had repaired themselves. The process is described in his 1990 book, *Dr. Dean Ornish's Program for Reversing Heart Disease.*

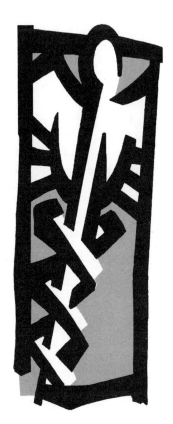

The medical therapies Ornish incorporated into his treatment represent the nucleus of what is called alternative, or holistic (whole body), medicine. Alternative medicine combines many different Eastern and Western medical specialties: Ayurvedic medicine, Chinese medicine, acupuncture and acupressure, nutrition, exercise, naturopathic medicine, homeopathic medicine, botanical medicine, chiropractic, and massage. However, just as there is no universal language, no single medical specialty—Eastern or Western, ancient or modern, scientific or unscientific—can provide the magic lantern that reveals all the mysteries of the human body. Each specialty has its strengths and weakness, its insights and limitations. Yet, taken together, the many specialties of alternative medicine offer great promise in helping people maintain optimal health.

That a vast number of people are seeking new ways to stay healthy outside of surgery and drugs was confirmed in a study reported in the *New England Journal of Medicine* which concluded that sixty million Americans used some type of unconventional medical therapy in 1992, spending more than $14 billion. Holistic options are increasing for those who wish to explore whole body therapies to maintain health and to prevent or treat chronic illness and disease. The following sections discuss major specialties of the alternative approach.

An old Chinese prayer says: "When you have a disease, do not try to cure it. Find your chi and you will be healed." Chinese medicine is based on the belief that humanity is part of a larger creation—the universe—and subject to the same laws that govern nature. All life and the entire material universe are said to originate from a single source called Tao—an integrated whole that is present in everything. Tao creates two opposing forces—yin and yang—archetypal opposites that are incomplete without the other and that combine to create all phenomena.

According to Dr. Yuan-Chi Lin, an associate professor of anesthesia and pediatrics at the Stanford University Medical Center, "Yin is present in the qualities of cold, rest, passivity, darkness, inwardness and decrease. Yang is associated with heat, activity, stimulation, light, outwardness and increase." In his book, *Pain in Infants, Children, and Adolescents,* written with John D. Yee and Paul A. Aubuchon, Lin says, "Health requires a balance of yin and yang within a given person, while disease is characterized by a disharmony or lack of balance between these two dynamic forces."

Within the body, the balance of yin and yang is manifest in the flow of an energy called chi (or the life force), which flows through the body in precise and orderly patterns called meridians. There are fourteen meridians, twelve associated with organs in the body and two that are responsible for unifying various systems. Each meridian, which runs vertically from the head to the feet, moving chi to specific parts of the body, is classified as yin or yang. Every part of the body is nourished with chi energy unless a meridian becomes blocked or stagnant, causing an imbalance in the flow of the life force. Certain organs, for example, can become excessive or hyperactive (yang), while others can become deficient or hypoactive (yin). There also can be excessive swelling or expansion (yang), or too much contraction (yin). Without adequate life force, tissues and organs can no longer efficiently eliminate waste from cells. As waste products accumulate, the blood-cleansing organs become stressed, and eventually lose their capacity to clean the blood. This accumulation of toxins (such as fat, cholesterol, ammonia, uric acid, triglycerides, and carbon dioxide) weakens the immune system to the point where a virus can take hold in the body. More specifically, according to Chinese thought, the accumulation diminishes the life force that is the foundation of health.

In Chinese medicine, all treatment is meant to bring about harmony between deficiency and excess, or between yin and yang. Foods, herbs, and other therapeutic techniques are used to restore this balance. Thus, a Chinese doctor might use acupuncture, acupressure, herbs, tai chi (a Chinese martial art like karate or judo which combines slow, balanced, and low-impact movements), moxibustion (heat applied to acupuncture points), or massage to increase or decrease the chi flow as needed.

Acupuncture and Acupressure

In his "Healing and the Mind" television series on the Public Broadcasting System (PBS), Bill Moyers visited a hospital in China where a thirty-five-year-old woman was undergoing an operation to remove a large tumor in her pituitary gland. Amazingly, the woman was conscious and able to talk to her doctor during the surgery. She reportedly felt no pain, despite being given only half the drugs that would be administered in the West, because her physician used acupuncture needles to help anesthetize her.

In China, acupuncture is most commonly applied for anesthesia. But it also is used to rebalance a chi disturbance in a patient—whether caused by an external influence such as coldness, an emotional influence such as excess anger, poor diet, or an organ imbalance. Acupuncture, like all Chinese medical therapies, seeks to diagnose a chi imbalance before a detectable physiological impairment occurs. Acupuncturists focus on helping patients balance the chi energy within and between the five major organ systems: the heart, lungs, liver, spleen, and kidneys.

To restore health, an acupuncturist uses tiny needles as antennas to direct chi to organs or functions of the body. The needles also can be used to drain chi where it is excessive, to warm parts of the body that are cool or stagnant, to decrease or increase moisture, and to reduce excessive heat. The acupuncturist does this by selecting points along the body's fourteen meridians that affect the functioning of specific organs and then using needles to slightly puncture and stimulate bodily tissue at these locations. The needles penetrate just below the epidermis and do not draw blood or cause discomfort. Sometimes heat is used, along with massage or electrical pulses.

The World Health Organization (WHO) currently recognizes more than forty medical problems, ranging from allergies to arthritis and AIDS, that can be helped by acupuncture treatment. According to Lin, acupuncture has become a respected therapy in American hospitals in the last twenty years, and is used to reduce pain in patients with sore throats, sickle-cell anemia, dysmenorrhea, dental surgery, hysterectomies, chronic back disorders, and migraine headaches. It has been used successfully to induce smoking cessation, and to treat alcoholism and opiate addiction (see Chapter 10). Lin's book contains a study which suggests that acupuncture can also effectively reduce pain in patients undergoing cancer chemotherapy.

Acupressure is a form of acupuncture in which fingers and thumbs rather than needles are used to press chi points on the surface of the body. Acupressure relieves muscular tension, which enables more blood—and therefore more oxygen and nutrients—to be carried to tissue throughout the body. This helps promote both physical calmness and mental alertness, and aids in healing by removing waste products. Many researchers now believe that, like acupuncture, acupressure triggers the release of endorphins, the neurochemicals that relieve pain.

Acupressure has been used successfully by both Eastern and Western practitioners to relieve mental tension and stress, tired and strained eyes, headaches, menstrual cramps, and arthritis. Acupressure also is used to promote general health care, relieve stiff necks and shoulders, prevent and combat colds, improve muscle tone, and boost energy levels.

More than fifteen million Americans have visited acupuncturists or acupressurists. Today, approximately nine thousand acupuncturists practice in the U.S. In most states, they must be medical doctors and have certification from the National Commission for the Certification of Acupuncturists. However,

---

Consulting An Acupuncturist

According to Dr. Yuan-Chi Lin, an associate professor of anesthesia and pediatrics at Stanford University Medical Center, these factors may be involved in a visit to an acupuncturist:

• The acupuncturist uses a history and physical examination of the patient in making a diagnosis.

• In addition to asking questions, attention also is focused on the character of the pulse and the appearance of the tongue.

• Unlike Western medicine, sophisticated biological testing is not employed.

• The goal of the history and the physical is to assess the balance of yin and yang in the patient, and to guide the acupuncturist in selecting the correct acupuncture points for a particular condition.

• Several treatments may be required over a period of weeks or months.

• The goal of therapy is to correct deficiencies or excesses of chi, thus restoring health.

---

some states do not regulate the practice at all, and it is advisable to check a practitioner's credentials.

Ayurvedic Medicine

In Boston, a thirty-nine-year-old woman whose cancer had traveled to her lymph nodes and twelve different sites in her bones consulted a well-known Ayurvedic doctor because her chemotherapy sessions left her without energy, her white blood cell count was consistently low, and her chances of survival were estimated to be only one percent. The physician prescribed a long-term Ayurvedic regimen that included meditation, revised diet and sleep patterns, massage, herbal preparations, yoga, and even exposure to certain sounds and aromas. After several years of treatment, her cancer went into remission, her general health was good, and her blood chemistry returned to the normal range, according to Craig Lambert in his article, "The Chopra Prescriptions," published in the September–October 1989 issue of *Harvard Magazine*.

This woman's case is far from an isolated one. While Westerners might consider her treatment to be "alternative," Ayurvedic medicine has been practiced in India for more than six thousand years. In Sanskrit, "Ayurveda" means the "science of life and longevity." The Ayurvedic approach treats the person, not just the disease, so each regimen is highly individualized. It is based on the premise that health is a state of balance among the body's systems—physical, emotional, and spiritual. Illness is seen as a state of imbalance.

Ayurvedic medicine has been popularized in the West by Dr. Deepak Chopra, whose best-selling books, *Perfect Health: The Complete Mind/Body Guide* and *Ageless Body/Timeless Mind,* clearly describe how it works. According to Chopra, "the guiding principle of Ayurveda is that the mind exerts the deepest influence on the body, and freedom from sickness depends upon contacting our own awareness, bringing it into balance, and then extending that balance to the body. This state of balanced awareness...creates a higher state of health."

Ayurvedic medicine stresses a holistic approach to health. It defines disease as the result of climatic extremes, bacterial attack, nutritional deviance, and stress, as well as other forms of emotional imbalance. Optimal health is achieved by cultivating mental and physical habits that are conducive to physical and spiritual well-being, and treatment often includes hatha yoga, diet, and the development of positive attitudes.

Biofeedback

For thousands of years, Eastern mystics have demonstrated the ability to control their heart rate, skin temperature, blood pressure, and other "involuntary" functions through concentration and willpower. Western physicians have begun experimenting with biofeedback machines to accomplish the same result. People suffering from migraine headaches, for example, can be connected to biofeedback machines that monitor bodily functions such as skin temperature, blood pressure, sweat, and electrical responses. Once hooked up to a machine, patients learn to consciously will a desired result, such as lowering their blood pressure. Electrodes attached to the body provide readings that give patients feedback to determine whether their mental powers are causing the desired physiological change.

Most health problems alleviated by biofeedback are related to stress and hypertension. This technique has proved particularly successful in the treatment of insomnia, asthma, menstrual cramping, irritable bowel syndrome, and pain symptoms involving chronically tight muscles.

Along with pelvic muscle exercises, biofeedback has been used to treat sphincteric incontinence in older women. Biofeedback also has been used as an adjunct therapy in physical training of people with spinal cord injuries, although exercise therapy has proven much more important.

Biofeedback offers promise as one method of partially treating schizophrenia and depression. It has been incorporated as a noninvasive technique for controlling parasympathetic cardiac arrhythmia. One Australian study suggests that biofeedback therapy can help patients recover from strokes. M.A. Benninga, in the January 1993 *Archives of Disease in Childhood,* and N.R. Binnie, in the September–October *World Journal of Surgery,* report how clinicians have used biofeedback to treat rectal ulcer syndrome, pediatric sickle-cell anemia, and cerebral palsy in children. R.E. Thomas, in the April 1993 issue of *Ergonomics* writes that it may prove helpful in treating carpal tunnel syndrome (CTS). Limited trials have shown the ability of biofeedback to control hyperactivity in children. Finally, it may offer a direct symptomatic treatment for reflex sympathetic dystrophy (RSD), an unusual debilitating chronic pain syndrome thought to be associated with continuous excessive discharge of regional sympathetic nerves. For a complete list of clinical trials using biofeedback and for more information and referrals, contact the Association for Applied Psychophysiology and Biofeedback.

Botanical Medicine

In China, when patients go to a clinic to pick up their medicine, they generally do not receive a pill. Instead, they are likely to be given a packet or pot containing a mixture of plants and herbs that a physician has prescribed for the patient's specific disorder. Some prescriptions are six hundred years old. Each has a written formula and may contain a combination of herbs, plants, plant roots, and, in some cases, a variety of animal parts such as oxen antlers or parts of a scorpion.

Many Western scientists assume that these botanical plants are effective because they contain chemicals that help a diseased part of the body to heal itself. However, Chinese doctors do not prescribe botanical medicines because of their active chemical ingredients, but because such medicines increase or decrease the patients vital life energy, or chi.

The World Health Organization estimates that 80 percent of the world's population relies primarily on traditional medicine for health care, including the use of plants. In the U.S., botanical plants were primary agents in medicine until the development of new pharmaceutical drugs in laboratories during the 1940s and 1950s. Even today, 25 percent of pharmaceutical drugs are derived directly from plants, according to Dr. Andrew Weil, author of both *Health and Healing* and *Natural Health, Natural Medicine*. Among the most important are the birth-control pill, originally derived from the Mexican yam; the heart medication digitalis, which comes from the foxglove plant; and the bark of the Pacific yew tree, which has yielded a promising new drug called taxol to treat ovarian and breast cancers. Beta-carotene, found in abundance in certain fruits and vegetables, is considered to be a powerful preventive agent against cataracts, high cholesterol, stress, and hypertension. Herbal preparations from leaves, seeds, stems, flowers, roots, and bark have proven very useful for chronic and mild conditions by aiding natural healing and stimulating the body's return to balanced health.

Natural botanical medicines taken wholly and directly from plants are widely available in the U.S., and sales of herbal medicines have grown as much as 20 percent a year for the last several years, according to an August 1993 article in *The Boomer Report*. However, most Americans take pharmaceutical medicines. Natural botanical medicines, including herbs, are not the same as the pharmaceutical

drugs that are synthesized from them. For example, botanicals are much milder in effect than drugs. Natural botanical drugs also release more slowly into the bloodstream when they are bound up with other inert components in the plant that prevent quick release into the digestive tract. As a result, Ayurvedic physicians only prescribe herbs extracted from whole plants because the herb's active ingredient is packaged along with other natural chemicals that offset possible undesirable effects. In addition, pharmaceutical drugs may lend themselves more easily to abuse, addiction, and toxicity, according to Weil.

Chiropractic Medicine

In 1895, Daniel David Palmer, a self-educated scientist and magnetic healer from Iowa, was waiting in his office for a patient, when his janitor, Harvey Lillard, who had been deaf for seventeen years, walked by. Noticing a small bump on the back of Lillard's neck, Palmer pushed it in and Lillard suddenly declared that he could hear.

From this event, Palmer deduced that the nervous system was the ultimate control mechanism of the body and that even minor misalignments of the spine, which he termed "subluxations," could significantly impact a person's health. And thus, the term chiropractic—literally, "done by hand"—a method of restoring wellness through adjustments of the spine, was coined. Palmer, however, credited the ancient Greeks with inventing the technique as early as 1250 B.C.

Palmer opened his own school of chiropractics in 1895. According to Thomas Weisman, a Novato, California-based "network chiropractor," the basis of Palmer's technique was that "as many as 31 different pairs of spinal nerves travel through openings in the vertebrae to and from the brain. If one of the vertebrae is partly displaced from its correct position, it can cause an impingement and pressure or irritate the surrounding nerves. As a result, essential nerve messages are distorted, which may cause damage to the surrounding muscles or tissues. Since the nervous system regulates all systems of the body, including the digestive, respiratory, circulatory, immune, muscular and elimination systems, subluxations can have far-reaching effects."

Today, an estimated fifty thousand chiropractors practice in the United States. The largest group consists of "broad scope" chiropractors who manipulate the spine to restore nerve flow and function, but whose goal is to diagnose, treat, and eliminate specific symptoms and conditions, usually associated with backaches and headaches. They sometimes incorporate other methods of treatment such as physical therapy, nutrition, and acupuncture.

The remaining American "straight" or "network" chiropractors, such as Weisman, practice in Palmer's tradition. Rather than diagnosing or treating specific conditions or symptoms, they treat subluxations (or partial dislocations of the spine) in an effort to restore normal nerve flow. Also, whereas "broad scope" chiropractic focuses entirely on physical stress and trauma to the spine, "network" chiropractic includes emotional, mental, and chemical factors that create tension in the spinal system and soft tissues.

Weisman states that "everybody is born with their own internal organizing power or innate intelligence. The chiropractor's sole function is to adjust the spine to eliminate any subluxations he is able to detect which are obstructing the expression of this innate intelligence through the nervous system."

"There are no diseases, only dis-ease," Weisman continues. "Diseases, symptoms, or conditions which are distressing our physical or emotional make-up are reflections of the mind-body being out of sync with its natural rhythm."

Many studies have documented benefits of chiropractic therapy. One published in 1990, for example, found that chronic low-back pain patients who were treated at chiropractic clinics ended up with less pain and more mobility than those treated at conventional hospitals. Another study published in 1991 concluded that people with acute low-back pain not caused by neurological complications could significantly boost their odds of recovering within three weeks by undergoing spinal manipulation.

Weisman related a 1986 study conducted at the University of Lund in Sweden which suggested that chiropractic treatment may significantly reduce the risk of immune breakdown and disease. Three different control groups were exposed to hazardous environmental chemicals linked to cancer: Group 1 consisted of healthy individuals who received long-term chiropractic care, Group 2 included healthy individuals who did not receive chiropractic care, and Group 3 consisted of people with cancer or other serious diseases who received no chiropractic treatment. Those individuals who received chiropractic care had 200 percent greater immunocompetence than Group 2, and 400 percent greater immunocompetence than Group 3. All chiropractic patients were "genetically normal"— that is, they had no obvious genetic reasons for increased resistance or susceptibility to disease. Ronald Pero, Ph.D., one of the investigators, concluded that "chiropractic may optimize whatever genetic abilities you have. I'm very excited to see that without chemical intervention...this particular group of patients under chiropractic care did show a very improved response."

In the U.S., chiropractors constitute the third largest medical profession after physicians and dentists. They are licensed to practice without supervision or referral from medical doctors in every state. They cannot, however, prescribe drugs or perform surgery. Those with a D.C. degree (Doctor of Chiropractic) have completed at least four years of training at an accredited chiropractic college.

Hospitals are increasingly adding chiropractors to their medical staffs, and their services are widely reimbursed by Medicare, Medicaid, workers' compensation, and private insurance. Surveys indicate that fifteen to twenty million Americans visited a chiropractor in 1992, the majority of them for treatment of low-back pain, according to Rick Weiss, in his article, "Bones of Contention," in the July/August 1993 issue of *Health.*

Exercise

In the Orient, there is an old expression: The body is like a hinge on a door. If it is not swung open, it will rust.

Virtually all cultures recognize the importance of regularly moving all parts of the body. In India, yogic exercise has played an important role in Ayurvedic medicine for over 6,000 years. Similarly, in China, exercise has been practiced for 2,500 years using martial arts such as tai chi.

Given the critical importance of regular exercise, it is surprising that an estimated 75 percent of all Americans, including children, do not exercise enough.

Many studies, as cited in Chapters 6 and 7, have shown that people who exercise regularly have fewer illnesses than sedentary persons. Vigorous exercise benefits the body both directly and indirectly by stimulating the immune system and enabling people to cope with a variety of stressors and toxins. The psychological benefits are equally as important, and exercise has been successfully used to treat disorders such as depression.

Regular exercise is usually part of any holistic medical program because, next to diet, it most effectively produces total body health. In fact, the American Cancer Society now recommends regular exercise as part of its ten-step program to prevent cancer. The many functions exercise plays in maintaining health and preventing disease are documented in Chapter 6.

Homeopathy

In *Health and Healing,* Weil describes how he once developed sudden attacks of pain that started in the center of his chest and eventually radiated to the middle of his back and his left shoulder, throat, and jaw. The pain was accompanied by difficulty in swallowing, as if something was lodged in the bottom of his esophagus. After consulting with several medical doctors, who could not relieve the pain, Weil visited a friend (previously an M.D.) who had become a homeopath. The friend asked him a number of questions not directly related to the specific pain, including questions pertaining to lifestyle and sleeping patterns.

The homeopath then diagnosed Weil as having symptoms provoked by elemental sulfur and gave him a vial of tiny white pellets that were lactose (milk sugar) covered with a drop of a dilute suspension of sulfur. After Weil took the pellets the pains completely disappeared and never returned. He describes the incident in his book, *Health and Healing,* published in 1983.

Homeopathy was founded in the late eighteenth century by the German physician Samuel Hahnemann, who became discouraged by prevailing medical techniques, such as bloodletting and blistering and the use of toxic substances such as mercury, to treat illness. He began experimenting with cinchona bark, which contains quinine, at that time a well-known remedy for fever and malaria. He found that while cinchona produced fever in healthy individuals, it relieved fever in people with malaria. Based on these experiments, Hahnemann stated in his *Organon of Medicine,* "A substance that produces a certain set of symptoms in a healthy person has the power to cure a sick person manifesting those same symptoms." He coined the name homeopathy, joining the Greek words "homoios," which means "like," and "pathos," for "suffering or sickness." Hahnemann maintained that the presence of an illness stimulates the body's defense system to combat the illness. The defensive reaction produces symptoms that are part of the body's effort to rid itself of the underlying disease. The symptoms are not the illness, Hahnemann claimed, but part of the curative process. This contrasts with the traditional view that symptoms are a manifestation of the disease itself.

Once a homeopath has diagnosed a disorder in a patient, a diluted solution to treat the problem is prescribed. This is done by matching or "proving" symptoms with the one substance that most closely reproduces these symptoms in a normal person.

Since Hahnemann's pioneering work, homeopaths have kept detailed clinical records of the results of giving small amounts of many different substances to volunteer subjects in good health. These substances contain chemicals, minerals, plant extracts, dilute preparations of animal and insect venoms, disease-causing germs, and some standard drugs. Matching the patient's symptoms with the substance that most closely reproduces them is crucial, because homeopaths assert that a single dose of that substance, highly diluted and properly prepared, has the capacity to cure the ailing patient.

To date, there have not been an extensive number of controlled clinical studies evaluating the effectiveness of homeopathic treatment. In 1991, however, three Dutch epidemiologists published an exhaustive review of 107 controlled experiments in which homeopathic remedies or placebos (dummy pills) were prescribed. The researchers concluded that the homeopathic remedies were more effective than the placebos in treating a variety of common problems including migraine headaches, dry cough, and ankle sprains, according to an article in the April 1991 issue of *HealthFacts.*

Since Hahnemann first published his findings in 1810, millions of people have relied exclusively on homeopathy for the treatment of all types of illnesses. According to the National Center for Homeopathy, sales of homeopathic medicine increased 50 percent between 1988 to 1990, reaching $150 million. Despite homeopathy's documented effectiveness, however, the American Medical Association (AMA) does not recognize homeopathic medicine because it believes the approach is not based on scientific principles. Currently, only three states (Arizona, Connecticut, and Nevada) license homeopaths and, as a result, a homeopathic practitioner may be licensed under other accepted forms of medicine, such as a medical doctor, acupuncturist, osteopath, or chiropractor.

Hypnosis

In *Beyond Biofeedback,* Elmer and Alyce Green of the Menninger Clinic describe the case of a patient with a painful pelvic cancer the size of a grapefruit. The patient was hypnotized and asked to find the room in his brain where valves controlled the blood supply to his body. He was told to turn off the valve that regulated the blood flow to his tumor. He did so, and during two months of sessions the tumor shrank to one-fourth its former size.

Hypnosis, like meditation, visualization, guided imagery, and spiritual exercises, is another method by which physicians can induce a positive mental state of healing in patients. According to the Office of Alternative Medicine at the National Institutes of Health, studies show that hypnosis can help patients heal faster and experience less pain. For example, many babies have been delivered by cesarean section using only hypnosis and no pain-relieving medications.

Through relaxation and concentration, hypnosis has proven successful in relieving such conditions as chronic back pain, ulcers, and morning sickness. In one study, documented by T.M. Laidlaw in the April 1993 *International Journal of Clinical & Experimental Hypnosis,* thirty-two patients with high hypnotizability recovered faster from cardiac surgery after being treated with formal hypnosis. Psychiatrists have also used hypnosis to treat diseases that manifest themselves as behavioral compulsions, such as phobias and eating disorders, and to help patients remember and deal with traumatic events. In most cases, patients learn self-hypnosis, which they can then apply themselves if the problem recurs.

In a University of Colorado Health Sciences Center study, hemophiliacs under hypnosis successfully reduced their need for blood transfusions. By reducing their need for blood transfusions, they significantly reduced their exposure to the AIDS virus and lowered their risk of liver and kidney damage. Self-hypnosis apparently provided the hemophiliacs with increased feelings of control and confidence and improved the quality of their lives. Hypnosis may also offer a powerful tool in helping patients with mental or dissociative disorders, reports W. LeBaw, in the 1992 issue of *Psychiatric Medicine.*

According to D. Spiegel in the July 1993 *American Journal of Psychiatry,* hypnosis has proven extremely effective in helping people to stop smoking. In one study of 226 smokers treated with self-hypnosis, 52 percent achieved complete abstinence only one week after the intervention. However, Dr. Roger Kennedy, internist and bioethicist at Kaiser Permanente Medical Center in Santa Clara, California, notes that people who use hypnosis to stop smoking have a high rate of relapse. Hypnosis is now recognized as a useful adjunctive treatment for excess weight, reports C. Kranhold in the March 1992 issue of *European Archives of Psychiatry and Clinical Neuroscience,* although very few controlled studies have been conducted on this topic.

Hypnotherapists are not regulated or licensed by the federal government or by state agencies, but many are licensed by the American Society of Clinical Hypnosis, whose members include medical doctors, dentists, psychiatrists, psychologists, nurses, and social workers.

Meditation

In his book, *Love, Medicine & Miracles,* Dr. Bernie Siegel defines meditation as "an active process of focusing the mind into a state of relaxed awareness. There are many ways of doing this. Some teachers recommend focusing attention on a symbolic sound or word (a mantra) or on a single image, such as a candle flame or a mandala. Others teach people to focus on the sound and flowing of the breath. The result of all meditation methods is ultimately the same: to induce a restful trance which strengthens the mind by freeing it from its accustomed turmoil."

In the last twenty-five years, a considerable body of research by Dr. Deepak Chopra, Dr. Bernie Siegel, Dr. Jon Kabat-Zinn, and others, has demonstrated how meditation benefits health. For example, blood chemistry reports have shown a lessening of lactate in the blood (lactate is related to high levels of anxiety). Also, electroencephalograms have shown an increase in alpha brain wave activity (alpha waves are present during states of deep relaxation and creativity). Meditation tends to lower or normalize blood pressure, pulse rate, and the levels of stress hormones in the blood. It also lowers abnormally high cholesterol levels and reduces mild hypertension. There is also evidence that with regular practice over a substantial period of time, meditation may increase concentration, memory, intelligence, and creativity.

Transcendental Meditation

Transcendental Meditation (TM) was introduced to the West in the 1960s by Maharishi Mahesh Yogi of India, and currently boasts more than three million practitioners in 110 countries. The aim of TM is to transcend normal thought processes to a heightened level of awareness called cosmic consciousness, producing in the body and mind a sense of profound rest and relaxation. The technique involves the mental repetition of a mantra, or Sanskrit sound, that is given to new practitioners by a TM instructor. TM's technique involves sitting comfortably in a chair with the spine erect, the body relaxed, and the eyes closed while the mantra is repeated silently for twenty minutes.

In 1975, Harvard professor Dr. Herbert Benson discovered that TM evoked a mechanism in the body that is the opposite of the "fight-or-flight response," the involuntary reaction to perceived danger that speeds up the body's processes (affecting heartbeat, blood pressure, and metabolic rate) while lowering immune system resistance. Benson called this opposite mechanism that the "relaxation response." The relaxation response can be evoked by sitting quietly and willing the body to relax and to assume its natural state of internal harmony. Two factors

The Medical Benefits of Meditation

- Lessens lactate in the blood (lactate is related to high levels of anxiety).
- Increases alpha brain wave activity (alpha waves are present during states of deep relaxation and creativity).
- Lowers or normalizes blood pressure, pulse rate, and the levels of stress hormones in the blood.
- Lowers abnormally high cholesterol levels.
- Reduces mild hypertension.
- May increase concentration, memory, intelligence, and creativity.
- Enhances immune system resistance.
- Induces the "relaxation response."

are vital: the repetition of a word or phrase and relaxation of the entire muscle system. According to Benson, the key to relaxation in all of these exercises is the passive disregard for intruding thoughts.

Naturopathic Medicine

The term "naturopathic" was first coined in 1895 by Dr. John Scheel to describe a combination of natural therapies that included nutritional therapy, herbal medicine, homeopathy, spinal manipulation, exercise therapy, hydrotherapy, electrotherapy, stress reduction, and natural cures. Naturopathy subsequently was popularized by a German-born healer named Benedict Lust, who in 1902 founded

A Naturopathic View of Disease

Dr. Ross Trattler, naturopath and author of *Better Health Through Natural Healing* (McGraw-Hill, 1988), summarizes the basic disease process and its causes as follows:

- Accumulation of toxic material within the body due to poor circulation, poor elimination, and lack of exercise.

- Unhealthy diet that is rich in harmful ingredients (fat, cholesterol, sugar, artificial ingredients, and excess protein) and low in essential vitamins, minerals, and fiber.

- Improper posture and body structure, including spinal misalignment, poor muscle tone, and blood and lymph stagnation.

- Destructive emotions including fear, stress, resentment, hatred, and self-pity, all of which have a debilitating effect on internal organs and the immune system.

- Suppressive drugs, such as antibiotics and vaccinations, which some studies have found depress the immune system.

- Excessive alcohol, coffee, and tobacco.

- Environmental agents in the soil, air, water, and workplace.

- Parasites, viruses, and infection.

- Genetic factors that create specific weaknesses, which allow accumulated toxins and these other factors to manifest as disease.

the American School of Naturopathy. Lust defined naturopathy as the use of nontoxic healing methods derived from Greek, Oriental, and European medical traditions. Naturopathy shares with these systems a belief in an underlying life force and views disease as the result of a healing effort of nature.

Naturopathic medicine assumes that the body is always striving for health. If an illness develops, the symptoms accompanying it are the result of the organism's intrinsic attempt to defend and heal itself. A naturopathic physician thus focuses on aiding the body in its effort to regain its natural health, rather than initiating a treatment that might interfere with this process.

Naturopathic doctors prefer nontoxic and noninvasive treatments that minimize the risks of harmful side effects. They are trained

to distinguish which patients they can treat safely and which need referral to other health care practitioners. Naturopaths currently are licensed to practice in all but seven states in the U.S. Naturopathic physicians who have attended an accredited four-year program are trained in most of the same scientific disciplines taught in conventional medical schools. Consequently, most naturopaths use medical tests, such as blood or urine analysis, for diagnosis. Many naturopaths may use modern medicine, including drugs and surgery in certain crisis situations, although they remain committed to using nontoxic and noninvasive methods. Currently, licensing for naturopathic physicians is available in seven states: Alaska, Arizona, Connecticut, Hawaii, Montana, Oregon, and Washington. There are two accredited colleges in the United States that offer degrees in naturopathic medicine: Bastyr College in Seattle,

Consulting a Naturopath

Naturopath Michael Murray, coauthor of the *Encyclopedia of Natural Medicine* and a member of the faculty of Bastyr College in Seattle, Washington, describes how naturopaths counsel patients:

• During the first visit, which normally lasts an hour, a naturopath uses history-taking, physical examination, laboratory tests, and other standard diagnostic procedures to learn as much as possible about the patient.

• Diet, environment, exercise, stress, and other aspects of lifestyle also are evaluated.

• Once a good understanding of the patient's health and disease is established (making a diagnosis of a disease is only one part of this process), the doctor and patient work together to establish a treatment and health-promoting program.

Washington, and Southwest College in Scottsdale, Arizona.

Nutrition

It is impossible to maintain optimal health without eating natural, nutritious foods. Many holistic physicians consider nutrition the most important aspect of alternative medicine. This is so because, like automobile engines, the human body cannot run without fuel—or energy. While certain people may be genetically strong, physically fit, and free of disease, if they ate strictly sugar, saturated fats, cholesterol, salt, and additives, the likelihood is that they would eventually become sick. If, on the other hand, they ate strictly natural, unprocessed foods, particularly fruits, vegetables, grains, beans, seeds, and nuts, they would probably live disability-free much longer.

Traditional medicine in China, Japan, and India has always stressed the key role of nutrition in health and healing. However, the importance of nutrition in maintaining health

was contested for many years by conventional doctors in the U.S. who argued that nutritional factors could not prevent (or cure) all chronic diseases. However, as discussed in Chapters 2, 3, and 4, a growing body of clinical evidence suggests that certain whole foods and nutritional supplements help maintain positive health and assist in the prevention or cure of a variety of diseases. In the last twenty years, a number of studies have shown that dietary factors play a role in at least five of the ten leading causes of death for Americans: heart disease, cancer, stroke, diabetes, and arteriosclerosis (hardening of the arteries).

The documented results of Ornish's "Reversal Program," described at the beginning of this chapter, also provide dramatic proof that ordinary people can reverse chronic illness with a combined program of nutrition, exercise, yoga, and group therapy. As a result, one major U.S. insurance company, Mutual of Omaha, now reimburses policyholders who enroll in Ornish's program.

Chapter 2 highlights a number of studies that detail specific food groups and foods that have been scientifically proven to enhance healthful living. Chapters 3 and 4 analyze the major vitamins, minerals, and trace elements and how they may be used in disease prevention and treatment.

Osteopathic Medicine

Osteopathy, or "bone treatment," was developed by Civil War healer and bone setter Andrew Taylor Still, who became frustrated with the unpredictability and ignorance involved in prescribing the toxic medications commonly used in the late 1800s. A deeply religious man, Still founded the American School of Osteopathy in Kirksville, Missouri, in 1892 after three of his children died of spinal meningitis, and dedicated himself to finding a way to enhance nature's own ability to heal.

As described by Weil in *Health and Healing,* "Still gave up the use of drugs completely and, instead, tried to promote healing by manipulating bones to allow free circulation of blood and balanced functioning of nerves. The technique he developed was the same used by generations of children to crack their knuckles: placing tension on a joint until an audible click or pop results." Still was able to find positions and motions to crack most of the larger joints of the body. He reportedly used his manipulations to treat conditions such as pneumonia, bacterial infections of the skin, typhoid fever, and diarrhea, Weil writes.

Osteopaths assume that the structure of organs, skeleton, and tissues directly affect the body's various functions. Thus the shape and position of the skeletal structure are central to maintaining optimal health. Osteopaths believe that the correction of posture problems, mobilization of joints, and alignment of the spine can improve health and aid in healing diseases.

Osteopathic medicine is very similar to chiropractic, with one important exception. Osteopaths focus more on the health of the arteries because they believe that when blood and lymphatics flow freely, the tissues can perform their physiological functions without restriction. When an individual suffers emotional or physical trauma, the tissues often contract, obstructing the fluid flow. Manipulation restores fluid flow throughout the impaired tissues and regenerates the body's inherent healing powers.

Osteopathic manipulation has been used successfully to treat children with genetic physiological disabilities. It also has been used to treat patients suffering from low-back pain, menstrual cramping, or dysmenorrhea. Recently, osteopathic manipulation has been introduced in clinical trials to help patients recover from coronary bypass graft surgery. In an October 1989 article in *INED,* J.L. Dickey reports that patients undergoing osteopathic manipulative treatment often perceive a sense of deep relaxation, tingling, energy flows, and relief of pain.

Most osteopaths are primary care physicians, and practice alternative medicine. Like M.D.s, osteopaths (Doctors of Osteopathy or D.O.s) provide comprehensive medical care, including preventive medicine, diagnosis, surgery, prescription medications, and hospital referrals. D.O.s are licensed in all fifty states in America.

Visualization Therapies

In *Love, Medicine & Miracles,* Siegel reported on a clinical trial in which a young boy with an inoperable brain tumor was taken by his parents to the Biofeedback and Psychophysiology Center at the Menninger Clinic in Topeka, Kansas. The staff taught him self-regulation techniques to help him to "control his body with his mind." He learned, for example, to imagine rocket ships, as in a video game, flying around in his head and shooting at the tumor. Several months later, he told his father, "I can't find my tumor any more." A CAT scan showed that the tumor had entirely disappeared.

The boy, in effect, was using visualization to eradicate his tumor. Visualization is a generic term that describes a variety of visual techniques used to treat disease. It is based on inducing relaxation in patients and having them visualize their medical problems, literally willing them away.

Visualization also has been used to treat cancer patients. In one clinical trial described in Siegel's book, a man with advanced throat cancer was given radiation treatment and told to visualize his white blood cells regenerating. His cancer dramatically disappeared within four months, and the patient subsequently cured both his arthritis and a twenty-one-year-old case of impotence using visualization techniques. In experiments conducted at the Stanford University Medical School, cancer patients who used guided imagery and other counseling techniques survived twice as long as patients who did not, according to an article by David Spiegel and others in the 1989 issue of *The Lancet.*

Therapists have used visualization or guided imagery to help heal patients suffering loss due to disease, altered body image, or the threat of death. Positive results have been documented even when a total cure may be out of the question. Writing in the December 1992 issue of *Perceptual and Motion Skills,* S. Hu states that many patients with phobias, for example, have been treated with visualization and positive thinking.

Yoga

As far back as the third century B.C., Patanjali, the father of classical yoga philosophy, defined yoga as "the cessation of the modification of the mind." Yoga, which in Sanskrit which means "union," focuses on altering the state of a person's mind and using the powers of the mind to generate healing within the body. By assuming a series of asanas (positions) and concentrating on breathing, people who practice yoga keep their spine supple and systematically exercise all of the body's major muscle groups. This in turn strengthens the organs by increasing respiration and blood flow.

The importance of breathing is central to all yogic teachings because the breath is considered to be the vehicle of "prana," or the vital life force. Prana enters the body when a person inhales. The method of breathing—whether shallow or deep, hurried or slow—controls how prana influences the body and mind. Indian yogis have long taught that to control the breath means to control the universal energy within, or to control the physical health and state of mind. According to Swami Rama, one of the most influential figures to demonstrate the authenticity of yoga to Western medicine, and reported by Tom Monte in *World Medicine: The EastWest Guide to Healing Your Body,* "All breathing exercises—advanced or basic—enable the student to control his mind through understanding prana."

An increasing number of traditional medical doctors, chiropractors, back specialists, and physical therapists recommend yoga to their patients both as a preventive and a remedial measure for the spine and as a stress-reduction technique. Many athletes find that yoga is an excellent adjunct to their training because it tones, stretches, and relaxes muscles and ligaments, which in turn improves their range of motion and helps prevent injury.

Guidelines for Evaluating a Physician's Background

The American Holistic Medical Association (AHMA) offers the following questions people may want to ask about physicians:

- Where and for how long did the physician train?
- Did the training include clinical experience?
- What conditions is the licensed or qualified to treat?
- What conditions is he or she not practitioner licensed to treat?
- How many people has the physician treated with the same condition that concerns you?
- What success has he or she had in treating that specific condition? Is there research or clinical studies that validate the treatment that has been suggested?
- What are the possible adverse reactions or side effects of the proposed treatment?
- How many visits will the treatment take?
- How much will it cost?

Other Alternative Medical Therapies

Many other therapies included in alternative medicine are not complete medical systems, but nevertheless have proven successful in treating or preventing specific ailments or diseases. Descriptions of several of the more popular therapies follow:

Hydrotherapy

Hydrotherapy is generally attributed to physician and spa advocate Vinzenz Priessnitz who, in the 1820s, collected data in Austria on the powers of water and temperature change to heal the body. Different methods of hydrotherapy use water and water immersion, including sitz baths, douches, spas and hot tubs, whirlpools, saunas, showers, immersion baths, poultices, and foot baths.

The healing properties of water include its buoyancy, which makes movement easier; its temperature, which promotes relaxation and decreases pain; its viscosity, which provides resistance so injured patients can maintain muscle tone and aerobic capacity; and its hydrostatic or circumferential pressure, which enhances blood circulation. One of hydrotherapy's most important benefits is that it allows therapists to treat patients sooner. After an injury or surgery, patients can begin an active program of stretching and conditioning right away instead of having their muscles atrophy. Recovery time can be reduced by as much as 50 percent in some cases, according to Wade Boyle and Andre Saine in *Lectures in Naturopathic Hydrotherapy.*

Hydrotherapy has proved particularly effective for discomforts associated with spinal stress. Clinical success has also been demonstrated on patients with steroid-dependent asthma, coughs, head colds, hoarseness, and burn injuries, reports Y. Tanizaki in the March 1993 issue of the *Japanese Journal of Allergology.* People with learning disabilities have benefited from spa therapy. Repeated water immersion has been used instead of medicine for patients with liver cirrhosis, arterial hypertension, rheumatoid arthritis, lumbar pain syndrome, pneumoconiosis and dust-induced bronchitis, and hypertension, reports A. Ader in the September 1993 issue of *Contributions to Nephrology.*

Massage

In China, every medical student must study massage for two years, and all doctors must complete at least a year of residency in massage and then pass an examination. Although in the West people tend to think of massage as a therapy for relaxation, the Chinese use it to treat chronic illness.

In Part One of Bill Moyer's "Healing and the Mind" PBS series, a thirty-seven-year-old Chinese woman with a lump in her breast was told she had fibrocystic disease. There currently is no effective treatment in the West for this disease. Instead of recommending surgery, a physician massaged her breast to move the blocked chi energy down her stomach and eventually out through the bottom of her feet. After a few treatments, the woman's cysts began disappearing, and she reported feeling virtually no pain. The doctor told Moyers that he had cured twenty-five of twenty-seven patients suffering from fibrocystic disease.

Massage also has proved very effective in treating back pain, and shows promise for depression. The Touch Research Institute (TRI) at the University of Miami Medical School studied the effect of massage on adolescent mothers and their infants, abused and neglected children in shelter care centers, adolescent psychiatric patients, anorexic and bulimic girls, and survivors of Hurricane Andrew. They found that after a 30-minute massage people had consistently lower levels of stress-related hormones—cortisol and norepinephrine—and were more alert, less restless, and better able to sleep, according to a November/December 1993 report in *Natural Health* by Meredith Gould Ruch.

Music Therapy

Most would not deny that beautiful music has a relaxing effect and makes people feel better. Today, many kinds of music are being used in hospitals and institutions across the United States to reduce the stress of surgery, cure physical and emotional depression, and stimulate communication with patients who have lost their ability to speak.

Music may be an effective therapeutic tool because it stimulates peptides and endorphins, natural opiates secreted by the hypothalamus that produce a pleasurable feeling. British osteopaths have claimed they can transmit the "correct" frequency of health to a diseased organ. While music therapy is not yet fully accepted in the United States, it has successfully been used to treat certain neuromuscular problems such as arthritis and degenerative bone condition.

American physicians now use music to treat patients recovering from grief and stress. In one clinical trial, the University of Massachusetts Medical Center in Worcester treated outpatients with Buddhist meditation and harp music. The program also taught patients how to pay attention to their bodies, their breathing patterns and their thoughts, according to Pamella Bloom's article in *New Age Journal*'s March/April 1987 issue.

Other Body Therapies

Alexander Technique

The Alexander technique was developed by an actor who concluded that bad posture was responsible for his own chronic voice loss. Practitioners teach simple, efficient physical movements designed to improve balance, posture, and coordination, and to relieve pain. Instructors offer gentle, hands-on guidance and verbal instruction to retrain students in the optimal use of their bodies. A session may focus on movements as basic as getting up from a chair properly.

Aston Patterning

Founded by Judith Aston, director of the Aston Training Center in Incline Village, Nevada, and former professor of dance and movement, this method is an integrated system of movement education, body work, and environmental evaluation. In specifically designed sessions, teacher and client work together to reveal and define the body's individual posture and movement patterns while training the body to move more efficiently and effortlessly.

Sessions can include any one or a combination of the following: movement education that teaches alternatives to stressful habits, massage-like body work that can relieve chronic physical and mental stress, and environmental consultation that modifies the individual's surroundings to reduce unnecessary stress and promote ease of movement.

The Feldenkrais Method

As part of his recovery after suffering a sports-related injury, nuclear physicist Moshe Feldenkreis developed a way to help people create more efficient movement by combining movement training, gentle touch, and verbal dialogue. Feldenkrais takes two forms. The first involves individual hands-on sessions (Functional Integration) where the practitioner's touch is used to improve the subject's breathing and body alignment. In the second form, in a series of classes of slow, nonaerobic motions (Awareness Through Movement), subjects "relearn" the proper ways to move their bodies. The method frequently is used to help reduce stress and tension, to alleviate chronic pain, and to help athletes and others improve their balance and coordination.

Hellerwork

Developed by former aerospace engineer Joseph Heller in the late 1960s, this technique combines deep-tissue muscle therapy and movement reeducation with counseling about the emotional issues that may underlie a physical posture. For example, feelings of insecurity may manifest themselves in stooped shoulders. Participants go through eleven 60- to 90-minute sessions. Hellerwork is used to treat chronic pain and to help "well" people learn to live more comfortably inside their bodies.

Kinesiology

Kinesiology is a diagnostic system based on the premise that individual muscle functions can provide information about a patient's overall health. Practitioners test the strength and mobility of certain muscles, analyze a patient's posture and gait, and inquire about lifestyle factors that may be contributing to an illness. Nutrition, muscle and joint manipulation, diet, and exercise are then incorporated into a treatment plan. Kinesiology is used by professionals licensed to diagnose, including chiropractors, dentists, medical doctors, and osteopaths.

Rolfing

Rolfing is a deep massage technique developed by biochemist Ida Rolf, who as a child benefitted from osteopathic manipulation of her spine and later studied hatha yoga. Rolfing uses deep manipulation of the fascia (connective tissue) to restore the body's natural alignment, which may have become rigid through injury, emotional trauma, and inefficient movement habits. The process typically involves ten sessions, each focusing on a different part of the body. Rolf practitioners are certified through the Rolf Institute in Boulder, Colorado, which was founded in 1970.

Choosing a Physician

The American Holistic Medical Association (AHMA) recommends that new patients ask the following questions when making a final decision about a holistic physician:

- Is the environment relaxed and supportive?

- Are appointments time honored, or do patients have to wait?

- Is the practitioner accessible?

- Is the practitioner concerned about patients' fears and anxieties about an illness or proposed treatment?

- Does the practitioner appear to represent a healthy lifestyle, or does he/she show signs of overweight, overwork, smoking, or drinking?

- Did the physician diagnose your condition fully?

- Did the physician order expensive tests?

- Did the practitioner prescribe prescriptions that have known side effects or cause adverse reactions?

- Do you trust both the physician's tone and the therapy outlined for you?

- Were you given a reasonable amount of time to evaluate the recommendations before beginning treatment, or do you feel you were rushed unnecessarily?

Choosing Alternative Care

As with conventional M.D.s, there is a wide variation in the background and training of holistic physicians and medical practitioners. Licensing regulations governing specific fields often vary from state to state. Therefore, it is important for patients to research a practitioner's background.

Summary

Alternative medicine emphasizes that health is a state of optimal well-being and not simply the absence of disease. The philosophy of holistic health emphasizes the unity of the mind, spirit, and body. The alternative approach focuses on the whole person, and emphasizes natural self-healing, the maintenance of health, and the prevention of illness, rather than the treatment of symptoms and disease.

Determining appropriate medical advice and treatment must be a combination of many factors. Each individual's needs will necessarily differ. All holistic physicians believe the body's inherent healing mechanism can be stimulated through natural means such as diet, nutrition, exercise, and botanical medicines, and by triggering the relaxation response through yoga, meditation, visualizations, biofeedback, or hypnosis. As further elaborated throughout this book, the goal of alternative medicine is to empower patients to participate in their own healing process.

Resources

References

Ader, A. "Water Immersion: Lessons from Antiquity to Modern Times." *Contributions to Nephrology* (1993): 171–86.

Benninga, M.A. "Biofeedback Training in Chronic Constipation." *Archives of Disease in Childhood* (January 1993): 126–29.

Binnie, N.R. "Solitary Rectal Ulcer: The Place of Biofeedback and Surgery in the Treatment of the Syndrome." *World Journal of Surgery* (September–October 1992): 836–40.

Bloom, Pamella. "Soul Music." *New Age Journal* (March/April 1987): 58–63.

"Boomers Are Biggest Users of Alternative Medicine." *The Boomer Report* (August 15, 1993): 6.

Boulter, P. "Learning Disabilities. Using Hydrotherapy: Maximizing Benefits." *Nursing Standard* (October 14–20, 1992): 5–7.

Boyle, Wade, and Andre Saine. *Lectures in Naturopathic Hydrotherapy.* East Palestine, OH: Buckeye Naturopathic Press, 1988.

Chopra, Deepak, M.D. *Perfect Health: The Complete Mind/Body Guide.* New York, NY: Harmony Books, 1991.

Dickey, J.L. "Postoperative Osteopathic Manipulative Management of Median Sternotomy Patients." *INED* (October 1989): 1319–22.

Eisenberg, D.M., et al. "Unconventional Medicine in the United States: Prevalence, Costs, and Patterns of Use." *New England Journal of Medicine* 328 (March 1993): 246–52.

Gould Ruch, Meredith. "Feeling Down? Study Shows Massage Can Lift Your Spirits." *Natural Health* (November/December 1993): 48–50.

Hahnemann, Samuel. *Organon of Medicine.* Translated by W. Boericke, M.D. New Delhi: B. Jain Publishers, 1992.

"Homeopathic Remedies: Safe, Inexpensive …And They Seem to Work." *HealthFacts* (April 1991): 1–2.

Hu, S. "Positive Thinking Reduces Heart Rate and Fear Responses to Speech-Phobic Imagery." *Perceptual & Motion Skills* (December 1992): 1067–73.

Kranhold, C. "Hypnotizability in Bulimic Patients and Controls: A Pilot Study." *European Archives of Psychiatry & Clinical Neuroscience* (1992): 72–76.

Laidlaw, T.M. "Hypnosis and Attention Deficits after Closed Head Injury." *International Journal of Clinical & Experimental Hypnosis* (April 1993): 97–111.

Lambert, Craig. "The Prescriptions." *Harvard Magazine* (September–October, 1989): 23–28.

LeBaw, W. "The Use of Hypnosis with Hemophilia." *Psychiatric Medicine* (1992): 89–98.

Monte, Tom, and the editors of *EastWest Natural Health. World Medicine: The EastWest Guide to Healing Your Body.* New York, NY: Putnam Berkley Group, Inc., 1993.

Ornish, Dean, M.D. *Dr. Dean Ornish's Program for Reversing Heart Disease.* New York, NY: Ballantine Books, 1990.

Siegel, Bernie, M.D. *Love, Medicine & Miracles.* New York, NY: Harper & Row Publishers, Inc., 1986.

Spiegel, D. "Predictors of Smoking Abstinence Following a Single-Session Restructuring Intervention With Self-

Hypnosis." *American Journal of Psychiatry* (July 1993): 1090–97.

Spiegel, David, et al. "Effect of Psychosocial Treatment on Survival of Patients with Metastatic Breast Cancer." *The Lancet* (1989): 888–91.

Tanizaki, Y. "Clinical Effects of Complex Spa Therapy on Patients with Steroid-Dependent Intractable Asthma." *Japanese Journal of Allergology* (March 1993): 423.

Thomas, R.E. "The Effects of Biofeedback on Carpal Tunnel Syndrome." *Ergonomics* (April 1993): 353–61.

Torem, M.S. "The Use of Hypnosis with Eating Disorders." *Psychiatric Medicine* (1992): 105–18.

Tredget, E.E. "Epidemiology of Infections with Pseudomonas Aeruginosa in Burn Patients: The Role of Hydrotherapy." *Clinical Infectious Diseases* (December 1992): 941–49.

Weil, Andrew, M.D. *Health and Healing.* Boston, MA: Houghton Mifflin Company, 1983.

Weiss, Rick. "Bones of Contention." *Health* (July/August, 1993): 44.

Yee, John D., Yuan-Chi Lin, and Paul A. Aubuchon. "Acupuncture," in *Pain in Infants, Children, and Adolescents.* Baltimore, MD: Williams & Wilkens, 1992: 341, 345.

Organizations

American Association of Acupuncture and Oriental Medicine.
4101 Lake Boone Tr., Ste. 201, Raleigh, NC 27607.

American Association of Homeopathic Pharmacists.
PO Box 2273, Falls Church, VA 22042.

American Chiropractic Association.
1701 Clarendon Blvd., Arlington, VA 22209.

American Institute of Homeopathic Education and Research.
5910 Chabot Crest, Oakland, CA 44018.

American Institute of Homeopathy.
1500 Massachusetts Ave. NW, Washington, DC 20005.

Association for Applied Psychophysiology and Biofeedback.
1200 W. 44th Ave., #304, Wheat Ridge, CO 80033.

British Institute of Homeopathy and College of Homeopathy.
520 Washington Blvd., Ste. 423, Marina Del Rey, CA 90292.

Council on Chiropractic Education.
44011 Westown Pky., Ste. 120, West Des Moines, IA 50265.

Homeopathic Educational Services.
2124 Kittredge St., Berkeley, CA 94704.

International Chiropractors Association.
1901 L St. NW, Ste. 800, Washington, DC 20036.

International Foundation for Homeopathy.
2366 Eastlake Ave. E., Ste. 30, Seattle, WA 98102.

National Center for Homeopathy.
801 N. Fairfax, Ste. 306, Alexandria, VA 22314.

National Commission for the Certification of Acupuncturists.
1424 16th St. NW, Ste. 601, Washington, DC 20036.

Office of Alternative Medicine, National Institutes of Health.
9000 Rockville Pke., Bethesda, MD 20892.

Additional Reading

Altman, Nathaniel. *Everybody's Guide to Chiropractic Health Care.* Los Angeles, CA: Jeremy P. Tarcher, Inc., 1989.

Brassard, C. "Biofeedback and Relaxation for Patients with Hypertension." *Canadian Nurse* (January 1993): 49–52.

Bricklin, Mark. *The Practical Encyclopedia of Natural Healing.* New York, NY: Penguin Books, 1990.

Carper, Jean. *The Food Pharmacy Guide to Good Eating.* New York, NY: Bantam Books, 1988.

Cerney, J.V. *Acupuncture Without Needles.* Parker Publishing Co., Inc. 1983.

Chopra, Deepak, M.D. *Ageless Body, Timeless Mind.* New York, NY: Harmony Books, 1993.

———. *Creating Health: How to Make Up The Body's Intelligence.* Boston, MA: Houghton Mifflin, 1987.

Cott, A. "Long-term Efficacy of Combined Relaxation: Biofeedback Treatments for Chronic Headache." *Pain* (October 1992): 49–56.

Cummings, Stephen, M.D., and Dana Ullman. *Everybody's Guide to Homeopathic Medicine.* New York, NY: St. Martin's Press, 1991.

Enomiya-Lassalle, Hugo. *The Practice of Zen Meditation.* HarperSanFrancisco: HarperCollins, 1992.

Frymann, V.M., and R.E. Carney. "Effect of Osteopathic Medical Management on Neurologic Development in Children." *Mimeo* (June 1992): 1–4.

Goodhart, R., and V. Young. *Modern Nutrition in Health and Disease.* Philadelphia, PA: Lea & Febiger, 1988.

Greenleaf, M. "Hypnotizability and Recovery From Cardiac Surgery." *American Journal of Clinical Hypnosis* (October 1992): 119–28.

Grundy, Scott, and Mary Winston, eds. *Low-Fat, Low-Cholesterol Cookbook.* Dallas, TX: American Heart Association, 1989.

Holmes, P. "Cranial Osteopathy." *INED* (May 29–June 4, 1991): 36–38.

Jin, P. "Efficacy of Tai Chi, Brisk Walking, Meditation and Reading in Reducing Mental and Emotional Stress." *Journal of Psychosomatic Research* (May 1992): 361–70.

Jordan, Sandra. *Yoga for Pregnancy.* New York, NY: St. Martin's Press, 1987.

Laffan, G. "Alternative Therapies: A New Holistic Science." *Nursing Standard* (January 13–19, 1993): 44–45.

Mills, Simon. *Out of the Earth: The Essential Book of Herbal Medicine.* New York, NY: Penguin Books, 1991.

Murray, Michael, and Joseph Pizzorno. *Encyclopedia of Natural Medicine.* Rocklin, CA: Prima Publishing, 1991.

National Research Council. *Diet, Nutrition and Cancer.* Washington, DC: National Academy Press, 1982.

Ng, R.K. "Cardiopulmonary Exercise: A Recently Discovered Secret of Tai Chi." *Hawaii Medical Journal* (August 1992): 216–17.

Ody, Penelope. *The Complete Medicinal Herbal.* London, England: Dorling Kindersley, 1993.

Porkett, Manfred, M.D. *Chinese Medicine.* New York, NY: Henry Holt & Co., 1992.

Reid, Daniel. *Chinese Herbal Medicine.* Boston, MA: Shambhala Publications Inc., 1993.

Sabatino, F. "Mind & Body Medicine: A New Paradigm?" *Hospitals* (February 1993): 66, 68, 70–72.

Saltman, Paul, Joel Gurin, and Ira Mothner. *The University of California San Diego Nutrition Book.* Boston, MA: Little Brown & Company, 1993.

Santillo, Humbart. *Natural Healing with Herbs.* Prescott, AZ: Hohm Press, 1991.

Stein, Diane. *The Natural Remedy Book for Women.* Freedom, CA: The Crossing Press, 1992.

Vishnu-devananda, Swami. *The Complete Illustrated Book of Yoga.* New York, NY: Harmony Books, 1988.

Weil, Andrew, M.D. *Natural Health, Natural Medicine.* Boston, MA: Houghton Mifflin, 1990.

Chapter 2

NATURAL NUTRITION

The human body is a complex organism that needs certain chemical constituents to stay alive. Since the body cannot produce most of these chemicals itself, it must get them from the environment. For example, because the human body is 60 percent water, it must replenish that water to continue functioning. Otherwise it becomes dehydrated and eventually dies.

Water, however, does not supply all the chemicals the body needs to grow, maintain its chemical structure, and rejuvenate itself. The other essential chemicals must be provided by nutrients found in foods. The combination and amount of foods people eat constitute their nutrition.

Nutrition is the most important factor in human life and health. Many people do not get enough food or water because of droughts, famine, poverty, and other adverse circumstances, and tragically become ill or die as a result.

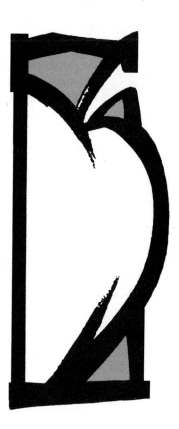

The absence of an essential nutrient in the body is called a nutritional deficiency, and diseases caused by lack of a specific nutrient are termed nutritional deficiency diseases. If the body contains too little iron, for example, it is said to have an iron deficiency, and one result is that the body will produce red blood cells that cannot carry a normal amount of oxygen. Without sufficient red blood cells, a person becomes weak and lacks energy, resulting in iron deficiency anemia.

Nutritional deficiencies are common in less developed parts of the world where finding enough food is a daily struggle for many people. In countries such as the United States, on the other hand, most people can easily supply themselves with the foods they need to live long, healthy lives. The challenge is rather in deciding which foods to eat and in what amounts.

Because the human body is a complex biochemical organism, scientists still do not know all of the nutritional chemical factors that contribute to optimal health. For one thing, every person's body is different—it is composed of a chemical structure of atoms and molecules. Even identical twins do not have exactly the same proportion of atoms and molecules in their bodies. In addition, every person's body continually changes as chemical constituents are used and replaced.

Required Nutrients

Scientists know that, in addition to water, everyone needs five basic types of chemical substances: carbohydrates, lipids (fats), minerals, proteins, and vitamins. How much of these substances people require depends on their age, sex, heredity (their unique genetic structure), the amount of exercise they get, and the amount of poisons (toxins) that exist in the body. Proteins and most carbohydrates and fats contained in foods are too large to be absorbed directly into the body. They first must be metabolized (broken down) into smaller chemical constituents before they can be utilized. On the other hand, vitamins and minerals (see Chapters 3 and 4) can be absorbed directly.

When a person eats a piece of meat, for example, it must be ground down by the teeth and mixed with saliva into smaller particles that can enter the gastrointestinal tract. As these particles reach the stomach and intestines, they are further broken down into proteins and fat that are absorbed directly into the blood. Elements of the meat that are not absorbed into the blood are eliminated later through the colon.

Each person's digestive system breaks down proteins, carbohydrates, and fats at slightly different rates. Some people eat faster than others; the amount of food consumed varies as well. What people eat and the speed and efficiency with which their bodies convert food into carbohydrates, fats, minerals, proteins, and vitamins, largely determines their energy level and the overall state of their health.

Calories

In addition to supplying the body's basic chemical materials, foods also provide a continuous source of energy. This energy is measured in calories, units of heat needed to raise the temperature of one kilogram of water one degree centigrade. As already discussed, the human body derives its energy from the breakdown of carbohydrates and fats. Carbohydrates and proteins supply approximately four calories per gram, while fats supply approximately nine calories per gram.

Carbohydrates

Carbohydrates are the chief source of the body's energy and are also used in the synthesis of some cell components such as DNA (acids found in the chromosomes of the nucleus of all cells). The two principal types of carbohydrates are simple sugars, found predominantly in fruit, and complex carbohydrates found in grains, fruits, and vegetables. Glucose, the most common of the simple sugars, is freely soluble in blood and cell fluids and supplies energy to all the body's tissues. Although only small amounts of glucose are ingested, most foodstuffs, with the exception of fatty acids, are converted to glucose before being utilized for energy in the body. Other simple sugars include fructose (one of the sweetest sugars) found in fruits and honey, sucrose (or common table sugar) harvested from sugar cane and sugar beets, and lactose, which is found almost exclusively in milk and milk products.

Sugar is not considered to be harmful when it is consumed in the proper amounts. Unfortunately, sugar flavors many manufactured food products and Americans tend to consume it to excess. The average American is estimated to take in almost a third of a pound of refined sugar each day in synthetic foods. Some scientists think that overconsumption of sugar may be related to several degenerative diseases and may cause a person's body to age more rapidly, according to a June 1990 article in *Longevity,* written by Peter Jarret.

Complex carbohydrates are found in such foods as grains (wheat, rice, corn, oats, and barley), legumes (peas and beans), plant roots, leaves and stems (most vegetables), and some animal tissue. They consist of two major classes: starch, which is digestible and is used to supply molecules for energy production and cellular structure; and fiber, which is not digestible but is nevertheless important for removing wastes from the body. Starch is present in granules within seeds, pods, or roots of plants. Glycogen, the animal form of starch, is found in muscle and liver. Most of the starch in an average person's diet comes from foods made from flour, such as bread, noodles, and pastries.

Cholesterol

Cholesterol helps produce hormones, contributes to development of the brain, and aids the functioning of the nervous system. Every person needs a certain amount of the right forms of cholesterol (HDL cholesterol), but it is not necessary to consume high levels of cholesterol in foods, because the liver manufactures all that the body needs.

Cholesterol is not soluble in water and, because it cannot mix with the blood, it is carried through the bloodstream in protein "packets" called lipoproteins. The two most common are low-density lipoproteins (LDL) and high-density lipoproteins (HDL). Blood cholesterol consists largely of LDL and HDL, although there are several other types of blood fats, including very low-density lipoproteins (VLDL), intermediate-density lipoproteins (IDL), and triglycerides.

Most of the cholesterol typically circulating in the bloodstream is carried by LDL. LDL is often called "bad" cholesterol because the portion not used by the body's normal functions tends to collect on the lining of blood vessels and can cause arteriosclerosis (buildup of fatty deposits, or plaque, in the arteries). Arteriosclerosis reduces the supply of blood carrying oxygen and other vital nutrients to the heart and other organs and may cause several heart disorders. Blood clots (thrombosis) that form around cholesterol deposits also can clog the arteries supplying the brain with oxygen and result in brain damage as well as strokes.

HDL cholesterol is usually called "good" cholesterol because it is more easily eliminated by the body. It also appears to help prevent the formation of fatty plaques in the arteries, and thus may protect against heart disease.

Cholesterol is highly concentrated in egg yolks and organ meats such as liver and is also found in milk, dairy products, poultry, and seafood. Only animal products contain cholesterol, although prepared foods including crackers or bakery goods may have high-cholesterol ingredients such as lard, eggs, or butter.

Many people find it difficult to determine whether their diet contains too much cholesterol, especially LDL cholesterol. Part of the problem is that many foods high in cholesterol are also high in saturated fat—meat, butter, cheese, whole milk, cream, and ice cream, for example. It is not clear whether cholesterol alone, especially "bad" cholesterol, is harmful, but a diet high in both LDL and saturated fats should be avoided.

Benefits of Fiber in the Diet

- Helps prevent constipation.
- Prevents diverticulosis by relieving stress on the colon wall.
- Increases enzyme secretion and activity.
- Lowers serum lipid levels (i.e., cholesterol and triglycerides) by preventing their manufacture in the liver.
- Maintains healthy bacterial flora in the colon.
- Is associated with a decreased incidence of most degenerative diseases including diabetes, irritable bowel syndrome, ulcerative colitis, appendicitis and cancer.

A simple blood test by a doctor or qualified health professional can tell people if their cholesterol levels are too high. If cholesterol numbers are borderline, the health professional will probably suggest starting on a cholesterol-lowering diet and redoing the test in a year. The doctor may recommend other lifestyle changes like exercising, quitting smoking, and limiting alcohol and coffee consumption to help reduce blood cholesterol levels and lower the risk of heart disease. If the LDL ratio is unusually high, and the person is at high risk of heart disease for other reasons, some physicians may prescribe cholesterol-lowering drugs to bring blood lipids down to normal levels.

Fiber

Fiber foods provide the other major form of complex carbohydrates in the human diet—cellulose—which is the primary constituent of all plant material. Cellulose is com-

posed of glucose molecules that humans cannot digest. However, it is extremely important because, along with bran and other fibers, cellulose helps in digesting food and preventing several disorders of the gastrointestinal tract, according to a 1991 article in the *Encyclopedia of Natural Medicine* by Michael Murray and Joseph Pizzorno. Fiber also adds bulk to the feces, thereby helping to prevent constipation and related disorders such as hemorrhoids. Fiber appears to lower the risk of appendicitis and of colon and rectal cancer by decreasing the time it takes for waste material and bacteria to pass through the gastrointestinal tract. Nutritionists recommend that people consume twenty to thirty grams of fiber daily. The best sources are vegetables, whole grains, fruits, and legumes.

Bran or uncooked oats are excellent ways to add fiber to the diet, as are pumpkin seeds and psyllium seeds.

Lipids (Fats)

Lipids are chemical substances that are relatively insoluble in water. The most familiar is triglyceride (body fat). Other lipids, including cholesterol and lecithin, are essential components of cell membranes. Vitamins A, D, E, and K are lipids, as are substances in the liver bile (bile acids) that help digest fats.

The lipids that most people eat in ordinary foods come in three principal forms: cholesterol; saturated fats, found primarily in animal products; and unsaturated fats—either polyunsaturated fats, as in sunflower oil and safflower oil, or monounsaturated fats like olive oil and canola oil. In general, saturated fats raise cholesterol levels in the blood, while unsaturated fats appear to reduce cholesterol, including LDL cholesterol, without adverse side effects.

Most Americans are now familiar with the danger of consuming too much fat, especially the saturated fats that are believed to contribute to heart disease. Saturated fats are found in animal foods (beef, pork, lamb, veal, egg yolks, whole milk, cream, cheese, ice cream, butter, and lard), chocolate, coconuts, and fats often used in processed foods, such as coconut, palm, and palm-kernel oils. Many studies have shown a relationship between dietary fat consumption and cancer of the breast, colon, and prostate gland, and nutritionists recommend eating no more than 10 percent of calories in the diet as saturated fat.

Proteins

Proteins are needed for survival because they are involved in virtually every bodily function. Approximately 20 percent of the human body consists of proteins, including the skeleton, muscle fiber, hair, skin, and nails.

When a protein-containing food such as meat is eaten, the protein is broken down in the stomach into amino acids. The human body needs twenty different amino acids to function, although it can manufacture only twelve of these itself. The other eight must be obtained from animal and plant protein foods. These essential amino acids, called phenylalanine, tryptophan, valine, threonine, lysine, isoleucine, leucine, and methionine, are required for optimum cell functioning. If they are not present, some normal body processes will be impaired. It is extremely important to eat the right amount of protein each day which, in turn, supplies the proper amount of the eight essential amino acids.

The difficulty for many people lies in knowing how much protein their bodies need each day and which foods contain the required amounts of amino acids. Nutritionists agree that adults need approximately fifty to sixty grams of protein daily, and most Americans eat enough meat, fish, eggs, and dairy products to fulfill their requirement for the essential amino acids.

Both meat and plant foods contain proteins, but meat is a better source because it contains all eight essential amino acids. Because most vegetables lack at least one essential amino acid, vegetarians usually must consume both grains and legumes to meet their amino acid needs. If people eat too little protein, they will develop symptoms of a protein deficiency. Children who do not eat enough protein, for example, will have retarded skeletal and muscle growth. Pregnant women may gain too little weight and be fatigued. Adults who lack protein often have weak immune systems that make them susceptible to infections and diseases. Proteins form a critical part of the antibodies that protect the body from viruses and bacteria.

Obtaining adequate amounts of high-quality protein is not a problem for most people in developed countries. In fact, many Americans eat twice the amount of protein they actually need, two-thirds of which comes from meat. Overconsuming protein at any one time is potentially dangerous because it cannot be fully absorbed by the body. The excess enters the bloodstream as partially digested protein (peptides), which are now thought to cause inflammation of some organs, tissues, and joints.

Scientists have begun to link eating too much meat protein with other health problems such as cancer and heart attacks. Americans who eat large amounts of meat tend to have higher rates of cancer of the colon, for example, although scientists are not sure precisely why. Most meat sold commercially also contains nonfood chemicals such as pesticide residues and hormone growth promoters that may be co-contributors to cancer, according to Gordon Edlin and Eric Golanty, in their 1992 book *Health and Wellness: A Holistic Approach*. Overconsumption of animal fat, especially the fat in red meat, also appears to increase men's risk for developing prostate cancer. Scientists at Harvard University and

Guidelines for Nutrition

The dietary guidelines published by these three U.S. agencies are summarized as follows:

- **General Recommendations:** Eat a diet rich in whole natural and unprocessed foods such as fruits, vegetables, grains, beans, seeds, and nuts. These foods contain valuable nutrients as well as dietary fiber.

- **Proteins:** Eat moderate quantities of protein, especially animal protein. Fish and many shellfish are excellent sources of low-fat protein.

- **Fats:** Maintain total fat intake at or below 30 percent of total caloric intake and saturated fats at less than 10 percent. Eat leaner cuts of meat, trim off excess fat, remove skin from poultry, and consume smaller portions.

- **Carbohydrates:** Carbohydrates should comprise between 60 and 70 percent of the total intake of calories. Only 10 percent of carbohydrates should be refined or concentrated sugars such as honey, fruit juices, dried fruit, sugar, or white flour. Foods high in calories from whole-grain cereals and bread are more healthful than foods or drinks containing sugar.

- **Dairy Products:** Eat dairy products for calcium, but avoid excessive amounts of whole milk, whole-milk cheeses, yogurt, ice cream, and other milk products that are high in saturated fats.

the Mayo Clinic compared the health records and eating habits of more than forty-seven thousand American men and divided them into two groups: those who ate large amounts of red meat and those who did not. The men whose diets included large quantities of red meat were more than 2 ½ times as likely to develop cancer as those who ate little red meat. And according to a study published in the *Journal of the American Medical Association (JAMA),* and cited in the October 6, 1993, *San Francisco Chronicle,* eating excessive amounts of protein-rich meat (which is also high in fats and cholesterol) can lead to heart disease.

Recommended Dietary Allowances (RDAs)

To help people determine the proper amounts of nutrients needed for optimum health, the Food and Nutrition Board (which operates under the National Academy of Sciences) has established the Recommended Dietary Allowances for protein, eleven vitamins, and seven minerals. The World Health Organization recommends a set of dietary standards very similar to the RDAs.

The RDAs generally are set about 30 percent higher than the average amount the body requires. On a statistical basis, this usually accommodates most healthy individuals. The RDAs are designed for people who are in good health, not suffering from clinical disease, and not under an unusual amount of stress. The RDAs also list nutrient requirements for children and for pregnant and lactating women. By eating a balanced diet of natural foods each day, most people are able to acquire the essential nutrients in amounts suggested by the RDAs.

Several other U.S. agencies have suggested general dietary guidelines that people can follow and modify, if necessary. For example, in 1990 the U.S. Department of Agriculture and U.S. Department of Health and Human Services urged Americans to adopt diets lower in fat (especially saturated fat) and higher in complex carbohydrates and fiber. They also recommended that Americans consume only moderate amounts of sugar, salt, and alcoholic beverages.

The American Council on Science and Health also issued a publication in 1990, entitled *Food and Life: A Nutrition Primer,* defining "a good diet" that it suggests all Americans follow. The council strongly recommends that Americans consume enough calories to maintain their optimal body weight, adequate carbohydrates and fats for energy needs, enough fat to absorb fat-soluble vitamins, essential fatty acids, and sufficient vitamins and minerals to facilitate enzyme processes.

The National Academy of Sciences (NAS) issued a report in 1990 suggesting virtually the same diet as the one detailed above. The academy also recommended that people maintain total fat intake at or below 30 percent of total caloric intake and saturated fatty acid at less than 10 percent. In addition, NAS urged Americans to consume only moderate amounts of meat protein and to obtain more calories from carbohydrates, especially whole-grain cereals and breads.

Nutrition for Children

Small children, particularly infants, need more of certain specific nutrients, including vitamins and minerals, than do adults. (The RDAs for vitamins and minerals for children are listed in Chapters 3 and 4.) All children need protein for energy, as well as some carbohydrates and fats, to ensure satisfactory growth and development. Many American children, along with American adults, however, consume significantly higher amounts of sugar and red meat than they need.

Many parents attempt to follow sound nutritional guidelines at home, but worry about the lunches and snacks their children eat at school. And indeed, American parents have good reason to be concerned. A fifteen-year study showed that American school lunches contribute less than one-third of total daily nutrient requirements, and that intakes of dietary components related to cardiovascular disease risk were excessive. Sixty to 80 percent of American children exceeded RDA amounts of daily total fat, saturated fat, cholesterol, and sodium. The study, reported in an article by R.P. Farris in the May 1992 *Journal of School Health,* concluded that schools should try to reduce the risk of cardiovascular disease by providing students with healthier foods and educational programs that promote positive lifestyles.

Nutrition for the Elderly

The elderly need to be especially conscientious about their daily nutrition. Illness, multiple medications, and the aging process itself can affect the type and quantity of food an older person eats. The elderly should pay particularly close attention to maintaining adequate caloric intake. With advancing age, people tend to need more calories to maintain their energy levels. If caloric intake is too low, it takes an older person longer to restore body cell mass, according to M.F. Martin, writing in the April 1992 issue of the *American Journal of Clinical Nutrition.*

The level of energy an older person expends also is important in maintaining good nutrition. One U.S. study compared energy requirements (listed in the RDAs) for healthy elderly men and the total energy the men used in daily activities. The study concluded that the RDAs for the elderly (55+) significantly underestimate their needs. The study, described by S.B. Roberts in the December 1992 *International Journal of Obesity,* also found that the low levels of nutrients suggested by the RDA may favor the buildup of unnecessarily high levels of body fat mass. Therefore, elderly persons may find they need to consume more than the RDAs recommend for their age group.

Overweight Americans

Holistically healthy people attempt to eat all the essential foods they need in the proper proportions. Unfortunately, 60 percent of Americans now consume excessive amounts of the wrong foods. According to a series of eight annual surveys conducted by Louis Harris and Associates in 1993 for *Prevention Magazine,* sixty-four million Americans are now overweight. Whether a person was overweight was determined by using insurance company tables that took into account age, sex, and body build. Interestingly enough, almost a third of those who were overweight did not know it, or at least did not admit it. Instead, they told interviewers that they were "at about the right weight." Overweight men were nearly twice as likely as women to feel their weight was acceptable. The survey also found that fewer Americans are trying to avoid eating too much sugar and sweets than they did in 1983. And fewer are making an attempt to consume enough vitamins and minerals or eat fish twice a week, according to *Prevention.*

Weight-Loss Programs

What should overweight people do to regain holistic health? Basically, they need to adopt a weight-loss program consistent with the major tenets of alternative medicine—

proper diet, adequate exercise, and a positive mental attitude. Generally, the basic equation for losing weight is the same whatever diet program is followed. To lose weight, energy intake must be less than energy expenditure. This can be accomplished by decreasing caloric intake (dieting), increasing the rate at which calories are burned (exercising), or a combination of the two.

As Murray and Pizzorno explain in their book, *Encyclopedia of Natural Medicine,* people must take in thirty-five hundred fewer calories than they expend in order to lose one pound of body weight. Therefore, to lose one pound in a week, they must reduce caloric intake by five hundred calories a day. This could be accomplished through exercise alone by jogging for forty-five minutes, playing tennis for an hour, or taking a brisk walk for one hour and fifteen minutes, assuming that caloric intake remained the same.

The most sensible approach to weight loss is to decrease calorie intake and increase energy expenditure. Most people will begin to lose weight if they keep their caloric intake below three thousand calories per day and do aerobic exercise for fifteen to twenty minutes three to four times per week. Starvation and crash diets usually result in rapid weight loss (largely muscle and water), but cause rebound weight gain. The most successful approach to weight loss is gradual weight reduction (half a pound to one pound per week) through adopting dietary and lifestyle modifications, according to Murray and Pizzorno.

Obesity

An estimated 1 to 2 million Americans are morbidly obese, or so overweight that their bodies cannot function normally. Because of many complications, these individuals may be putting themselves at a high risk for death. An additional 1.24 million people fall into the category of medically significant obesity. Obesity can lead to diabetes, heart disease, and cancer. In men, for example, obesity has been directly linked to cancer of the colon, prostate, and rectum. A February 1990 article in *Consumer Reports Health Letter* reports that obesity in women is directly associated with cancer of the breast, gall bladder, ovaries, and uterus. Obese people also have higher incidences of arthritis, gallstones, and gout.

There is no single reason why obese people obsessively overeat. Genetic, psychological, and dietary factors may all contribute to the condition. Data suggest that if the obese person has one parent with a weight problem, the chance of developing morbid obesity is 60 percent. If both parents have a weight problem, the probability rises to 90 percent, according to Armour Forse, Peter N. Benotti, and George Blackburn in an article in the September–October 1989 *Nutrition Today.*

In addition, obesity is influenced by a person's metabolism and the interactions between appetite, metabolic rate, adipose tissue, and brain neurochemicals. Diet, of course, always contributes to obesity because even people with poor metabolism would not become obese unless they ate too much. Overeating compounded by the fact that obese people usually get very little cardiopulmonary exercise.

Traditional Treatments for Obesity

How do health practitioners attempt to treat obesity? There are several basic approaches for helping obese people lose weight and not regain it. One is to psychologically condition an obese patient to stop eating excessive amounts. Another approach is to use gastric bypass surgery to make the stomach smaller and thus less capable of storing large amounts of food. This typically involves

applying stainless steel staples across the top of the stomach which shortens the stomach and results in early satiety. Although somewhat extreme, gastric bypass surgery generally works, and obese patients normally achieve a twenty-pound weight loss, according to Forse, Benotti, and Blackburn.

Conventional physicians also use toxic drugs such as dexfenfluramine (dF) to decrease hunger in obese patients. Further experiments with dF are needed, however, to test for toxicity, drug tolerance morbidity, and mortality from obesity. Very Low Calorie Diets (VLCDs) in conjunction with prolonged use of dF have also been shown to be effective, according to Michelle Holmes in the January 1990 *American Family Physician.*

Alternative Treatments for Obesity

It is extremely difficult to help obese patients lose a large amount of weight. Can a holistic weight-loss program help obese patients? The answer is yes—some diet programs have been successful in a limited number of clinical trials, but they must be total mind/body programs that combine treatments involving nutritional counseling, VLCDs, exercise, and group therapy.

VLCDs clearly produce rapid weight loss in the first several weeks of a treatment program. However, obese patients tend to regain the same amount of weight—or even more—unless their lifestyles are altered through behavior modification. Holistic physicians attempt to educate patients to monitor their own health and eating habits and dramatically alter the amount and pattern of what they eat. The patients must also exercise to increase their energy expenditure and be trained in self-awareness and assertiveness. In one clinical trial, 10 percent of obese patients who were given two weeks of behavior modification (BMOD) prior to a VLCD regained weight, whereas 33 percent who were not given the BMOD prior to the VLCD regained weight, reports R.O. Kramath in the *American Journal of Clinical Nutrition's* July 1992 issue.

Anorexia Nervosa

Individuals with anorexia nervosa are usually people of normal or slightly above normal weight who start on an "innocent" diet and eventually begin suppressing hunger sensations to the point of self-starvation, according to the California Medical Association's July/August 1989 *Health Tips*. They may subsist on as few as 250 calories a day. The causes of anorexia nervosa are primarily psychological, although some people with the disorder may have a genetic predisposition that is triggered by psychological factors. Psychological factors are suspected because the vast majority of anorexics are white North American women between the ages of thirteen and twenty-two. Many are starting to menstruate or have just graduated from high school. The widespread pressure on these women to diet and stay thin just as they enter adult society may contribute to anorexia.

Treatments for Anorexia Nervosa

Treatment for anorexia typically involves reducing patients' fears of a normal body weight by encouraging them to gradually regain their natural body weight. Group support and medication play an important role in reducing their anxiety about eating. Some nutrient supplements and nasogastric or intravenous feeding also have proven successful. Nutritional supplements alone usually are insufficient, because the underlying psychological factors must be treated as well.

Bulimia

An increasing number of young Americans, particularly females, overconsume enormous amounts of food and then make themselves vomit. This is a chronic eating disorder called bulimia with both short- and long-term complications. The condition usually begins in conjunction with a diet and, once the binge-purge cycle begins, bulimics cannot stop themselves from either eating excessive amounts or vomiting. The average meal for a normal nonbulimic person contains approximately a thousand calories. People with bulimia may eat from five thousand to as many as fifty thousand calories in one extended meal and then vomit once the binge is over. Some bulimics may be underweight and a few may be obese, but most tend to maintain a fairly normal weight. In some bulimic women, the menstrual cycle becomes irregular and the desire for sexual intercourse usually declines.

There are two potentially fatal aspects of bulimia. If people dramatically increase their body weight in a short amount of time, they may develop heart problems and high blood pressure. In addition, vomiting for extended periods of time can cause chloride and potassium deficiencies that often lead to heart arrhythmias and heart damage. Most bulimics have very low self-esteem and are often depressed, according to an article by Dixie Farley in the May 1986 *FDA Consumer Reports*.

Treatments for Bulimia

Some bulimic patients have been treated successfully with behavioral modification. Patients with severe cases, however, sometimes require intensive treatment, in an inpatient unit at a hospital, for example. Medication may be useful in certain circumstances, including antidepressants, but to date there is no antibulimia drug per se, report

D.B. Woodside and P. Garfinkel in *Nutrition Today* (June 1989).

The nontraditional approach to bulimia recognizes that while genetic and physiological factors may contribute to the disorder, successful treatment must involve rebuilding the patient's self-esteem. Holistic physicians usually avoid prescribing antidepressant drugs because they have side effects, and do not eliminate the underlying psychological causes of bulimia. A controlled pharmacological approach, however, can prove useful, particularly in the early stages. For example, a study conducted at the University of Pittsburgh School of Medicine found that bulimic women eat more when supplies of the brain chemical serotonin (a neurotransmitter that causes narrowing of the lumen of blood vessels) are depleted. Small doses of natural or synthetic serotonin might help prevent binge eating, and hopefully further study will lead to a more successful treatment, according to an article by A. James Giannini in the April 1990 *American Family Physician.*

Psychological approaches may also prove effective. For example, many bulimic patients mistakenly think that vomiting helps them lose weight quickly. In fact, calories are retained in the gastrointestinal tract even after vomiting. Several studies have shown that bulimic patients eat more slowly than control groups, and they also take significantly longer to start eating. If these patients are placed in support groups that stress exercise and that intervene before binge eating begins, it may possible to eventually cure the patients' disorder.

Summary

Eating wholesome natural foods is the most important factor in maintaining optimum holistic health. Everyone needs to daily consume the essential nutrients of water, proteins, carbohydrates, fats, vitamins, and minerals in their correct amounts and proportions so that the body will function smoothly and maintain its natural balance. Eating less than the minimum daily recommended amounts of foods can cause severe physiological disorders, and overconsuming unnecessary foods also can result in serious medical complications. Some people may need to take certain vitamins, minerals, and other botanical substances to maintain good health and well-being. These are described in the chapters that follow.

Resources

References

American Council on Science and Health. *Food and Life Primer* (July 1990): 34–35.

California Medical Association. *Health Tips* index 435 (July/August 1989): 1.

Edlin, Gordon, and Eric Golanty. *Health and Wellness: A Holistic Approach.* Boston, MA: Jones and Bartlett Publishers, Inc., 1992.

Farley, Dixie. "Eating Disorders: When Thinness Becomes an Obsession." *FDA Consumer Reports* (May 1986): 20–21.

Farris, R.P. "Nutrient Contribution for the School Lunch Program." *Journal of School Health* (May 1992): 180–84.

Forse, Armour, Peter N. Benotti, and George Blackburn. "Morbid Obesity: Weighing The Treatment Options." *Nutrition Today* 24 (September–October 1989): 10–11, 14–15, 87.

Giannini, A. James. "Anorexia and Bulimia." *American Family Physician* 41 no. 4 (April 1990): 1175.

"Health Risks of Overweight." *Consumer Reports Health Letter* (February 1990): 11.

Holmes, Michelle. "Current Therapies for Obesity." *American Family Physician* (January 1990): 317.

Jarret, Peter. "Are We Slowly Dying From Pollution Overload?" *Longevity* (June 1990): 64.

Kamrath, R.O. "Repeated Use of VLCD in a Structured Multidisciplinary Weight Management Program." *American Journal of Clinical Nutrition* (July 1992): 288S–89S.

Martin, M.F. "The Effect of Age on the Caloric Requirement of Malnourished Individuals." *American Journal of Clinical Nutrition* (April 1992): 783–89.

Murray, Michael, and Joseph Pizzorno. *Encyclopedia of Natural Medicine.* Rocklin, CA: Prima Publishing, 1991.

"Red Meat Linked to Fatal Prostate Cancer." *San Francisco Chronicle* (October 6, 1993): 5, 14.

Roberts, S.B. "What Are the Dietary Energy Needs of Elderly Adults?" *International Journal of Obesity* (December 1992): 969–76.

"2 Out of 3 Americans Are Overweight, Survey Finds." *San Francisco Chronicle* (May 3, 1993): A4.

U.S. Department of Agriculture and U.S. Department of Health and Human Services. "Nutrition and Your Health: Dietary Guidelines for Americans." *Home and Garden Bulletin* (November 1990): 3–4.

Woodside, D.B., and P. Garfinkel. "An Overview of the Eating Disorders Anorexia Nervosa and Bulimia Nervosa." *Nutrition Today* (June 1989): 27–29.

Organizations

American Anorexia/Bulimia Association, Inc.
133 Cedar Ln., Teaneck, NJ 07666.

American Dietetic Association
208 S. LaSalle St., Ste. 1100, Chicago, IL 60604.

American Nutritionists Association
PO Box 34030, Bethesda, MD 20817.

American Society of Bariatric Physicians
5600 S. Quebec, Ste. 310B, Englewood, CO 80111.

American Society for Clinical Nutrition
9650 Rockville Pke., Bethesda, MD 20814.

Center for the Study of Anorexia and Bulimia
1 W. 91st St., New York, NY 10024.

Food and Nutrition Information Center
National Agricultural Library, Beltsville, MD 20705.

National Anorexic Aid Society, Inc.
PO Box 29461, Columbus, OH 43229.

National Association of Anorexia Nervosa and Associated Disorders
PO Box 7, Highland Park, IL 60035.

National Institute of Mental Health, Eating Disorders Program
Bldg. 10, Rm. 3S231, Bethesda, MD 20892.

National Research Council, National Academy of Sciences
2101 Constitution Ave. NW, Washington, DC 20036.

Additional Reading

Blundell, J.E. "Dietary Fat and the Control of Energy Intake: Evaluating the Effects of Fat on Meal Size and Postmeal Satiety." *American Journal of Clinical Nutrition* (May 1993): 55–57.

Brody, Jane. *The Good Food Book.* New York, NY: Bantam Books, 1990.

Buery, V.J. "Across-the-day Monitoring of Mood and Energy Intake Before, During and After a Very-Low-Calorie Diet."

American Journal of Clinical Nutrition (July 1992): 277S–78S.

Carper, Jean. *Food—Your Miracle Medicine: How Food Can Prevent & Cure over 100 Symptoms & Problems.* HarperSanFrancisco: HarperCollins, 1993.

Hamilton, M. *The Duke University Medical Center Book of Diet and Fitness.* New York, NY: Ballantine Books, 1990.

Hirschman, Jane. *Overcoming Overeating.* Reading, MA: Addison-Wesley, 1988.

Ikeda, Y. "Comparison of Clinical Usefulness of VLCD and Supplemental LCD." *American Journal of Clinical Nutrition (July 1992): 275S–76S.*

Leibel, R.L. "Energy Intake Required to Maintain Body Weight Is Not Affected by Wide Variation in Diet Composition." *American Journal of Clinical Nutrition* (February 1992): 350–55.

McDougall, John. *The New McDougall Cookbook.* Boston, MA: Dutton, 1992

National Institute of Mental Health. *Facts About Anorexia Nervosa.* Bethesda, MD: National Institute of Mental Health, Public Inquiries Branch, November 1990.

National Research Council, National Academy of Sciences. *Diet and Health:Implications for Reducing Chronic Disease Risk.* Washington, DC: National Research Council, National Academy of Sciences, 1989.

Ornish, Dean, M.D. *Eat More, Weigh Less.* HarperSanFrancisco: HarperCollins, 1993.

Pauling, Linus. *How to Live Longer and Feel Better.* New York, NY: W.H. Freeman and Co., 1986.

Phinny, S.D. "Exercise During and After VLCD." *American Journal of Clinical Nutrition* (July 1992): 190S–94S.

Pope, H. *New Hope for Binge Eaters.* New York, NY: Colophon, 1985.

Public Health Service. *The Surgeon General's Report on Nutrition and Health.* Public Health Service, 1988.

Sadur, C.N. "Body Composition and Weight Maintenance with a Very Low Calorie Diet for the Treatment of Moderate Obesity." *American Journal of Clinical Nutrition* (July 1992): 286S–87S.

Siegel, M. *Surviving an Eating Disorder.* New York, NY: Harper & Row Publishers, Inc., 1988.

Spalter, A.R. "Thyroid Function in Bulimia Nervosa." *Biological Psychiatry* (March 1993): 408–14.

Urbain, W. *Food Irradiation.* New York, NY: Academic Press, 1986.

Chapter 3

VITAMINS

In 1976, Linus Pauling, the late Nobel Prize-winning chemist, announced that vitamins (especially vitamin C) could help prevent strokes, mental illness, heart disease, cancer, and infection. With "optimal intake," he claimed, people could extend their lives an extra twelve to eighteen years. (Pauling defined "optimal intake" as falling somewhere between 3,200 and 12,000 milligrams a day, or what a person could obtain from consuming 45 to 170 oranges.) Pauling's dramatic claim, although subsequently challenged by many scientists, set off international studies of possible links between vitamins and disease prevention. By the late 1980s, one of every three Americans was taking vitamin C supplements, and today Americans spend $2 billion a year on vitamins, according to David Zimmerman, author of *Zimmerman's Complete Guide to Nonprescription Drugs*. A growing body of evidence gathered from both underdeveloped and fully industrialized countries now strongly reinforces Pauling's once-maverick contention that vitamins play a significant role in maintaining good health and in helping to treat infection and disease.

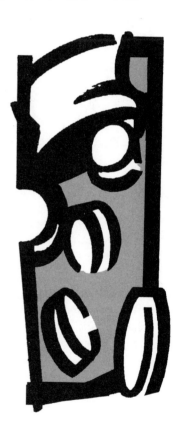

The Role of Vitamins

Vitamins are chemical compounds that must be included in the human diet to ensure growth and health. They are needed only in small amounts to build, maintain, and repair tissues and usually are available in a balanced diet that features a variety of fresh fruits and vegetables.

Recommended Dietary Allowance (RDA) for Vitamin A

	RE
Infants (0–1 year)	375
Children (1–10 years)	600
Males (11–24 years)	1,000
Males (25–51+ years)	1,000
Females (11–24 years)	800
Females (25–51+ years)	800
Pregnant Females	800
Breast-feeding Females	1,300

Note: RDA for vitamin A is expressed in RE (Retinol Equivalents). 1 mcg. equals 1 RE.

To obtain sufficient vitamins, most nutritionists recommend that a daily diet include multiple servings of: cereal or bread; dairy products (milk, cheese, ice cream, cottage cheese); meat, fish, or eggs; and vegetables and fruits. Several vitamins are recommended as supplements, either because they are deficient in the diet or because the body does not produce them.

However, vitamins alone will not take the place of a good diet, nor will they provide energy. The human body needs substances found in food such as protein, minerals, carbohydrates, and fats, and vitamins themselves often cannot work without the presence of various foods.

There is substantial controversy as to whether people should take vitamin supplements and whether such supplements can prevent chronic diseases. Individuals should be fully informed of the supplements' potential levels of toxicity because they are medicines

and can cause either desirable or undesirable changes in the body's physiology or internal anatomy. Some vitamins, when taken in excessive doses, can cause side effects, adverse interactions with other drugs, and other problems.

This chapter analyzes each of the essential vitamins and describes its chemical composition, its physiological functions, its occurrence in natural foods or supplements, and the current Recommended Dietary Allowance (RDA). The RDA for each vitamin represents the best current assessment of safe and adequate intakes and serves as the basis for information that appears on product labels. Each section discusses concerns about deficiency and toxicity and concludes with results of clinical trials of vitamin therapies.

Vitamin A

Vitamin A is a fat-soluble, solid terpene alcohol essential for skeletal growth, testicular and ovarian function, embryonic development, and differentiation of tissues. It is crucial for the normal functioning of the eye, by combining with the red pigment of the retina (opsin) to form rhodopsin, which is necessary for sight in partial darkness. In addition, vitamin A is required for adequate immune system response, builds the body's resistance to respiratory infections, and helps form and maintain healthy skin, hair, and mucous membranes.

Vitamin A is available in several forms. Retinols are a derivative of vitamin A found in foods that come from animals (meat, milk, and eggs), as well as fish liver oils, cheese, and butter. Beta-carotene, a pre-vitamin found in leafy green vegetables and yellow fruits, is converted by the body into vitamin A.

Symptoms of vitamin A deficiency include lack of tear secretion, dry or rough skin, weight loss, poor bone growth, weak tooth enamel, night blindness, changes in mucous membranes, susceptibility to respiratory infections, and diarrhea. Many months of a vitamin A deficient diet are required before any adverse symptoms develop, however, and most healthy individuals have a two-year supply of vitamin A stored in the liver.

Vitamin A deficiency is a major health problem in many developing countries where it can cause several major eye diseases. One of these diseases, xerophthalmia, characterized by conjunctival dryness with hardening of the tissue, is contracted by approximately 500,000 people each year in India. Half of these cases reportedly to lead to blindness, and only 30 percent of children with severe xerophthalmia are likely to survive, according to a report by K. Vijayaraghavan in the December 1, 1990, issue of *The Lancet.*

Overdoses of vitamin A can lead to hypervitaminosis A, resulting in fatigue, abdominal upset, brittle nails, and other adverse side effects.

Vitamin A and Cancer. Vitamin A and its derivatives (beta-carotene, retinol) represent one class of anticarcinogenic phytochemicals. Vitamin A has been demonstrated to reduce cancerous tumors in animals and may reduce the risk of lung cancer in humans. In a study published in March 1992 by the *New England Journal of Medicine,* researchers reported that high doses of a derivative of vitamin A, marketed as the acne drug Accutane, prevent lung, throat, and mouth cancers in people who are at high risk of developing them.

Researchers at the M.D. Anderson Cancer Center of the University of Texas in Houston also successfully treated patients with head and neck cancer using Accutane. Because these patients' tissues already were primed to become cancerous, they were very likely to grow new, separate cancers that were more life-threatening than the first. Accutane prevented new cancers from forming in most

> ## The Benefits of Vitamin A
>
> - Builds resistance to infections, especially of the respiratory tract and mucous membranes.
> - Counteracts night blindness and weak eyesight.
> - Promotes healthy skin.
> - Helps prevent lung, throat, and mouth cancers in people who are high risk of developing them.
> - Helps prevent head and neck cancer.
> - Strengthens pregnancy (when taken in conjunction with iron) by combatting a deficiency of red blood cells in anemic women.

patients in the study for nearly three years. However, the drug did not prevent the recurrence of the original tumors, as reported by Frank Murray in *Today's Living,* October 1992.

Accutane has serious side effects when administered in high doses, but researchers reported that if lower doses also work, the stage will be set for giving Accutane to people who smoke or drink heavily and are therefore at relatively high risk for head or neck cancers. The findings strongly indicated that other cancers might also be preventable.

Vitamin A and Pregnancy. Malnourished pregnant women often suffer from anemia because they lack the nutrient iron that is crucial for carrying oxygen in the blood. A 1993 study suggests that pregnant women have a much better chance of combatting anemia by ingesting vitamin A and iron supplements, instead of iron pills alone. The study, conducted in West Java, Indonesia,

B Vitamins

The B family consists of thiamine (B1), riboflavin (B2), niacin (B3), pantothenic acid (B5), pyridoxine (B6), biotin, folic acid (B9), and cobalamin (B12). The B vitamins tend to be interdependent, so that excess intake of any one of them may generate a need for equivalent amounts of the others. B vitamins consumed in excess of the body's need are normally excreted in urine.

included 251 malnourished women who were between sixteen and twenty-four weeks pregnant. One group of women received 2.4 milligrams of vitamin A and sixty milligrams of iron, a second group was given vitamin A and a placebo, a third group received iron and a placebo, and a fourth took two dummy pills. Anemia was eliminated in 97 percent of the women who received both vitamin A and iron pills. By comparison, anemia was eliminated in 68 percent of those who took only iron, 35 percent who took vitamin A alone, and 16 percent who took only the placebos. Dr. D. Suharno, writing in the November 27, 1993, issue of *The Lancet,* warned that extremely high doses of vitamin A can be toxic, however, and cause fetal malformations during the first three months of pregnancy.

Vitamin B1

Vitamin B1 (thiamine), is a water-soluble nutrient important for growth, digestion, and normal functioning of the nervous system, muscles, and heart. Vitamin B1 keeps mucous membranes healthy and replaces deficiency caused by alcoholism, cirrhosis, overactive thyroid, infection, breast-feeding, absorption diseases, pregnancy, prolonged diarrhea, and burns.

Natural sources of vitamin B1 include brewer's yeast, rice, bran, brown rice, wheat germ and whole-grained products, oatmeal, beef kidney and liver, dried beans (garbanzo, navy, and kidney), salmon, soy beans, and sunflower seeds.

People deficient in vitamin B1 commonly experience a loss of appetite, weakness and lassitude, nervous irritability, insomnia, weight loss, muscle aches and pains, mental depression, and constipation. Alcoholics usually are deficient in most of the B vitamins, including B1.

Vitamin B1 has been used to treat certain types of depression associated with alcoholism. One study conducted in New Zealand concluded that alcoholics, who exhibit many of the symptoms of beriberi (including fatigue, diarrhea, weight loss, and paralysis), also may benefit from vitamin B1 supplements containing at least 200 mg. of thiamine. The study concluded that thiamine is a therapeutic agent that "is literally lifesaving in a significant proportion of patients," according to J. Cade's report in the February 1986 *Australian-New Zealand Journal of Psychiatry.*

Vitamin B2

Vitamin B2 (riboflavin) aids in the release of energy from food and preserves the integrity of the nervous system, eyes, and skin. It acts as a component in two coenzymes (flavin mononucleotide and flavin adenine dinucleotide), both of which are needed for normal tissue growth. Vitamin B2 maintains healthy mucous membranes lining the respiratory, digestive, circulatory, and excretory tracts when used in conjunction with vitamin A. In their *Encyclopedia of Natural Medicine,* Murray and Pizzorno report that vitamin B2 appears to decrease a craving for sugar and thus may help prevent diabetes, and improves vision, especially in elderly people. It aids in treating infections, stomach problems, burns, alcoholism, and liver disease.

Natural sources of vitamin B2 include almonds, liver, kidney, beef, brewer's yeast, cheese, chicken, and most B1 sources. Vitamin B2 deficiencies may result in itching and burning of the eyes, cracking of the skin, inflammation of the mouth, and bloodshot eyes. A deficiency of riboflavin also is believed to be linked with cataract formation.

The use of oral contraceptives has been associated with inducing several nutrient deficiencies, including riboflavin, pyridoxine, ascorbic acid, and zinc, while iron, copper, and vitamin A levels typically are increased. These findings suggest decreased liver metabolism of riboflavin. Females who suffer from premenstrual syndrome, or PMS (see Chapter 13 for a complete discussion), may benefit from B2 supplements administered under the care of a health practitioner.

The administration of large doses of B vitamins, especially riboflavin, has been shown to be quite effective in the treatment of acute acne (rosacea), according to the *Encyclopedia of Natural Medicine*.

Vitamin B3

Two chemicals have vitamin B3 properties: nicotinic acid (niacin) and niacinamide (nicotinamide adenine dinucleotide). Both are necessary for releasing energy from foods, for the utilization of fats, and for tissue respiration. Niacin helps control blood fat levels and is important for the proper functioning of skin and nerves. It also promotes growth, maintains normal functioning of the gastrointestinal tract, and is necessary for metabolism of sugar. Vitamin B3 reduces cholesterol and triglycerides in the blood; dilates blood vessels; treats vertigo (dizziness), pellagra, and

Recommended Dietary Allowance (RDA) for Vitamin B1 (Thiamine)

	mg.
Infants (0–1 year)	0.4
Children (1–10 years)	0.8
Males (11–24 years)	1.4
Males (25–51+ years)	1.4
Females (11–24 years)	1.1
Females (25–51+ years)	1.1
Pregnant Females	1.5
Breast-feeding Females	1.6

ringing in the ears; and prevents premenstrual headaches. Niacinamide is generally used in treatment because, unlike niacin, it does not cause burning, flushing, or itching of the skin.

Niacin can be made in the body from the amino acid tryptophan. Natural sources of vitamin B3 include chicken, beef liver, lean meat such as turkey or veal, brewer's yeast, wheat products, yeast, green vegetables and beans, halibut, salmon, swordfish, tuna, peanuts, pork, and sunflower seeds. Strict vegetarians who eat no animal foods must rely on nuts and legumes for niacin. Niacin found in some cereals and in vegetables such as corn may be present in chemically unusable forms.

Signs of vitamin B3 deficiency include pellagra, inflammation of the skin and tongue, gastrointestinal disturbances, nervous system dysfunctions, muscle weakness, headaches, fatigue, mental depression, irritability, loss of appetite, neuritis, nausea, dizziness, weight loss, and insomnia.

Recommended Dietary Allowance (RDA) for Vitamin B2 (Riboflavin)

	mg.
Infants (0–1 year)	0.4
Children (1–10 years)	1.1
Males (11–24 years)	1.6
Males (25–51+ years)	1.5
Females (11–24 years)	1.3
Females (25–51+ years)	1.3
Pregnant Females	1.6
Breast-feeding Females	1.8

Vitamin B5

Vitamin B5 (pantothenic acid) is another B vitamin essential for normal growth and development. It aids in the release of energy from foods and helps synthesize numerous body materials.

Recommended Dietary Allowance (RDA) for Vitamin B3 (Niacin)

	mg.
Infants (0–1 year)	6
Children (1–10 years)	12
Males (11–24 years)	19
Males (25–51+ years)	17
Females (11–24 years)	15
Females (25–51+ years)	14
Pregnant Females	17
Breast-feeding Females	20

Vitamin B5 is found in blue cheese, brewer's yeast, corn, eggs, lentils, liver, lobster, peanuts, peas, soybeans, sunflower seeds, wheat germ, whole-grain products, and meats of all kinds.

There are no known deficiency symptoms for vitamin B5 alone. However, a deficiency in one B vitamin is usually associated with an overall lack of B nutrients. Pantothenic acid usually is given with other B vitamins if symptoms of any vitamin B deficiency exist, including excessive fatigue, sleep disturbances, loss of appetite, and nausea. Anyone with inadequate caloric or nutritional dietary intake may be vitamin B5-deficient. Vitamin B5 is recommended by physicians for people with a chronic wasting illness, those suffering excess stress for long periods, or those who have recently undergone surgery. Vitamin B5 supplements are sometimes recommended for those who participate in vigorous physical activities, such as athletes and manual laborers. No RDA has been established for vitamin B5.

Vitamin B6

Vitamin B6 (pyridoxine) is a water-soluble B vitamin critical for the metabolism of amino acids. Along with niacinamide, vitamin B6 aids in the absorption of proteins, helps the body use fats, and assists in the formation of red blood cells. It helps the normal functioning of the brain, maintains chemical balance among body fluids, regulates excretion of water, and helps in energy production and resistance to stress.

Vitamin B6 can be found in avocados, bananas, bran, brewer's yeast, carrots, whole-wheat flour, hazelnuts, lentils, rice, salmon, shrimp, soybeans, sunflower seeds, tuna, and wheat germ. A pyridoxine deficiency results in depressed immunity, noted by a reduction in the quantity and quality of antibodies produced, shrinkage of lymphatic tissues including the thymus gland, decreased thymic hormone activity, and a reduction in the number and activity of lymphocytes. Factors contributing to a vitamin B6 deficiency include low dietary intake, excess protein intake, and alcohol and oral contraception use.

Vitamin B6 and Asthma. Vitamin B6 may be of direct benefit to asthmatic patients, since it is involved in the synthesis of all major neurotransmitters. In one study, plasma and red cell pyridoxal phosphate (the active form of vitamin B6) levels in fifteen adult patients with asthma were significantly lower than in sixteen controls. In his 1975 book, *Meganutrients for Your Nerves,* H. Newbold said that all patients reported a dramatic decrease in frequency and severity of wheezing and asthmatic attacks while taking the supplements.

Vitamin B6 and Cancer. Vitamin B6 is one of the most promising B vitamins for cancer treatment. Hans Ladner and Richard Salkeld, German and Swiss researchers, respectively, conducted a clinical trial treating cancer patients with vitamin B6 in addition to radiotherapy. Three hundred milligrams of B6 were given over a seven-week period to 105 endometrial cancer patients, aged forty-five to sixty-five. These patients had a 15 percent improvement in five-year survival rates compared to 105 patients who did not receive the B6 supplements. No side effects from the B6 supplementation were observed. Another study suggested that B6 supplementation to correct metabolic abnormality might prevent recurrence of bladder cancer.

Ladner and Salkeld also confirmed the beneficial effects of B6 on radiation-induced symptoms (nausea, vomiting, and diarrhea) in gynecological patients treated with high-energy radiation. They subsequently gave B6 to sixty-three hundred patients with cervical, uterine, endometrial, ovarian, and breast cancers and concluded that both quality of life

Recommended Dietary Allowance (RDA) for Vitamin B6 (Pyridoxine)

	mg.
Infants (0–1 year)	0.5
Children (1–10 years)	1.4
Males (11–24 years)	2.0
Males (25–51+ years)	2.0
Females (11–24 years)	1.5
Females (25–51+ years)	1.6
Pregnant Females	2.2
Breast-feeding Females	2.1

and survival rates significantly improved. This clinical trial was cited in 1991 by Robert D. Reynold in a chapter in *Essential Nutrients in Carcinogenesis.*

Vitamin B6 also has proved effective in inhibiting melanoma cancer cells. One research team developed a topical B6 pyri-

Recommended Dietary Allowance (RDA) for Vitamin B9 (Folic Acid)

	mcg.
Infants (0–1 year)	30
Children (1–10 years)	75
Males (11–24 years)	200
Males (25–51+ years)	200
Females (11–24 years)	180
Females (25–51+ years)	180
Pregnant Females	400
Breast-feeding Females	280

Recommended Dietary Allowance (RDA) for Vitamin B12 (Cobalamin)

	mcg.
Infants (0–1 year)	0.4
Children (1–10 years)	1.0
Males (11–24 years)	2.0
Males (25–51+ years)	2.0
Females (11–24 years)	2.0
Females (25–51+ years)	2.0
Pregnant Females	2.2
Breast-feeding Females	2.6

doxal that "produced a significant reduction in the size of subcutaneous cancer nodules and complete regression of cutaneous papules." While the results were considered preliminary, they may lead to a more successful topical B6 treatment for several forms of skin cancer, according to Reynold.

Vitamin B9 (Folic Acid)

Folic acid is an acid which helps promote normal red blood cell formation. It acts as a co-enzyme for normal DNA synthesis and functions as part of a co-enzyme in amino acid and nucleoprotein synthesis. It also maintains nervous system integrity and intestinal tract functions. In pregnant mothers, vitamin B9 helps regulate embryonic and fetal development of nerve cells.

Most people obtain sufficient amounts of folic acid in their daily diet. Natural sources include barley, beans, brewer's yeast, calves' liver, fruits, garbanzo beans (chickpeas), green and leafy vegetables, lentils, orange juice, oranges, peas, rice, soybeans, sprouts, wheat, and wheat germ.

Folic acid deficiency is the most common vitamin deficiency in the world. Unlike vitamin B12, the body does not maintain a large surplus of folic acid; folic acid stores in the liver and kidneys will sustain the body for only one to two months.

Alcoholics frequently are deficient in B9 because alcohol impairs folic acid absorption, disrupts folic acid metabolism, and causes the body to excrete folic acid. In addition to alcohol, anticancer drugs, drugs for epilepsy, and oral contraceptives also cause a folic acid deficiency.

Folic acid deficiency is common in pregnant women. Vitamin B9 is vital to cell reproduction within the fetus. Without a constant source of vitamin B9 for the fetus, birth defects will result. In November 1992, the FDA recommended that food, preferably enriched flour, be fortified with folic acid to prevent neural tube defect, a common birth defect that occurs when the spinal column fails to close completely during the first six weeks of pregnancy.

Folic acid deficiencies are frequently found in patients with chronic diarrhea, coeliac disease, and Crohn's disease. Vitamin B9 deficiency may result in anemia, depression, and a swollen, red tongue.

Vitamin B9 and Gum Disease. Studies have shown that folic acid, administered either topically or internally, produces significant reduction of gingival inflammation (gum disease) by binding toxins secreted by plaques. The use of folate mouthwash is particularly recommended for pregnant women, oral contraceptive users, those using antifolate drugs (e.g., phenytoin and methotrexate), and people suffering from other conditions associated with an exaggerated gingival inflammatory response.

B Vitamins and Disease Prevention

- Vitamin B1 helps treat certain types of depression and alcoholism.

- Vitamin B2 may help prevent diabetes and improves vision, especially in elderly people.

- Vitamin B3 helps control blood fat levels.

- Vitamin B6 helps treat endometrial cancer and may prevent recurrence of bladder cancer.

- Vitamin B6 reduces radiation-induced symptoms such as nausea, vomiting, and diarrhea.

- Vitamin B6 has proved effective in inhibiting melanoma cancer cells.

- Vitamin B9 helps prevent birth defects, and can regress precancerous cells in the cervix.

- Vitamin B9 prevents some psychological disorders and helps treat gum disease.

- Vitamin B12 may help treat schizophrenia.

Vitamin B12 (Cobalamin)

Vitamin B12 maintains the health of all body cells by production of nucleic acid. It also helps preserve nerve tissue and enhances blood formation and the production of DNA (which is found in the chromosomes of the nucleus of all cells) and RNA (which carries gene data from the nucleus to the cytoplasm).

Vitamin B12 is found only in animal sources such as beef and beef liver, clams, flounder, herring, liverwurst, mackerel, sardines, blue and Swiss cheese, eggs, and milk. Strict vegetarians must therefore take a B12 supplement such as nutritional yeast. Large amounts of folic acid can mask a B12 deficiency, and large doses of vitamin C are known to increase the need for B12. B12 requires absorption of a special protein that some individuals are unable to produce, necessitating B12 injections.

There have been few studies of how vitamin B12 therapies might aid in preventing certain chronic diseases. However, research has shown that when schizophrenics with low vitamin B12 levels are given B12 supplements, their symptoms improve, according to an article by E. Reynold in the *British Journal of Psychiatry* in March 1970. Vitamin B12, along with several other nutrients and plant compounds, has also been used in therapeutic trials to rebuild weak immune systems.

Although B12 deficiency is less prevalent in psychiatric patients than that of folic acid deficiency, determining B12 levels in the blood is considered a useful screening measure for psychiatric patients. Patients with severe mania and psychosis secondary to B12 deficiency have had complete remission after B12 supplementation, E. Reynold reported. An improvement is usually noted within four to seven days with virtually no side effects.

Vitamin C

Vitamin C, also known as ascorbic acid, is a water-soluble, white crystalline that is essential for the formation of collagen and fibrous tissue; for normal intercellular matrices in teeth, bones, cartilage, connective tissue, and skin; and for the structural integrity of capillary walls. It aids in fighting bacterial

Recommended Dietary Allowance (RDA) for Vitamin C

The optimum dose level for vitamin C is one thousand to five thousand milligrams (mg.) per day, depending upon the age and physical condition of the person taking it. To reduce the frequency and severity of colds, for example, Pauling recommended that individuals take at least three thousand mg. per day, although it has been estimated that an average of eight thousand mg. per day is required to prevent colds in 95 percent of the population.

	mg.
Infants (0–1 year)	35
Children (1–10 years)	45
Males (11–24 years)	60
Males (25–51+ years)	60
Females (11–24 years)	60
Females (25–51+ years)	60
Pregnant Females	70
Breast-feeding Females	95

infections, interacts with other nutrients, and has been shown to relieve emotional and environmental stress and depression and to protect the circulatory system from fat deposits. Vitamin C is a key factor in many immune functions as well, including white blood cell function, interferon levels, increasing antibody levels and response, and increasing the secretion of thymic hormones. Vitamin C has been used as part of aggressive treatment programs for people with AIDS, cancer, and other diseases in which optimizing immune function is a critical therapeutic goal.

Vitamin C is present in citrus fruits, tomatoes, berries, potatoes, and fresh, green, leafy vegetables such as broccoli, brussel sprouts, collards, turnip greens, parsley, and cabbage. Relative to other nutrients, it is one of the safest substances known.

Vitamin C also is available in tablets, extended-release capsules, oral solutions, and injections. Tablets and capsules are sold in most health food stores. Vitamin C injections are available only from a physician.

Vitamin C deficiency symptoms include shortness of breath, digestive difficulties, easy bruising, swollen or painful joints, nosebleeds, anemia, frequent infections, and slow healing of wounds. Conversely, while massive daily doses of vitamin C are not necessarily toxic because the body expels what it cannot use, they can cause stomach upset and diarrhea.

Vitamin C and Cataracts. Cataracts are caused, in part, by changes in proteins located in the eye, and research studies suggest that vitamin C can prevent these changes. In one study, reported in the July 1992 *Environmental Nutrition,* people who took several vitamin supplements, including vitamin C, had four times less risk of developing cataracts than those who took no supplements. Research on vitamin C's role in preventing cataracts is still inconclusive, however, as other antioxidant nutrients such as vitamin E and beta-carotene help prevent cataracts as well.

Vitamin C and Cholesterol. Studies have demonstrated that vitamin C lowers LDL ("bad") cholesterol levels in the blood because it attacks free radicals—the highly unstable oxygen molecules that damage (or oxidize) body tissues and blood fats. The free radicals' effect on LDL is similar to what happens to a steak when it is exposed to the air too long: it oxidizes and turns brown. Scientists now think that vitamin C and other antioxidants prevent the oxidation process caused by free radicals. According to Jeffrey Frei, assistant professor of nutrition at Harvard School of Public Health, in the October 1991 issue of *Prevention Magazine,* "Vitamin C traps free radicals in the surrounding environment before they can attack the LDL particle. As long as there is vitamin C, free radicals cannot attack LDL because the C forms a very tight, protective shield around it." Furthermore, vitamin C strengthens HDL cholesterol (the good form) by making it more resistant to free-radical damage. Lowering blood cholesterol levels is still the only proven way to reduce heart disease. As a result, many physicians now recommend foods rich in vitamin C, E, and beta-carotene (such as fruits and vegetables) as a way of lowering cholesterol. In addition, many experts suggest that the current RDA for vitamins C and E may be too low, and that beta-carotene (a form of vitamin A) should be added.

Vitamin C and Disease Prevention. Many studies have shown that increased vitamin C intake can produce a number of beneficial effects, including reducing the risk of cancer, strengthening the immune system, protecting against the effects of pollution and cigarette smoke, enhancing wound repair, and increasing life expectancy.

Pauling first postulated the theory that moderate doses of vitamin C (250 to 1,000 mg.) effectively prevented the spread of viral and bacterial infections, and that large doses of one gram or more may cure those infections.

A growing body of scientists now believes that vitamin C also reduces the risk of cancer. In 1991, Dr. Gladys Block, professor of nutrition at the University of California at Berkeley, reviewed more than 100 studies linking vitamin C or vitamin C-rich foods (primarily fruit) and cancer prevention. Block

Vitamin C and Cholesterol

- Increases the rate at which cholesterol is removed by its conversion to bile acids and excretion via the intestines.
- Increases high density lipoprotein (HDL) cholesterol levels. High HDL levels are correlated with low risk of heart disease.
- Through its laxative effect, accelerates elimination of waste, thereby decreasing the reabsorption of bile acids and their reconversion to cholesterol.

VITAMIN C

found that vitamin C's protection is most convincing for cancers of the throat, mouth, pancreas, and stomach. In an article in the *American Journal of Clinical Nutrition,* published in January 1991, she also suggested that vitamin C has a protective effect against cancers of the cervix, rectum, and breast. A 1992 National Cancer Institute study, reported in the July 6, 1992, issue of *Cancer Weekly,* found that the protective effect of vitamin C against breast cancer was as great, if not greater, than the effect of reducing saturated fat intake.

Vitamin C performs several functions that explain why it may be important in preventing cancer. It acts as an antioxidant that protects cells and tissues from damage caused by free radicals, significantly influences immune function, and may inhibit the spread of tumors. Vitamin C was directly associated with "a significant protective effect" against cancer in thirty-three out of forty-six studies that Block analyzed. Several of the studies also showed a positive correlation between fruit intake and protection against cancer.

Vitamin C and Disease Prevention

- Reduces the risk of some cancers.
- Diminishes the side effects of radio-therapy and chemotherapy.
- Halts the spread of viral and bacterial infections.
- Reduces the risk of developing high blood pressure.
- Lessens the risk of heart disease.
- Protects the skin against ultraviolet A (UVA) and ultraviolet B (UVB) light exposure thereby preventing premature aging and wrinkles.
- Reduces cholesterol levels.
- Helps prevent cataracts.

However, while these studies indicate vitamin C "reduces the risk of cancer," they do not prove that vitamin C "cures" it.

The importance of vitamin C-rich diets was further confirmed in a broad-based study of esophageal cancer in China. In 1983, blood samples were collected from 100 adults (aged twenty-five to sixty-four years), and then analyzed. Both men and women who took vitamin C had significantly lower death rates from esophageal cancer. Death rates for people who did not take vitamin C were more than three times higher, according to a June 1984 report by Wande Guo and others in *Nutrition and Cancer.*

Vitamin C levels (as ascorbic acid) also inhibit skin tumors. A 1992 study carried out at Duke University Medical Center strongly suggests that vitamin C protects the skin against ultraviolet A (UVA) and ultraviolet B (UVB) light exposure. The January 1992 *Harvard Health Letter* said that the Duke investigators concluded that vitamin C acts as an antioxidant and prevents UVA and UVB oxidative damage to collagen, elastin, proteo-glycan, and cell membranes. Some scientists now think that vitamin C will eventually be shown to prevent premature aging, wrinkles, and skin cancer.

Vitamin C and Hypertension. Medical surveys have found that people whose vitamin C levels are low tend to have high blood pressure. A recent study published in *Environmental Nutrition* found that 1,000 mg. a day of supplemental vitamin C significantly reduced systolic blood pressure (the top number in a blood pressure reading) in a group of twenty women, twelve of whom had borderline hypertension. The vitamin C–blood pressure connection deserves further research.

Vitamin C and Increased Longevity. Adding substantially larger amounts of vitamin C to ordinary diets may prolong life by lessening the risk of heart disease and cancer. A large U.S. survey conducted by the National Center for Health Statistics (NCHS) demonstrated a strong correlation between vitamin C intake and decreased mortality. Between 1971 and 1974, the NCHS collected extensive diet and nutrition information from 11,348 adults aged twenty-five to seventy-four. Investigators at the UCLA School of Public Health subsequently reviewed the participants' estimated daily vitamin C intake and divided them into three groups: less than 50 mg.; 50 mg. or more from dietary sources; and 50 mg. or more from food, plus regular vitamin C supplementation, usually in the form of pills containing several hundred milligrams.

For men with the highest vitamin C intake, the total number of deaths was 35 percent lower than predicted, mortality due to cardiovascular diseases was 42 percent lower, and cancer deaths were 22 percent less.

Benefits were not as apparent for women in the high-C group: there was an overall drop in expected mortality of 10 percent, with a 25 percent decline in deaths caused by heart disease, and a 15 percent reduction in those due to cancer, according to a report published in the July 1992 issue of *Environmental Nutrition*. Many of the participants also took vitamins A and E, which act to block the oxidation of cholesterol and other molecules thought to play important roles in the development of cancer and heart disease. Although the UCLA study does not prove that vitamin C supplements will guarantee a longer life, the findings do suggest that substantial amounts of vitamin C provide greater protection against fatal diseases.

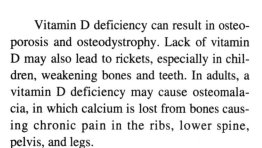

Recommended Dietary Allowance (RDA) for Vitamin D

	mcg.
Infants (0–1 year)	10
Children (1–10 years)	10
Males (11–24 years)	10
Males (25–51+ years)	5
Females (11–24 years)	10
Females (25–51+ years)	5
Pregnant Females	10
Breast-feeding Females	10

Vitamin D

Vitamin D is a fat-soluble vitamin chemically related to steroids. It is essential for the normal formation of bones and teeth and for the absorption of calcium and phosphorus in the gastrointestinal tract. Vitamin D is also called cholecalciferol and is available from both natural and synthetic sources.

Small amounts of vitamin D are present in natural foods, especially milk and dairy products. Other natural foods containing vitamin D include saltwater fish, especially salmon, sardines, and herring; organ meats; fish-liver oils; and egg yolks. Vitamin D is also obtained through exposure to sunlight. Ultraviolet rays activate a form of cholesterol in an oil of the skin and convert it to a type of vitamin D, which is then absorbed. In some cases, vitamin D cannot be absorbed without the presence of other foods such as fat.

Ten micrograms per day, or 400 International Units (IU), is the recommended amount of vitamin D to ensure normal development in babies. When a normal diet does not supply sufficient vitamin D, supplements are often recommended.

Vitamin D deficiency can result in osteoporosis and osteodystrophy. Lack of vitamin D may also lead to rickets, especially in children, weakening bones and teeth. In adults, a vitamin D deficiency may cause osteomalacia, in which calcium is lost from bones causing chronic pain in the ribs, lower spine, pelvis, and legs.

Like vitamin A, vitamin D can accumulate in the body, causing such serious side effects as kidney failure and kidney stones. Symptoms that indicate a person has consumed too much vitamin D include nausea, weakness, and widespread aches, usually followed by more serious problems, such as high blood pressure and irregular heartbeat.

Vitamin D and Disease Prevention. Vitamin D analogs may offer a potential endocrine therapy for breast cancer. In a study reported in the September 23, 1991, issue of *Cancer Weekly,* patients with advanced breast cancer were treated daily with 1 gram of calcitrol ointment for six weeks; 21 percent subsequently showed partial slowing of the

Vitamin D and Disease Prevention

- Helps treat hypoglycemia and certain types of bone disease.
- Is an effective topical treatment for psoriasis.
- Offers a potential endocrine therapy for breast cancer.
- Reduces the rate of colon cancer.

spread of cancer. Several other studies have shown that colon cancer is less common in people who have high levels of vitamin D in their blood. One study, conducted over a nineteen-year period, reported that a daily intake of more than 3.75 micrograms of vitamin D reduced the incidence of colon cancer by 50 percent. A daily intake of at least 1200 mg. of calcium was reported to reduce the risk of colon cancer by 75 percent. Based on the results of these studies, daily intakes of 1500 mg. of calcium for women and 1800 mg. of calcium for men, as well as at least 5 micrograms of vitamin D, are recommended to reduce the risk of colon cancer, according to an article by Frank Garland in the July 1991 *American Journal of Clinical Nutrition.*

Vitamin D and the Elderly. Food and sunlight are primary sources of vitamin D, and because many elderly people do not get enough of either one, they are often vitamin D-deficient. Older people also manufacture vitamin D more slowly, and the resulting deficiency can cause their bones to weaken and grow brittle. As a result, researcshers have urged that the RDA for vitamin D be raised for this age group. Some preliminary findings suggest that taking vitamin D supplements may delay bone mass loss.

The importance of vitamin D in the bone formation of infants and bone preservation in the elderly is directly related to its role in controlling the body's ability to absorb phosphorous and calcium. Apparently, the human requirement for the essential mineral calcium changes dramatically throughout the life cycle. The need for calcium rises during growth in childhood, pregnancy, lactation, and menopause, and is lower between the ages of twenty-five and fifty-one—thus the daily dietary requirement ranges from 5 to 10 micrograms.

Vitamin D Supplements. Dihydrotachysterol, a form of vitamin D, is used to treat hypoglycemia, which occurs when there is insufficient calcium in the blood or when calcium is not used properly by the body. Calcitrol, another form of vitamin D available only by prescription, is used to treat hypoglycemia and certain types of bone disease that occur in patients who are undergoing renal dialysis for kidney disease. A third form of vitamin D, calciportiol, has been shown to be an effective topical treatment for psoriasis, according to L. May in *Drug Information,* published in 1993.

Vitamin E

Vitamin E is a co-factor in many enzymes that promote normal growth and development, including the formation of red blood cells. Along with vitamin C, it helps prevent the corrosive oxidation of free radicals in the body,

Natural sources of vitamin E include wheat germ, liver, sunflower seeds, whole grains, walnuts, hazelnuts, almonds, butter, eggs, turnip greens, asparagus, spinach, peas, peanuts, cashews, soy lecithin, and vegetable oils. Salad oils, margarine, and shortening provide about 64 percent of vitamin E in the

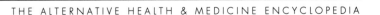

average U.S. diet, fruits and vegetables about 11 percent, and grains and grain products about 7 percent.

A diet high in polyunsaturated fats is a major cause of vitamin E deficiency. In *How To Live Longer and Feel Better,* Pauling suggests that "a diet high in unsaturated fatty oils, especially the polyunsaturated ones, can destroy the body's deposits of vitamin E, and cause muscular lesions, brain lesions, and degeneration of blood vessels. Care must be taken not include a large amount of polyunsaturated oil in the diet without a corresponding intake of vitamin E." Pauling recommends that the RDA of vitamin E for adults be raised.

Vitamin E and Alzheimer's Disease. Patients with Alzheimer's disease have been found to have high levels of two enzymes linked to damage of nerve cells, and vitamins A, E, and beta-carotene may slow down the disease's progression. Researchers at Central Middlesex Hospital in London measured serum levels of vitamins A and E and four major carotenoids (any of various yellow to red pigments found in foods) in ten patients with Alzheimer's disease, ten with dementia, and twenty nondemented elderly individuals. Plasma concentrations of vitamin E and beta-carotene were significantly lower in patients with Alzheimer's and dementia than in the control group. Since vitamins A and E and carotenoids act as free radical scavengers, their deficiency may accelerate the degenerative processes in the brain that cause Alzheimer's disease, according to an article in the June 1992 *Nutrition Research Newsletter.*

Vitamin E and Angina. A study conducted in Edinburgh, Scotland, tested the hypothesis that low plasma concentrations of vitamin E may be related to the risk of angina. Plasma concentrations of vitamins A, C, E, and beta-carotene were measured in six thousand Edinburgh men aged thirty-five to fifty-five.

Recommended Dietary Allowance (RDA) for Vitamin E

	mg.
Infants (0–1 year)	4
Children (1–10 years)	7
Males (11–24 years)	10
Males (25–51+ years)	10
Females (11–24 years)	8
Females (25–51+ years)	8
Pregnant Females	10
Breast-feeding Females	12

Note: One mg. equals 1 IU (International Unit), and labels may list either.

Plasma concentrations of vitamins C, E, and carotene were inversely related to the risk of angina, while vitamin A showed no relationship. The researchers emphasized that their findings, obtained in a population with a high heart disease risk and low intakes of fruit and green vegetables, may not apply to other communities but their evidence strongly suggests that populations with a high incidence of coronary heart disease may benefit from eating diets rich in natural antioxidants, particularly vitamin E. The study was reported by R.A. Riemersma and others in the January 5, 1991, issue of *The Lancet.*

Vitamin E and Bypass Heart Surgery. Vitamin E may prevent the formation of free radicals during the final phase of bypass surgery—an operation to improve blood flow to the heart. Free radicals often form while surgeons briefly flood the heart with richly oxygenated blood, but until recently surgeons

Vitamin E and Disease Prevention

- Prevents cardiovascular ailments including ischemic heart disease (IHD).
- Guards lungs against air pollutants such as ozone, nitrous oxide, and cigarette smoke.
- Prevents the breakdown of the immune system in older people, decreasing the likelihood of infectious disease and tumors.
- Reduces the risk of cataracts, cardiovascular disease, and other problems associated with aging.
- Helps prevent epileptic seizures.
- Reduces the risk of cancer.
- May slow down Alzheimer's disease.
- Prevents the formation of free radicals during the final phase of bypass surgery.
- Relieves joint inflammation in rheumatoid arthritis.

had no way of shielding the heart from this process. Dr. Terrence Yau of the University of Toronto reported that presurgical supplementation with vitamin E improved the heart's ability to pump during the risky five-hour postoperative period. He and his colleagues gave fourteen patients 300 mg. of highly purified vitamin E daily for two weeks prior to their bypass operations, and achieved successful, though preliminary, results, according to an article by Kathy A. Fackelmann in *Science News* of November 24, 1990.

Vitamin E and Cancer. Several studies conducted in Finland found that, on average, patients who developed cancers had less vitamin E in their bloodstreams than did healthy patients. The Finnish studies of 21,172 men and 15,093 women preliminarily support the premise that higher vitamin E levels in the blood help reduce the risk of cancer, according to an article in the June 1992 *Nutrition Research Newsletter.*

A 1992 National Cancer Institute study involving more than eleven hundred patients found that, while several supplements appeared to lessen the risk of oral cancers, only vitamin E cut the risk in half. The study, reported in the July 6, 1992, *Cancer Weekly,* confirmed that vitamin E helped protect the fatty acids in cell membranes against free radicals.

Vitamin E and Cardiovascular Disease. Vitamin E helps prevent cardiovascular ailments including blood clots, protects against cell damage by oxidation, and guards lungs against air pollutants such as ozone, nitrous oxide, and cigarette smoke. Approximately eighty studies have found that children of smokers are more prone to bronchitis, pneumonia, hospitalizations, and missed school days. When they are given a daily intake of at least 5,000 to 10,000 IU of vitamin A, along with 400 to 800 IU of vitamin E, their lungs and mucous membranes are less prone to damage, reports S. Langer in the September 1990 issue of *Better Nutrition.*

It is now widely accepted that vitamin E keeps the blood free-flowing without causing profuse bleeding by exerting a powerful anti-clotting effect in veins and arteries. A study described by Frank Murray in the August 1990 *Better Nutrition* showed that 1,476 patients with general arteriosclerosis (thickening of the lining of the arteries, which limits blood flow) who were given vitamin E for ten years had a significantly higher survival rate than patients who had not taken this vitamin. Dr. Gnut Haeger, a prominent Swedish surgeon, has successfully used high doses of vitamin E to treat elderly patients with poor blood circulation in the legs, according to the same article.

Vitamin E and Epilepsy. Preliminary evidence suggests that vitamin E may be helpful in preventing epileptic seizures. Using controlled dosages of vitamin E, doctors at the University of Toronto reduced the frequency of seizures by more than 60 percent in ten of twelve children who took 400 IU daily for three months in addition to their regular medication. When children taking a placebo were switched to vitamin E, seizure frequency was reduced 70 to 100 percent. A 1989 report in *Epilepsia* said that the researchers noted there were no adverse side effects. Because the results are based on only one study, however, additional research is needed to confirm whether vitamin E supplements can help reduce or prevent epileptic seizures.

Vitamin E and Ischemic Heart Disease (IHD). According to a 1991 World Health Organization (WHO) study, low blood levels of vitamin E are the most important risk factor in deaths from IHD. IHD is known to occur when blood circulation to the heart is inadequate, usually because of coronary artery damage, resulting in pains or spasms. While not conclusive, this study tentatively suggests that vitamin E may play a protective role against IHD.

The WHO study also showed that vitamin E blood levels were more significant in predicting death than high cholesterol, elevated blood pressure, or smoking. Forty participants consisted of men aged forty to forty-nine from sixteen European cities; some of the men were smokers. Low blood levels of vitamin E were linked with death in 62 percent of the cases. The highest death rate

The Benefits of Vitamin E

- Maintains adequate pulmonary capacity.
- Helps prevent blood clots in the arteries and veins.
- Dissolves existing clots.
- Increases available oxygen in the blood.
- Increases the heart's efficiency by reducing its need for oxygen.
- Facilitates circulation by dilating capillaries and developing collateral blood vessels.

occurred when patients had a combination of low vitamin E, low vitamin A, high total cholesterol, and high blood pressure, as reported by J. de Keyser in the June 27, 1991, issue of *The Lancet.*

Two major studies conducted by the Harvard School of Public Health, and reported in the November 19, 1992, *New York Times,* concluded that taking daily doses of vitamin E may cut the risk of heart disease by one-third to one-half. The studies lend further support to the theory that vitamins and other substances that retard oxidation are good for the heart. In the first study, 87,245 female nurses in the U.S. were surveyed, 17 percent of whom took vitamin E. After eight years of follow-up, the researchers found that nurses who had taken vitamin E for at least two years had a 46 percent lower risk of heart disease than those who did not take the supplement. The other study surveyed 51,529 male health professionals. A 37 percent lower risk of heart disease was reported among the men who took regular vitamin E supplements. Both studies concluded that the amount of vitamin

E in vitamin-rich food such as lettuce was not sufficient to produce the benefit. That occurred only when people took at least 100 IU of vitamin E daily, the amount in a single vitamin supplement.

Vitamin E and Longevity. As discussed earlier, free radicals contribute to the gradual development of chronic diseases, such as hardening of the arteries, cancer, cataracts, Parkinson's disease, Alzheimer's disease, arthritis, and other complications of aging. Vitamin E is now believed to reduce the damage caused by free radicals and to help prevent or delay the onset of these diseases, thereby potentially increasing life span.

Langer's article in *Better Nutrition* also quotes Dr. Jeffrey Blumberg of the USDA Human Nutrition Research Center on Aging: "If we really want to increase our life span, we need to decrease our caloric intake, add vitamin E, vitamin C and beta-carotene supplements to our diet, and pay closer attention to the protein, fatty-acid composition and trace mineral content of our diet. As to the ideal vitamin E intake, I would suggest 100, 200, or 300 mg. daily."

Blumberg adds: "Traditionally it was accepted that a decline in various body systems, such as heart, lung and immune functions, was a natural part of aging. But new evidence leads us to believe that the rate of decline may be governed more by environmental factors, that is, nutrition and lifestyle, than by aging per se. Age-related losses in lean body mass and bone, as well as increases in fat, may be slowed or even reversed, regardless of a person's age."

Murray also describes a study of the nutritional status of more than a thousand volunteers by Dr. Judith Hallfrisch, principal investigator for the Gerontology Nutrition Study at the National Institute on Aging. Hallfrisch found that even those volunteers who ate healthy foods "had inadequate intakes of vitamins E and B6, magnesium, zinc, iron and calcium." Along with adequate intake of vitamin E and other nutrients, Hallfrisch believes that healthy, low-stress lifestyles will eventually lead to longer lifespans. "For those committed to extending their life span and remaining in relatively good health," she concludes, "an adequate intake of such antioxidants as vitamin E, vitamin C, and beta-carotene is essential."

Vitamin E supplements also may prevent the breakdown of the immune system in older people, thereby decreasing the likelihood of infectious disease and tumors. The antioxidant defense system remains strong in most people throughout youth and the middle years, but the body's ability to produce antibodies decreases with aging. Additional research is required to determine if people who take vitamin E supplements develop more antibodies as result.

Vitamin E and Ozone Protection. Vitamin E also may protect humans against the dangerous effects of ozone, which causes a stiffening and accelerated aging of lung tissue. In preliminary studies, vitamin E has been shown to protect humans against the effects of ozone in smog. According to the research, described by W. Pryor in the March 1991 *American Journal of Clinical Nutrition,* ozone interacts with polyunsaturated fatty acids to form free radicals, and vitamin E apparently delays this reaction.

Vitamin E and Parkinson's Disease. Parkinson's disease is a progressive disease of the brain that results in tremor, joint rigidity, muscle weakness, and slow movement. As the disease progresses, higher brain functioning is disabled and motor control deteriorates. It is believed to be caused by the pathological destruction of specific cells in the basal ganglia of the brain, particularly in the substantia nigra. These cells are responsible for a particular neurotransmitter, dopamine, which in turn controls communication between cells.

Currently, patients with Parkinson's disease are treated with levodopa and other compounds related to dopamine. Unfortunately, levodopa has severe side effects and many physicians prescribe it only as a last resort. According to a report in the November 16, 1989, *New England Journal of Medicine,* one form of vitamin E, tocopherol, seems to postpone the disability of Parkinson's disease, thereby delaying the need for treatment with levodopa. Results are preliminary, however, and more research is needed to determine if tocopherol is effective as a long-term therapy.

Vitamin E and Rheumatoid Arthritis.
Patients with rheumatoid arthritis (RA) have derived significant relief from inflammatory pain when given fish oil rich in vitamin E. In one European study, described by Jacob E. Tulleken, Pieter C. Limberg, and Martin van Rijswijk in their 1990 book, *Arthritis and Rheumatism,* RA patients who received fish oil for three months suffered substantially less joint inflammation. The results suggest, however, that this effect may have been more related to fatty acid consumption than vitamin E intake, although vitamin E probably enhances the effects of the fish oil.

Summary

Vitamins, like minerals, herbs, and food supplements, are medicines and people need to be aware of their effects and the minimum and maximum amounts recommended for optimal health. A balanced, natural diet of healthy foods normally provides an adequate supply of the daily recommended dose of vitamins. Not everyone, however, receives the RDA for each vitamin, and a number of diseases are associated with vitamin deficiencies. For this reason, people diagnosed with any of these diseases (or having symptoms associated with them), or who think their diet is not nutritionally adequate, should consult a physician to determine if vitamin supplements are advisable.

Resources

References

Block, Gladys. "Vitamin C and Cancer Prevention: The Epidemiological Evidence." *American Journal of Clinical Nutrition* (January 1991).

Bower, M. "Topical Vitamin D Analogs in Advanced Breast Cancer." *Cancer Weekly* (September 23, 1991): 20.

Cade, J. "Massive Thiamine Dosage in the Treatment of Acute Alcoholic Psychoses." *Australian-New Zealand Journal of Psychiatry* (February 1986).

"Calciportiol: Advice for the Patient." *Drug Information in Lay Language* (1990): 294.

"Can Vitamins Protect Your Arteries?" *Prevention* (October 1991): 33.

de Keyser, J. "Serum Concentrations of Vitamins A and E and Early Outcome After Ischaemic Stroke." *The Lancet* (June 27, 1991): 1562.

"Depressed Plasma Peridoxal Phosphate Concentration in Adult Asthmatics." *American Journal of Clinical Nutrition* (1985): 684–88.

"Effect of Deprenyl on the Progression of Disability in Early Parkinson's Disease." *New England Journal of Medicine* (November 16, 1989): 1364.

Epilepsia (Vol. 30, No. 1, 1989).

Fackelmann, Kathy A. "Vitamin E May Safeguard Bypass Hearts." *Science News* (November 24, 1990): 333.

Garland, Frank, and Edward D. Gorham.

"Can Colon Cancer Incidence and Death Rates be Reduced with Calcium and Vitamin D?" *American Journal of Clinical Nutrition* (July 1991): 193.

Guo, Wande, et al. "Correlations of Dietary Intake and Blood Nutrient Levels with Esophageal Cancer Mortality in China." *Nutrition and Cancer* (June 1984): 121–27.

Harvard Health Letter (January 1992).

Langer, S. "Vitamin E: The Anti-clogging Antioxidant." *Better Nutrition* (September 1990).

May, L. *Drug Information.* St. Louis, MO: Mosby Year Book, Inc., 1993.

Murray, Frank. "Vitamin A Fights Cancer." *Today's Living* (October 1992): 8.

———. "Vitamin E May Delay Aging." *Better Nutrition* (August 1990).

Murray, Michael, and Joseph Pizzorno. *Encyclopedia of Natural Medicine.* Rocklin, CA: Prima Publishing, 1991.

New York Times (November 19, 1992): A10.

Newbold, H. *Meganutrients for Your Nerves.* New York, NY: Peter H. Wyden, 1975.

Pauling, Linus. *How to Live Longer and Feel Better.* New York, NY: W.H. Freeman and Co., 1986: 204.

———. *Vitamin C and the Common Cold.* New York, NY: W.H. Freeman and Co., 1971.

Pryor, W. "Can Vitamin E Protect Humans Against the Pathological Effects of Ozone in Smog?" *American Journal of Clinical Nutrition* (March 1991): 702.

Reynold, E. "Folate Deficiency in Depressive Illness." *British Journal of Psychiatry* (March 1970): 121, 287–92.

Reynold, Robert D. "Vitamin B6 Deficiency and Carcinogenesis," in *Essential Nutrients in Carcinogenesis.* New York, NY: Plenum Press, 1986.

Riemersma, R.A., et al. "Risk of Angina Pectoris and Plasma Concentrations of Vitamins A, C, and E and Carotene." *The Lancet* (January 5, 1991): 337.

Rivard, C. "Folate Deficiency Among Institutionalized Elderly, Public Health Impact." *Journal of American Geriatric Society* (1986): 211–14.

Soharno, D., et al. "Supplementation With Vitamin A and Iron for Nutritional Anaemia in Pregnant Women in West Java, Indonesia." *The Lancet* (November 27, 1993): 1325–28.

Tulleken, Jacob E., Pieter C. Limburg, and Martin van Rijswijk. *Arthritis and Rheumatism* (September 1990).

U.S. National Cancer Institute. *Cancer Weekly* (July 6, 1992): 12.

Vijayaraghavan, K. "Effect of Massive Dose Vitamin A on Morbidity and Mortality in Indian Children." *The Lancet* (December 1, 1990): 1342–43.

"Vitamin A Strengthens Pregnancy." Associated Press (November 26, 1993).

"Vitamin C: A Secret to a Long Life and a Healthy Heart." *Environmental Nutrition* (July 1992): 3.

"Vitamin E Prevents Oral Cancers." *Cancer Weekly* (July 6, 1992): 12.

"Vitamin Levels in Alzheimer's Disease." *Nutrition Research Newsletter* (June 1992): 77.

"Vitamins and Minerals." *Nutrition Research Newsletter* (June 1992): 77.

Whitehead, N., F. Reyner, and J. Lindebaum. "Megaloblastic Changes in the Cervical Epithelium Association with Oral Contraceptive Therapy and Reversal with

RESOURCES

Folic Acid." *Journal of the American Medical Association* (1973): 226.

Zimmerman, David. *Zimmerman's Complete Guide to Nonprescription Drugs.* Detroit, MI: Gale Research Inc. and Visible Ink Press, 1993.

Additional Reading

Chopra, Deepak, M.D. *Quantum Healing: Exploring the Frontiers of Body, Mind, Medicine.* New York, NY: Bantam Books, 1993.

Davidson, Michael, M.D. "Vitamin E and Cardiovascular Disease." *Vitamin E Symposium* (June 1990).

Gannon, Kathi. "The Role of Free Radicals in the Aging Process." *Drug Topics* (February 18, 1991).

Hallfrisch, Judith, Ph.D. "Nutrition Components of the Baltimore Longitudinal Study in the Aging Process" *Harvard Health Letter* (January 1992).

Kutsky, Roman J., Ph.D. *Handbook of Vitamins, Minerals and Hormones.* New York, NY: Van Nostrand Reinhold Co., 1973.

London, R.S., et al. "Vitamin E: Healing for PMS." *Journal of the American College of Nutrition* (February 1983).

Muller, D.P.R., M.D., et al. "Vitamin E in Brains of Patients with Alzheimer's Disease and Downs Syndrome." *The Lancet* (May 10, 1986).

Riggs, Maribeth. *Natural Child Care: A Complete Guide to Safe & Effective Herbal Remedies & Holistic Health Strategies for Infants & Children.* New York, NY: Crown Publishing Group, 1992.

Siegel, Bernie, M.D. *Love, Medicine & Miracles.* New York, NY: Harper & Row Publishers, Inc., 1986.

———. *Peace, Love & Healing.* New York, NY: Harper & Row Publishers, Inc., 1989.

Sokol, Ronald J., M.D. "Improved Neurologic Function After Long-Term Correction of Vitamin E Deficiency in Children with Chronic Cholestiasis." *New England Journal of Medicine* (December 19, 1985).

Sommera, Tarwotjo, G. Hussaini, and D. Susanto. "Increased Mortality in Children with Mild Vitamin A Deficiency." *The Lancet* (1983): 585–88.

"Vitamin A and Malnutrition/Infection Complex in Developing Countries." *The Lancet* (December 1, 1990): 139.

Chapter 4

MINERALS AND TRACE ELEMENTS

Minerals and trace elements are essential parts of enzymes involved in many of the body's biochemical and physiological processes, including the transportation of oxygen to the cells. If the human body requires more than one hundred milligrams of the element daily, the substance is labeled a mineral. If less than one hundred milligrams are needed each day, the substance is termed a trace element.

Unlike most vitamins, minerals are inorganic substances that usually are not destroyed by cooking, food processing, or exposure to air or acid. However, they sometimes combine with other substances in food to form insoluble salts that cannot be absorbed by the human digestive tract. The body utilizes at least eighty-four minerals and trace elements. If there is a deficiency or an absorption interference for any one of the eighty-four, malfunctions may result in the part of the body that depends on that mineral.

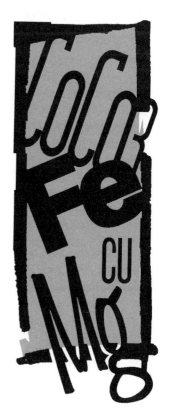

Most minerals and trace elements are widely available in foods, especially fresh fruits and vegetables, and severe deficiencies are unusual. However, iron deficiency occurs frequently in infants, children, and pregnant women. Zinc and copper deficiencies are also common among the elderly.

In the following sections, each essential mineral and trace element is discussed, including its chemical composition, physiological functions, availability in natural foods or supplements, and current Recommended Dietary Allowance (RDA), as issued by the Food and Nutrition Board of the National Academy of Sciences. The RDA for minerals and trace elements, as in the

Recommended Dietary Allowance (RDA) for Calcium

	mg.
Infants (0–1 year)	500
Children (1–10 years)	800
Males (11–24 years)	1,200
Males (25–51+ years)	800
Females (11–24 years)	1,200
Females (25–51+ years)	800
Pregnant Females	1,200
Breast-feeding Females	1,200

case with vitamins, represents the best current assessment of safe and adequate intakes.

Symptoms of deficiencies and excessive intake also are described. Mineral supplements should be used only with the approval of a physician or health practitioner. Like vitamins, some minerals in excessive doses are known to cause side effects, adverse interactions with other drugs, and other problems.

Minerals

Calcium

Calcium, the major constituent of the structural framework of bones, is the body's most prevalent mineral. Approximately three pounds of a 160-pound man's weight are calcium. For both men and women, 98 percent of the body's calcium is found in the bones, 1 percent in the teeth, and the remaining 1 percent in soft body tissues, where it performs a variety of essential functions.

In addition to supporting the growth and continued strength of bones and teeth, calcium helps maintain cell membranes and the "cement" that holds cells together. It is essential to proper blood clotting, and it assists in regulating the transport of ions in and out of cells, thus making muscular contractions and relaxation possible.

The bones act as a calcium deposit for the rest of the body. Although they are commonly thought of as fixed, solid objects, bones continually lose and regain calcium. A network of hormones keeps the calcium level in blood and other bodily fluids at a constant level, depositing temporary excesses in the bones and removing calcium from the bones if it is needed elsewhere.

The richest food sources of calcium are milk and dairy products, including yogurt and hard cheeses. Canned sardines and salmon, caviar, almonds and Brazil nuts, molasses, shrimp, soybeans, tofu, and green, leafy vegetables (particularly collard and dandelion greens and spinach) also are good sources, but oxalic acid in spinach renders much of the vegetable's calcium insoluble and nonabsorbable.

A persistent calcium shortage leads to distorted bone growth in children and a softening and deterioration of bones in adults. Osteoporosis, a weakening of the bones, affects one in four women after menopause. An inadequate calcium supply occurs when too little is consumed, too much is lost, or not enough is absorbed. At the other extreme, an excess of calcium in the body has been shown to depress nerve function, cause drowsiness and extreme lethargy, and decrease iron levels.

A vitamin D deficiency interferes with the absorption of calcium through the intestinal tract. Calcium absorption also is impaired by excessive dietary fat and continued use of corticosteroids, the synthetic equivalent of hormones made in the adrenal gland. Patients with irritable bowel syndrome (IBS), for example, have been shown to be at risk of developing calcium deficiency due to malabsorption, cortisoid use, and vitamin D deficiency. As a result, IBS patients are at risk for metabolic bone diseases.

Lack of dietary calcium in adults can result in a condition known as osteomalacia, or softening of the bone. In contrast, those suffering from osteoporosis have a deficiency of both calcium and other minerals, as well as a decrease in the nonmineral framework (organic matrix) of bone. Taking calcium supplements has proved effective in reducing age-related bone loss. Currently, calcium citrate appears to be the best form of calcium supplement, both in terms of better absorption and decreased risk of developing kidney stones.

Calcium deficiencies also may be indirectly related to hypertension. Several studies show that people with hypertension consume a smaller amount of daily calcium than nonhypertensive people, and may benefit from calcium supplementation. Clinical studies have demonstrated that calcium supplementation may also lower blood pressure. According to Dr. Leon Chaitow in *The Mind/Body Purification Program,* people living in areas with a soft-water supply (water with increased lead levels) are at risk for hypertension, and this may be partly due to the fact that soft water is normally low in calcium and magnesium. Coffee, alcohol, and smoking reduce calcium levels in the body and are associated with an increased risk of developing osteoporosis.

Along with other nutrients, calcium has been used with moderate success to reduce the risk of angina and heart disease. It also is routinely prescribed by naturopaths for mild allergies. In addition, calcium has been used to reduce cholesterol. In one study, reported in the *Encyclopedia of Natural Medicine,* a daily administration of two grams of calcium carbonate (eight hundred milligrams of elemental calcium) resulted in a 25 percent decrease in serum cholesterol in men with high cholesterol levels, over a period of one year.

Chloride

Chloride, which enters the body primarily through table salt, is a constituent of acid in the stomach (hydrochloric acid). It interacts with sodium, potassium, and carbon dioxide to maintain an acid-base balance in body cells and fluids and is vital for normal health.

Most people consume more than adequate amounts of chloride in salt substitutes (potassium chloride), sea salt, and table salt (sodium chloride). Only people on a severely salt-restricted diet need to be concerned about how much chloride they consume, and should consider using potassium chloride as a salt substitute. As noted, excessive consumption of dietary sodium chloride in ordinary table salt, coupled with diminished dietary potassium, may increase the risk of hypertension.

Magnesium

Magnesium catalyzes hundreds of metabolic reactions in the body's soft tissues. It plays an essential role in the release of energy from glycogen (stored muscle fuel), the manufacture of proteins, the regulation of body temperature, and the proper functioning of nerves and muscles. Its specific physiological function is to aid bone growth and the proper functioning of nerves and muscles, including regulation of a normal heart rhythm. It also strengthens tooth enamel, keeps metabolism steady, and, in larger doses, works as a laxative.

Good sources of magnesium include nuts (particularly almonds and cashews), fish, molasses, soybeans, sunflower seeds, wheat germ, and green, leafy vegetables.

Recommended Dietary Allowance (RDA) for Magnesium

	mg.
Infants (0–1 year)	500
Children (1–10 years)	120
Males (11–24 years)	350
Males (25–51+ years)	350
Females (11–24 years)	290
Females (25–51+ years)	280
Pregnant Females	320
Breast-feeding Females	345

Magnesium deficiency has been linked to several forms of mental illness. In a February 1992 article in *Prevention Magazine,* Mark Bricklin reported that doctors at the Albert Einstein College of Medicine had found that patients who displayed symptoms of depression, agitation, and hallucinations were deficient in magnesium. A follow-up study revealed that antipsychotic medications often decrease magnesium levels in patients. It is now believed that some patients who do not respond well to medication show mental symptoms that may be caused partly by low magnesium levels. Replication studies will be necessary to confirm if magnesium supplements can improve mental functioning, and, in severe cases, to help treat schizophrenia and depression.

Magnesium supplementation also may help people with osteoporosis, who typically have lower magnesium levels than people without this condition. Magnesium deficiency is cross-linked with high intakes of dairy foods fortified with vitamin D. People with osteoporosis may therefore require higher lev-

els of magnesium, as well as calcium supplements that are not derived from dairy products.

Magnesium deficiency has been linked to premenstrual syndrome (PMS). Red blood cell magnesium levels in women with PMS have been shown to be significantly lower than in women who do not have PMS. In one clinical trial, magnesium supplements given to PMS patients resulted in a reduction of nervousness (in 89 percent), of breast tenderness (96 percent), and of weight gain (95 percent), according to R.S. London in the October 1991 issue of the *Journal of the American College of Nutrition.*

A magnesium deficiency is common in alcoholics, due primarily to alcohol-induced loss of this mineral through the kidneys, a process that continues during alcohol withdrawal.

Magnesium deficiency may play a major role in some cases of angina. It has been observed that men dying suddenly of heart attacks have significantly lower levels of heart magnesium, as well as potassium, than matched controls. Magnesium supplements have proven helpful in the management of irregular heartbeats, and several studies suggest that it could be a partial treatment for angina caused by coronary artery spasm, according to a report by P. Turlapaty in the March 1980 issue of *Science.*

Magnesium is beneficial in treating patients experiencing acute attacks of bronchial asthma. One clinical study, reported by E. Brunner in the September 1985 *Journal of Asthma,* confirmed that magnesium significantly improves breathing in asthmatics. The degree of improvement directly correlates with serum magnesium levels.

In some regions of the world, the rate of heart disease is related to the magnesium content of the water supply. The Inuit in Greenland, for example, have very little heart disease, which has been attributed partially to high levels of serum magnesium in their water supply. Magnesium is known to contribute significantly to the strength of contraction of the heart muscle.

Magnesium deficiency is prevalent in patients with irritable bowel syndrome. Patients with low magnesium levels often have symptoms of muscle weakness, anorexia, low blood pressure, confusion, and hyperirritability. Magnesium levels are significantly lower in diabetics, and magnesium supplements are commonly used in treatment, according to A. Careiello in *Diabetes Care,* published in 1982.

Phosphorus

Phosphorus acts with calcium as a partner in bone and teeth formation and is found in every cell of the body as a component of nucleic acids. It is vital for the metabolism of carbohydrates and the functioning of several B vitamins, and is used to transport fats throughout the body.

Good sources of phosphorous include meat, fish, poultry, milk, nuts, legumes, and whole-grain cereals and breads. Most people take in more than enough phosphorus from the large amount of meat they eat and from phosphorus salts used in processed foods. Prolonged use of antacids can lead to a harmful loss of phosphorus, and frequent consumption of carbonated drinks (which contain phosphorus) can distort the crucial ratio of calcium to phosphorus. If a diet contains too much phosphorus, calcium is not utilized efficiently.

A low-calcium, high-phosphorus diet has been linked with the development of osteoporosis, a condition in which the bones lose mass and become brittle. In contrast, vegetarian diets are associated with a lower risk of osteoporosis, although bone mass in vegetarians does decrease in the fourth and fifth

Recommended Dietary Allowance (RDA) for Phosphorus

	mg.
Infants (0–1 year)	400
Children (1–10 years)	800
Males (11–24 years)	1,200
Males (25–51+ years)	800
Females (11–24 years)	1,200
Females (25–51+ years)	800
Pregnant Females	1,200
Breast-feeding Females	1,200

decades. Several factors probably account for this slower decrease in bone mass. Most important is a lowered intake of protein and phosphorus. A high-protein diet or a diet high in phosphates is associated with increasing the excretion of calcium in the urine.

Potassium

Potassium is important for the proper functioning of muscles, including the heart. Potassium is a crucial regulator of the amount of water in cells, which determines their ability to function properly. It helps in the transmission of nerve impulses, is a buffer for body fluids, and catalyzes the release of energy from carbohydrates, proteins, and fats. Potassium also may help prevent high blood pressure.

Natural sources include avocados, bananas, citrus fruits, dried fruits, lentils, milk, molasses, nuts, parsnips, potatoes, raisins, canned sardines, fresh spinach, and whole-grain cereals. No Recommended Dietary Allowance for potassium has been established. However, too much sodium in the diet can compromise the body's supply of potassium, and potassium deficiencies can occur following severe diarrhea and the use of diuretics.

Symptoms of potassium deficiency include weakness, paralysis, low blood pressure, and irregular or rapid heartbeat that can lead to cardiac arrest and death.

People with low levels of potassium may be susceptible to high blood pressure. Dr. Gopal Kirshna of Temple University found that putting male patients on a potassium-deficient diet for only nine days led to significant increases in blood pressure. Similar experiments in Japan have confirmed Kirshna's findings. High blood pressure is even more common in Japan because of the culture's typically high sodium diet. According to Kirshna, quoted in Bricklin's article in the February 1992 issue of *Prevention Magazine* previously cited in this chapter, Americans should consume at least three grams of potassium every day. "And there is some experimental evidence that taking more would be better. The best thing to do is to incorporate potassium-rich foods into the diet. The ideal way is to choose sources that do not give you too many calories, or too much fat or cholesterol. The most desirable sources are fruits and vegetables."

The loss of potassium ions through stress may contribute to fatigue and exhaustion. When the body's cells lose potassium, they function less effectively and eventually die. The effects of stress also can be reduced by maintaining and supplementing potassium levels. Exercise and relaxation techniques such as meditation, biofeedback, and self-hypnosis are probably more important components of a stress management program, however.

Sodium

Sodium is present in all the cells of the body. Its most important function is to regulate the balance of water inside and outside the cells. Sodium also plays a crucial role in maintaining blood pressure, aids muscle contraction and nerve transmission, and regulates the body's acid-base balance.

Natural sources of sodium include bacon and ham, beef, milk, margarine and butter, bread, clams, green beans, and canned sardines and tomatoes. Most people consume sodium as sodium chloride in ordinary table salt.

No RDA for sodium has been established, although nutritionists suggest that three thousand milligrams is adequate for normal body function. Sodium deficiencies occur almost entirely in people ill with dehydration, patients recovering from surgery, or persons experiencing excessive sweating due to overexercising in a hot climate. Symptoms of a sodium deficiency include muscle and stomach cramps, nausea, fatigue, mental apathy, and appetite loss.

A typical American diet contains three thousand to twelve thousand milligrams of sodium a day. People who consume more than three thousand milligrams of sodium run the risk of high blood pressure and hypertension. Excessive intake of sodium chloride (salt), coupled with diminished dietary potassium, has been shown to increase blood fluid volume and result in hypertension in susceptible individuals. Conversely, a low-sodium, high-potassium diet reduces the rise in blood pressure during periods of mental stress by reducing the blood-vessel constricting effect of adrenaline. However, sodium restriction alone does not improve blood pressure control; there also must also be a high intake of potassium, writes F. Skrabal in the October 1981 issue of *The Lancet*.

Sulfur

Sulfur is important because it binds protein molecules, and therefore is a crucial constituent of proteins in hair, fingernails, toenails, and skin. It also plays a role in oxidation-reduction reactions and aids the secretion of bile in the liver. No recommended daily dietary amount has been established, and deficiencies in humans are unknown since sulfur is widespread in protein foods. The best natural sources include cabbage, clams, dried beans, eggs, fish, lean beef, milk, and wheat germ.

Trace Elements

Chromium

Chromium is necessary to maintain normal metabolism of glucose (blood sugar) and may be important in preventing diabetes. A small amount of chromium helps insulin regulate blood sugar and improves glucose tolerance of some people with maturity-onset diabetes.

Only a small amount of dietary chromium is absorbed by the body. Beef, fish, dairy products, whole-grain products, fresh fruits, chicken, potatoes, oysters, and brewer's yeast are good sources of chromium. Some Americans, particularly the elderly, pregnant women, and malnourished people, are often chromium deficient.

No RDA for chromium has been established, although .05–.20 milligrams has been established as a safe amount to take daily. A basic high-quality multivitamin and mineral supplement high in B-complex vitamins normally contains the daily requirement for chromium.

Chromium and Disease Prevention. Chromium is believed to prevent some forms

of dental cavities and may help protect against cancer of the esophagus. Chromium chloride supplementation (200 milligrams per day) results in a decrease in serum triglycerides and total cholesterol, while increasing HDL levels and improving glucose tolerance.

Cobalt

Cobalt, a trace element stored primarily in the liver, is necessary to manufacture vitamin B12 in the body. It helps promote normal red blood cell formation and acts as a substitute for manganese in the activation of several enzymes. It also replaces zinc in some enzymes.

Natural sources of cobalt include beet greens, cabbage, clams, figs, kidney, lettuce, liver, milk, oysters, spinach, and watercress.

Cobalt deficiencies can lead to anemia, with symptoms including weakness (especially of the arms and legs), a sore tongue, nausea and appetite loss, bleeding gums, numbness and tingling in the hands and feet, difficulty maintaining balance, shortness of breath, depression, headache, and poor memory.

Excessively toxic amounts of cobalt can cause goiter (by blocking iodine intake) and a red blood cell disorder called polycythemia.

No RDA has been established for cobalt, but deficiencies of this trace element are extremely rare.

Copper

Copper is an essential component of several respiratory enzymes and is needed for the development of normal red blood cells. It acts as a catalyst in the storage and release of iron to form hemoglobin for red blood cells and promotes connective tissue formation and central nervous system function. It is normally used as a nutritional supplement for anyone who is undergoing prolonged intravenous feeding.

The richest dietary sources of copper include barley, nuts, honey, lentils, mushrooms, mussels, oats, oysters, salmon, and wheat germ.

No daily requirement for copper has been established, but most diets exceed needed amounts. Copper deficiencies contribute to health problems such as anemia; faulty development of bone and nervous tissue; loss of elasticity in the tendons and major arteries, possibly causing rupture of the blood vessels; abnormal development of the lung's air sacs, possibly predisposing people to emphysema; and abnormal pigmentation and structure of the hair. There is preliminary evidence that a copper deficiency may eventually lead to senility.

A deficiency of copper has been linked to marked elevation of cholesterol levels, and it has been suggested that the deficiency plays a role in the development of arteriosclerosis. Copper supplements may be helpful for patients with Crohn's disease, an inflammatory disease of the small intestine. In studies reported by C.O. Morain in the 1984 *British Medical Journal,* patients with Crohn's disease have been found to display one or more nutrient deficiencies, including copper, vitamin K, niacin, and vitamin E.

Adult psychotic patients have an excess of copper that may produce a schizophrenic syndrome or depression. Copper excess also is connected to learning and behavior disorders in children.

High copper levels appear to have the same toxic effects as other heavy metals. Several studies have associated high copper levels with learning disabilities in children. Other related metals were cadmium, lead, and manganese. High levels of copper also have been directly associated with periodontal (gum) disease.

Fluoride

Small amounts of fluoride, starting before birth and continuing throughout life, are essential for the development and maintenance of strong, decay-resistant teeth. Fluoride contributes to solid bone and tooth formation by helping the body retain calcium. In addition, it interferes with the growth of bacteria that cause dental plaque.

Food sources of fluoride include tea, apples, cod, eggs, kidneys, canned salmon and sardines, and plants grown in areas where fluoride is present in the water. There is no reliable evidence to support contentions that water fluoridation causes or contributes to cancer. However, in high doses, fluoride is just as toxic as the other trace elements and may cause mottling of the teeth.

No RDA for fluoride has been established, and most humans consume adequate amounts in their daily diet.

Fluoride and Osteoporosis. Fluoride may help prevent bone loss in the elderly and the debilitating fractures which often accompany it. There is also some evidence that fluoride, along with calcium and vitamin D, helps in treating osteoporosis, according to H. Winter Griffiths in the 1988 book, *Vitamins.* However, its use should be carefully monitored by a physician.

Germanium

Germanium is naturally found in sea algae, aloe vera, Siberian ginseng, garlic, and comfrey. Its properties have been extensively analyzed in Japan. In *Miracle Cure: Organic Germanium,* Dr. Kazuhiko Asai reports that organically bound germanium acts as a biological transmitter between the brain and the nervous system. Clinical case studies in Japan, where the use of germanium is widespread, have shown it to be effective in the controlled reversal of chronic allergies, hepatitis, cancer, leukemia, cataracts, and cardiovascular disorders, according to R. Ornstein's publication, *The Human Ecology Program*.

Germanium also has been used successfully to treat numerous ailments ranging from headaches to allergies. The compound is considered an "immunostimulant," a substance that activates the body's defense system. A number of animal experiments conducted by Asai strongly indicate that Ge-132 (one form of germanium) inhibits tumors in a variety of cancers in mice.

Iodine

Iodine is an integral component of two important thyroid hormones (thyroxin and triiodothyronine) that regulate metabolism. It is essential for normal reproduction and cell functioning. Iodine keeps skin, hair, and nails healthy, and prevents goiter.

Seafoods, including cod, herring, lobsters, oysters, canned salmon, seaweed, and shrimp, are nature's richest sources of iodine. However, the majority of iodine is derived from the use of iodized salt (70 micrograms of iodine per gram of salt). Except for seafood and seaweed, most foods contain extremely small amounts of iodine. Some foods contain substances that prevent the utilization of iodine, such as turnips, cabbage, mustard, cassava root, soybeans, peanuts, pine nuts, and millet.

Foods high in iodine should be eliminated from the diets of those who are iodine-sensitive. At one time, it was necessary to add iodine to salt to help prevent goiter in certain parts of the U.S. where little seafood was consumed and the soil was iodine-deficient. However, because iodine is now in many processed foods, most Americans receive the minimum RDA.

Iodine deficiency leads to a shortage of

Benefits of Germanium

- Increases the production of gamma-interferon, a potent antiviral, anti-cancer agent.
- Dramatically increases the oxygen capacity of the blood.
- Helps reverse chronic allergies, hepatitis, leukemia, cataracts, and cardiovascular disorders.

thyroid hormones and goiter (an enlargement of the thyroid gland). If this deficiency occurs before or shortly after birth, it may result in cretinism, or retarded growth.

Hypothyroidism and/or iodine deficiency are associated with a higher incidence of breast cancer. Research has shown that thyroid supplementation decreases breast pain, serum prolactin levels, and breast nodules in thyroid patients. These results suggest that unrecognized hypothyroidism and/or iodine deficiency may be a factor in fibrocystic breast disease (FBD). Iodine may be very important in the treatment and prevention of FBD because it has significant anti-inflammatory and antiscarring effects, according to Z. Mielen's article in *Texas Biological Medicine*, published in 1968.

Iron

Iron is an essential ingredient in all cells, particularly the oxygen-carrying cells of the blood and muscles, which use two-thirds of the iron requirement. Without iron, hemoglobin (the oxygen transport pigment of red blood cells) and myoglobin (the hemoglobin of muscle cells) cannot be formed, nor can certain vital enzymes.

Recommended Dietary Allowance (RDA) for Iodine

	mg.
Infants (0–1 year)	45
Children (1–10 years)	80
Males (11–24 years)	150
Males (25–51+ years)	150
Females (11–24 years)	150
Females (25–51+ years)	150
Pregnant Females	175
Breast-feeding Females	200

Iron found in animal foods such as beef, liver, fish, and poultry is more readily absorbed than that found in milk, eggs, cheese, or vegetables such as spinach. Eating foods containing iron along with foods rich in vitamin C, such as citrus fruits, tomatoes, or green peppers, can enhance iron absorption. Several foods and beverages contain substances that inhibit iron absorption, including tea, coffee, wheat bran, and egg yolks. Overuse of antacids and calcium supplements also decreases iron absorption. These items should be restricted in the diets of individuals with iron deficiencies.

Iron deficiency, or anemia, can produce such symptoms as fatigue, listlessness, irritability, pallor, and shortness of breath, which reflect a lack of oxygen being delivered to tissues and a buildup of carbon dioxide. The problem most commonly occurs in infants, young children, adolescents, and women of child-bearing age, some of whom may need to take iron supplements.

Iron supplements are routinely given to pregnant and nursing women. However, they should not be taken without a physician's recommendation based on one or more blood tests. Since iron is stored in the body and lost only through bleeding, it is possible to accumulate an excess of iron that can damage the liver, pancreas, and heart.

A 1986 study by the U.S. Department of Agriculture (USDA) has found that women who have below-normal iron supplies may start feeling cold before they experience tiredness, the usual side effect of iron-deficiency anemia. The USDA study concluded that all women of childbearing age (roughly ages 19 to 50) have iron intakes of only 61 percent of the Recommended Dietary Allowance. Additionally, E. Pollitt, in the April 1976 *Journal of Pediatrics,* noted that iron deficiency is the second most common nutritional problem for all Americans after obesity.

Iron and Detoxification. Iron supplements are included in most detoxification diets. This is because iron, along with many other nutrients, helps combat heavy-metal poisoning. Normally a high potency multiple vitamin supplement is recommended, along with minerals such as iron, calcium, magnesium, zinc, copper, and chromium. Iron deficiency can contribute to immune dysfunction, due to the body's diminished ability to produce T-cells that fight off infection.

Iron is an important nutrient for bacteria as well as humans. During infection, one of the body's defense mechanisms to limit bacterial growth is to reduce plasma iron. There is much scientific evidence to support the conclusion that iron supplementation is not recommended during acute infection, especially for young children. However, in patients with impaired immune function, chronic infections, and low iron levels, adequate supplementation is essential.

Iron and Learning Disabilities. Virtually any nutrient deficiency can result in impaired brain function, and insufficient iron is the nutrient deficiency found most often in

American children. Iron deficiency is associated with markedly decreased attentiveness, shorter attention span, decreased persistence, and decreased voluntary activity—all of which are usually responsive to iron supplementation, according to D. Wray, writing in the May 1975 *British Medical Journal.*

Iron and Mouth Ulcers. A study of 330 patients with recurrent mouth ulcers found that 47 (14.2 percent) were deficient in iron, along with folic acid or vitamin B12. A. Hoffer states in *Orthomolecular Nutrition* that these deficiencies were corrected by iron and vitamin B supplementation, and the majority experienced complete remission.

Lithium

Lithium has no known role in the body's internal metabolism. Lithium ointment, however, is used topically to treat certain types of herpes (such as herpes zoster), as reported by G. Skinner in *Medicine, Microbiology and Immunology,* published in 1980.

Lithium has also been successfully used to treat manic-depressive psychosis in large doses of approximately a thousand milligrams per day. Physicians regularly use up to three hundred milligrams of lithium per day to increase energy levels, diminish fatigue, eliminate depression, and alter mood changes associated with multiple food allergies, according to Skinner.

Manganese

Manganese is concentrated in cells of the pituitary gland, liver, pancreas, kidney, and bones. It stimulates production of cholesterol by the liver and helps many body enzymes generate energy. It is essential for blood clotting, bone formation, development of other connective tissues, cholesterol synthesis, and the metabolism of proteins, fats, carbohy-

Recommended Dietary Allowance (RDA) for Iron	
	mg.
Infants (0–1 year)	8
Children (1–10 years)	10
Males (11–24 years)	12
Males (25–51+ years)	10
Females (11–24 years)	15
Females (25–51+ years)	15
Pregnant Females	30
Breast-feeding Females	15

drates, and nucleic acids.

Good natural sources of manganese include avocados, barley, dried beans, blackberries, bran, buckwheat, nuts, coffee, ginger, oatmeal, peas, seaweed, and spinach. Symptoms of manganese deficiency include difficulty in walking, blurred speech, tremors of the hands, and involuntary laughing.

Manganese functions in the antioxidant enzyme superoxide dismutase (manganese SOD), which is deficient in patients with rheumatoid arthritis. Manganese supplementation has been shown to increase SOD activity (increased antioxidant activity).

Manganese and Disease Prevention. Manganese may be useful in treating diabetes because of its important co-factor role in glucose metabolism. Diabetics tend to have only half the manganese found in normal individuals. Low magnesium levels also appear to be a significant risk factor in the development of cardiovascular disease, particularly coronary artery spasm. Magnesium supplementation may be warranted for these diseases, according to A.

Recommended Dietary Allowance (RDA) for Selenium

	mg.
Infants (0–1 year)	15
Children (1–10 years)	25
Males (11–24 years)	60
Males (25–51+ years)	70
Females (11–24 years)	50
Females (25–51+ years)	55
Pregnant Females	65
Breast-feeding Females	75

Mooradian in the October 1987 *American Journal of Clinical Nutrition.*

Manganese and Epilepsy. Hoffer, who studied the role manganese may play in epileptic seizures, found that one group of people with epilepsy had abnormally low manganese blood levels. Certain substances in the diet, including magnesium, calcium, and iron, may prevent manganese from being absorbed properly. Women with PMS, for example, also have low manganese levels (77 percent less than normal), and manganese supplements may provide temporary relief.

Molybdenum

Molybdenum forms part of the enzyme system responsible for the development of bones, liver, and kidneys. It helps convert nucleic acid to uric acid, a waste product eliminated in the urine.

Natural sources of molybdenum include beans; cereal grains; dark green, leafy vegetables; organ meats (liver, kidney, sweet-breads); peas, and other legumes. It should be noted that dietary concentration of molybdenum may vary according to the status of the soil in which grains and vegetables are grown.

No RDA for molybdenum has been established. A balanced natural diet of unprocessed foods provides all the molybdenum necessary for a healthy child or adult. However, most American diets are thought to be deficient in molybdenum as they are in chromium, because modern food processing tends to remove this mineral nutrient from the average diet.

Selenium

Selenium is a trace element that even in small amounts enhances the immune system by helping to prevent free radical formation. It acts synergistically with vitamin E and possibly with vitamin A.

Dietary sources of selenium include seafood, chicken, egg yolks, milk, garlic, wheat germ and whole-grain products, and vegetables such as broccoli, cabbage, celery, cucumbers, mushrooms, and onions.

In *Selenium in Biology and Medicine,* published in 1991, Larry Clark reports that researchers suggest that large doses of selenium are safe and may prove effective in cancer prevention. For example, researchers in Finland found that people whose diets are low in selenium increase their risk of developing cancer, especially of the stomach and lungs. This conclusion was based on blood samples from nearly forty thousand people whose health had been tracked for ten years.

Even the best planned diets may be selenium deficient, depending partially on where the food is grown. In China, selenium is virtually absent in the soil, and, as a result, children commonly suffer from a heart condition called Kershan's disease. In the early 1970s, Chinese physicians studied more than thirty-six thousand children whose diets were supplemented with selenium. Of these, only twenty-one developed Kershan's disease. Among 9,642 other children from the same area who did not receive any selenium supplement, 107 contracted the disease and 53 died, according to an article by J. Mitchell in the July–August 1991 issue of *Health News & Review.*

Selenium and Disease Prevention. Selenium currently is prescribed to treat yeast infection. It may help treat cataracts, several forms of skin cancer, and cervical dysplasia. Because food allergies have been associated with immune system dysfunction, selenium— along with zinc, B-complex vitamins, and thymus extract—has been prescribed to treat specific allergies. Selenium functions synergistically with vitamin E in the treatment of gout. It has been used (200 micrograms a day along with cod liver oil and vitamin E) to treat multiple sclerosis, reports J. Wikstrom in *Acta Nerulogie Scandinavia,* published in 1976. The antioxidant activities of selenium and vitamin E also deter periodontal disease (as free radicals are extremely damaging to the gums), as well as psoriasis.

Serum selenium levels are low in patients with rheumatoid arthritis (RA), probably because selenium serves as a mineral co-factor in the free radical scavenging enzyme glutathione peroxidase, the enzyme important in reducing the production of inflammatory prostaglandins and leukotrines. Free radicals, oxidants, prostaglandins, and leukotrines cause much of the damage to tissues observed in RA. Clinical studies have not yet clearly demonstrated that selenium supplementation alone improves the signs and symptoms of RA; however, one clinical study indicated that selenium combined with vitamin E had a positive effect, according to an article by U. Tarp in the September 1985 *Scandinavian Journal of Rheumatology.*

Benefits of Selenium

- Protects against the toxic effects of the heavy-metal poison cadmium, predominantly found in cigarette paper and paint.
- Protects against high mercury content taken into the body through seafood and other sources.
- Increases the effectiveness of vitamin E, thus improving the oxygen-carrying capacity of the blood.
- Prevents chromosomal damage that causes birth defects and cancer.
- Reduces the risk of stomach and lung cancer and heart disease.

Silicon

Silicon plays an important role in connective tissue, especially bones and cartilage. Vegetal silica, a form of silicon, is extracted from the herb horsetail and sold in health food stores. Silica (silicon dioxide), the most abundant silicon compound, is also available in supplement form. No RDA has been established for this trace element.

Zinc

Zinc is a component of the molecular structure of nearly a hundred human enzymes involved in major metabolic processes, most of which work with the red blood cells to move carbon dioxide from the tissues to the lungs. Zinc functions as an important antioxidant; promotes normal growth and development; aids in wound healing; enhances cell division, repair, and growth; maintains normal levels of vitamin A in the blood; and helps synthesize DNA and RNA.

Recommended Dietary Allowance (RDA) for Zinc

	mg.
Infants (0–1 year)	5
Children (1–10 years)	10
Males (11–24 years)	15
Males (25–51+ years)	15
Females (11–24 years)	12
Females (25–51+ years)	12
Pregnant Females	15
Breast-feeding Females	17

Natural sources include lean beef, egg yolks, fish, lamb, milk, oysters, pork, sesame and sunflower seeds, soybeans, turkey, wheat bran and germ, and whole-grain products. Diets heavily dependent on grains, which contain large amounts of phytates that block zinc absorption, may result in zinc deficiencies. Symptoms of zinc deficiency include retarded growth, rashes and multiple skin lesions, psoriasis, low sperm count, delayed wound healing, and diminished learning capacity. Prenatal zinc deficiency also interferes with the maturation of the brain.

Zinc deficiencies have been linked to prostatic hypertrophy (prostate enlargement) and prostate cancer. Dr. Andre Voison, in his 1988 book *Grass Productivity,* claims that when a 35 percent drop in normal zinc levels occurs, a mild enlargement of the prostate is observed. A 38 percent drop in zinc levels leads to chronic prostatitis. Cancer often develops when zinc levels are reduced by 66 percent. Voison's work is cited by Ornstein in *The Human Ecology Program,* published by the San Francisco Medical Research Foundation in 1987.

Prostate problems are virtually unknown in areas where pumpkin seeds are regularly eaten, such as eastern Europe. Pumpkin seeds are high in zinc, essential amino acids, magnesium, and the polyunsaturated fatty acids found in lecithin.

Zinc and AIDS. Both zinc and copper are known to be important in the functioning of the immune system, and deficiencies in either may predict vulnerability to AIDS. In one study, zinc and copper levels were examined in fifty-four homosexual men who were infected with the human immunodeficiency virus (HIV) and later developed AIDS. Zinc blood levels were lower in men who were infected and progressed to AIDS compared with those who were infected but did not develop to AIDS. Zinc deficiency predicted the progression to AIDS independently of other factors, such as the number of CD4+ lymphocyte levels or age, reports A. Sherman in *History of Nutritional Immunology,* published in March 1992.

Zinc and Diabetes. Zinc deficiencies may play a role in diabetes because it is essential for the production of insulin, the hormone responsible for maintaining normal glucose levels in the blood. Abnormally fluctuating glucose levels, called hypoglycemia, lead to unstable mental and emotional conditions due primarily to overconsumption of refined sugar. As a result, the pancreas must produce greater amounts of insulin to balance an inordinate amount of sugar absorbed into the bloodstream. Zinc appears to help restore normal insulin levels and is being used to help treat hypoglycemia and diabetes.

Zinc and Head Injuries. A study reported by Bricklin in the February 1992 issue of *Prevention Magazine* found that zinc is effective in promoting recovery from serious head injury. A medical group at the University of Kentucky conducted a three-year study in which sixty head-injury patients were given either the normal amount of zinc found in intravenous formulas and hospital food, or about five times that much in zinc supplements. A standard test, the Glasgow Coma Scale, was used by neurosurgeons to assess mental functioning after head injury. Results revealed that a month after their accidents, the zinc-supplemented patients scored significantly higher on the test, indicating faster recovery from injury. The results suggest that zinc may play an important role in several areas of cognition and neurotransmission.

Zinc is highly concentrated in the hippocampus of the brain, which is responsible for the coordination of thoughts, feelings, and emotions. Extensive research by orthomolecular (nutritional) physicians has demonstrated that sufferers of schizophrenia and manic depression are depleted in zinc, L-ascorbic acid, vitamin B, and essential amino acids. Adequate levels of these substances appear to be prerequisites for proper neurological functioning, according to Bricklin's article.

Zinc and Immune System Diseases. Zinc is instrumental in many immune system processes, thymus gland function, and thymus hormone action. When zinc levels are low, the number of T-cells (which kill bacteria and viruses) is significantly reduced. Thymic hormone levels also are lower and many white blood cell functions critical to the immune response are severely impaired. All of these effects are reversible with adequate zinc absorption. In addition, zinc has been shown to inhibit the growth of several viruses including herpes simplex.

Adequate zinc levels are particularly important in the elderly and young children. Zinc supplementation in the elderly results in the production of a higher number of T-cells and enhanced cell-mediated immune re-

The Benefits of Zinc

- Promotes recovery from serious head injury.
- May play an important role in cognition and neurotransmission.
- Helps maintain normal glucose levels in the blood.
- May help treat hypoglycemia and diabetes.
- May help relieve inflammation from rheumatoid arthritis.
- Used to treat advanced hardening of the arteries.
- May help relieve PMS symptoms.

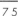

ZINC

sponses. Children prone to upper respiratory tract infections typically have low levels of zinc and other trace minerals.

Zinc and Premenstrual Syndrome (PMS). Many women experience anxiety, bloating, and other premenstrual symptoms that can disrupt their professional and personal lives for a few days each month. Several tentative experiments show that zinc may help relieve PMS by regulating the secretion of several key hormones, including progesterone, during menstruation. Dr. C. James Chuong of the Baylor College of Medicine found significantly lower zinc blood levels in women with PMS than in control samples, according to a report by K. Fackelmann in the October 27, 1990, issue of *Science News*. Chuong emphasizes that further work needs to be done to confirm the proposed link between PMS and zinc.

Zinc and Rheumatoid Arthritis. Some preliminary evidence suggests that zinc supplements may relieve rheumatoid arthritis. In *Wellness Medicine,* published in 1990, Dr. Robert Anderson reports on one study in which 220 milligrams per day of zinc were added to existing therapy for 12 weeks in 24 patents with rheumatoid arthritis. According to Anderson, "There were significant improvements in flexibility (less stiffness), their sense of well-being, and increasing walking time with decreased swelling." Anderson cites another study in which 24 patients with advanced hardening of the arteries received 150 milligrams of zinc daily, which resulted in a distinct improvement in eighteen of the patients.

Summary

Despite the documented role minerals and trace elements play in ensuring the healthy functioning of the body, many people still underestimate the importance of consuming enough of them in the daily diet. The small amounts of the essential minerals needed for human health can be obtained from foods, especially fresh fruits and vegetables. It is important that people monitor whether they are consuming adequate amounts through their diet alone by following the RDAs. If individuals believe they are deficient in a particular mineral or trace element, they should consult their physician or health practitioner to determine whether or not supplements are advisable.

Resources

References

Anderson, Robert A., M.D. *Wellness Medicine.* New Canaan, CT: Keats Publishing, Inc., 1990.

Asai, Kazuhiko, Ph.D. *Miracle Cure: Organic Germanium.* Tokyo, Japan: Japan Publications, Inc., 1978.

Bricklin, Mark. "New Respect for Nutritional Healing." *Prevention* (February 1992): 3.

Brunner, E. "Effect of Parenteral Magnesium on Pulmonary Function, Plasma cAMP, and Histamine in Bronchial Asthma." *Journal of Asthma* (September 1985): 3–11.

Careiello, A. "Hypomagnesium in Relation to Diabetic Retinopathy." *Diabetes Care* (1982): 558–59.

Chaitow, Leon, M.D. *The Body/Mind Purification Program.* New York, NY: Simon & Schuster, Inc., 1990.

Clark, Larry. *Selenium in Biology and Medicine.* New York, NY: Van Nostrand Reinhold Co., 1991.

Fackelmann, K. "PMS: Hints of a Link to Zinc." *Science News* (October 27, 1990): 263.

Griffith, H. Winter. *Vitamins.* Tucson, AZ: Fisher Books, 1988.

Hoffer, A. *Orthomolecular Nutrition.* New Canaan, CT: Keats Publishing, Inc., 1978.

London, R.S. "Effect of a Nutritional Supplement on Premenstrual Symptomatology in Women With Premenstrual Syndrome: A Double-Blind Longitudinal Study." *Journal of the American College of Nutrition* (1991): 494–99.

Mielens, Z. "The Effect of Oral Iodides on Inflammation." *Texas Biological Medicine* (1968): 117–21.

Mitchell, J. "Many Riches From Selenium." *Health News & Review* (July–August 1991): 7.

Mooradian, A. "Micronutrient Status in Diabetes Melitus." *American Journal of Clinical Nutrition* (October 1987): 646–53.

Morain, C.O. "Elemental Diet as Primary Treatment of Acute Crohn's Disease."

British Medical Journal (September 1984): 1859–62.

Murray, Michael, and Joseph Pizzorno. *Encyclopedia of Natural Medicine.* Rocklin, CA: Prima Publishing, 1991.

Ornstein, R. *The Human Ecology Program.* San Francisco, CA: San Francisco Medical Research Foundation, 1987.

Pollitt, E. "Iron Deficiency and Behavior." *Journal of Pediatrics* (April 1976): 372–81.

Sherman, A. "Zinc, Copper and Immunity." *History of Nutritional Immunology* (March 1992): 604.

Skinner, G. "The Effect of Lithium Chloride on the Replication of Herpes Simplex Virus." *Medicine, Microbiology and Immunology* (1980): 139–48.

Skrabal, F. "Low Sodium/High Potassium Diet for Prevention of Hypertension." *The Lancet* (October 1981): 895–900.

Tarp, U. "Selenium Treatment in Rheumatoid Arthritis." *Scandinavian Journal of Rheumatology* (September 1985): 249–55.

Turlapaty, P. "Magnesium Deficiency Produces Spasms of Coronary Arteries." *Science* (March 1980): 199–200.

Voison, Andre. *Grass Productivity.* Washington, DC: Island Press, 1988.

Wikstrom, J. "Selenium, Vitamin E and Copper in Multiple Sclerosis." *Acta Nerulogie Scandinavia* (1976): 287–90.

Wray, D. "Recurrent Apthatae: Treatment with Vitamin B12, Folic Acid and Iron." *British Medical Journal* (1975): 490–93.

Additional Reading

American Dietetic Association. *Handbook of Clinical Dietetics.* New Haven, CT: Yale University Press, 1981.

American Medical Association. *Drug Evaluations.* Chicago, IL: American Medical Association, 1986.

Butler, Kurt, and Lynn Rayner. *The Best Medicine: The Complete Health and Preventive Medicine Handbook.* New York, NY: Harper & Row Publishers, Inc., 1985.

Edmunds, Marilyn. *Nursing Drug Reference.* Bowie, MD: Brandy Communications Company, 1985.

Hendler, Sheldon, M.D. *The Complete Guide to Anti-Aging Nutrients.* New York, NY: Simon & Schuster, Inc., 1985.

Lerch, Sharon. "Memory Booster (Iron and Zinc)." *American Health* (March 1992): 129.

Marshall, Charles W. *Vitamins and Minerals: Help or Harm?* Philadelphia, PA: George F. Stickley Company, 1983.

Mills, Collins. "Zinc in Human Biology." *Journal of the American Dietetic Association* (May 1990): 756.

Murray, Frank. "Zinc Helps the Immune System." *Better Nutrition for Today's Living* (May 1991): 10.

Neil, M., et al. "Relationship of Serum Copper and Zinc Levels to HIV-1 Seropositivity to AIDS." *Journal of Acquired Immune Deficiency Syndromes* (October 1991): 976.

"Nutrition and Your Health: Dietary Guidelines for Americans." *Home and Garden Bulletin.* U.S. Department of Agriculture, 1992.

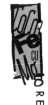

Chapter 5

BOTANICAL MEDICINES

Botanical (plant) medicines have been the basis of all known medical traditions. Throughout history, various cultures have handed down their accumulated knowledge of botanical medicines to successive generations. In the last 150 years, chemists and pharmacists have isolated and purified the "active" compounds in many plants in an attempt to produce reliable pharmaceutical drugs. Approximately 5,000 botanical plants have been extensively tested for possible use as medicines. Currently, 25 percent of all prescription drugs are directly or indirectly derived from herbs, shrubs, or trees. Some pharmaceutical drugs are extracted directly from plants, while others are synthesized to duplicate the properties of natural plant compounds.

Extensive research is under way in the United States, Europe, and Asia to investigate the chemical properties of another 5,000 botanicals for possible use in treating cancer, AIDS, diabetes, heart disorders, and many other diseases. This chapter discusses the more widely used botanical medicines whose effects have been studied in clinical trials. The English common name or popular name in the U.S. is given first, followed by the plant's botanical name.

Warnings about the use of prescription drugs mentioned in other sections of this book also apply to botanical medicines. Some botanicals contain toxic compounds in addition to the pharmacologically useful substances. Therefore, it can be harmful to take a botanical without being aware of all of its potential side effects. Also, certain people may be at high risk of intoxication including chronic users, children, the elderly, the sick, the malnourished or undernourished, and those on long-term medications. For these reasons, botanical medicines should be taken

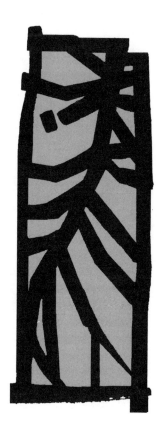

Choosing a Botanical Medicine

Encapsulated. Many botanical medicines are finely ground into powder and enclosed in capsules. These can be easy to use and are probably the best form for people who need to know the precise dosage. However, they can be less potent than whole dried herbs because, once they are powdered, their components have greater exposure to air and degrade faster.

Fomentation. A fomentation is an external application of herbs, generally used to treat swelling, pain, colds, and flu. Fomentations usually are prepared by soaking a towel or cloth in the desired botanical tea and then applying the towel (as hot as possible) over the affected area.

Freeze-Dried Extracts. These are produced by freezing the plant material to remove water or alcohol, and then exposing them to flash evaporation (using low absolute pressure and controlled heat).

Fresh Plants. The fresh plant may be an ideal form of botanical medicine, although people should first consult with an herbalist to identify the right species and to understand all the chemical properties of an herb or plant. The potency and toxicity of each plant species vary according to what part of the plant is used—the leaves, roots, or flowers—and what combination of chemical compounds it contains.

Infusion. Infusion was once the most common way of preparing herbs. A teaspoon of leaves, blossoms, or flowers is boiled in water and steeped for three to five minutes. Honey often is added as a sweetener.

Plaster. A plaster is similar to a poultice, except that the herbal materials are placed between two pieces of cloth and applied to the affected surface. This is a desirable alternative when the skin is irritated, because plasters help prevent the herb from coming in direct contact with the skin.

Poultice. A poultice may be used to reduce swelling by applying a warm paste of powdered herbs directly to the skin.

Solid Extracts. Some botanical medicines are available in solid extract forms that are made by first preparing a tea or tincture and then evaporating it until a gummy residue remains. The residue is mixed with other substances and sold as capsules. This is the most expensive of all botanical medicine forms, as well as the most reliable and potent.

Standardized Extracts. These are liquid or solid extracts of botanicals that have been standardized for content or one or several components.

Teas. Many botanical medicines are available as teas—either as single plants or in combinations of plants. Teas lose some of the properties of whole plants because any constituents that are not soluble in water are lost. Heating also evaporates some of the plant's medicinal components.

Tincture. A tincture is an extract of a plant in a solution of water and alcohol. It is easy to use and can retain its potency for several years.

only under the supervision of a physician, herbalist, or health practitioner. The following table highlights the major forms in which botanical medicines are available.

Algae (Spirulina)

Algae and micro-algae have been growing wild in the oceans (seaweed) and alkaline lakes (blue-green algae) for thousands of years. According to Helen C. Morgan and Kelly J. Moorhead's *Spirulina: Nature's Superfood,* spirulina grew wild in the great lakes of Central Mexico and was prized by the Aztecs as a food source. The Aztecs collected spirulina from the surface of the lakes with fine-meshed nets, dried the plant in the sun, and made it into a thick paste that they formed into cakes.

There are more than 30,000 known species of algae. Blue-green algae, the most primitive, is the most commonly used as food. It contains no nucleus and its cell walls are soft and easily digested, unlike other algae plants that contain hard cellulose. In the last 10 years, seaweed and blue-green algae have been harvested and made available commercially as food sources. They contain extremely high concentrations of calcium, potassium, manganese, copper, silicon, zinc, and lithium.

The best known form of blue-green algae, spirulina, is now sold in powder, tablet, or supplement fruit drink forms. Robert Henrikson, president of the Earthrise Company in San Rafael, California (which produces Earthrise spirulina), documents in *The Ultimate Guide to Health & Fitness* that spirulina is currently being used in Third World countries to treat malnutrition. In Togo, for example, spirulina is called "green medicine." Malnourished infants taking 3 to 15 grams of spirulina per day show rapid weight gain. In China, Nanjing Children's

Hospital uses spirulina in a baby-nourishing formula to help infants recover from a variety of nutritional deficiencies. Spirulina's high protein level, easy digestibility, and concentration of vitamins, minerals, and essential fatty acids make it ideal for therapeutic feeding.

According to Henrikson, spirulina has a higher concentration of protein (60 percent), amino acids, beta-carotene, vitamin B12, gamma-linoleic acid (GLA), trace minerals, and natural pigments than any other natural food source. Morgan and Moorhead state that spirulina is the only natural food containing all the essential and nonessential amino acids. With extra iron and trace minerals added to commercial growing ponds, spirulina has been found to have an iron concentration 10 times higher than any other conventional food—and Henrikson claims studies have shown that iron in spirulina is 60 percent more absorbable than a typical iron supplement such as iron sulfate. Spirulina growing projects are under way in Peru, India, Senegal, Vietnam, China, Mexico, Thailand, Japan, southern California, Oregon, and Hawaii.

Henrikson states that spirulina also contains phycocyanin, a blue-green pigment (found only in blue-green algae) that may help prevent some cancers. He cites a Japanese patent application that states that daily ingestion of a small dosage of phycocyanin accelerates normal cell growth and inhibits the growth of malignant tumors in cancer patients. M. Boyd reports in the 1989 *Journal of the National Cancer Institute* (Volume 16) that glycolipids extracted from blue-green algae have been found to inhibit the AIDS virus in experimental studies.

Henrikson also cites a 1986 Japanese study that found men with hypertension and hyperlipidemia had lower serum cholesterol, triglyceride, and LDL levels after consuming nine spirulina tablets daily for eight weeks.

He suggests that the cholesterol reduction may be partially due to the very high gamma GLA content in spirulina. Spirulina and mother's milk are the only natural foods that contain GLA which have successfully treated several inflammatory disorders, including arthritis, according to J. Belch, writing in the *Annals of the Rheumatic Diseases.*

It has also been inferred that spirulina increases the strength of the immune system. Henrikson cites a 1987 Japanese research study that proved that taking spirulina supplements increased lactobacillus flora in laboratory animals. He suggests that humans consuming spirulina supplements can improve their digestion and stimulate their immune systems as well. Because spirulina improves the absorption of minerals and maintains proper intestinal flora, which prevent some types of infections, this botanical is being extensively studied in clinical trials.

Aloe Vera

There are at least 120 known species of aloe, many of which have been used as botanical medicines. The sap and rind portions of the aloe vera leaf contain healing components such as analgesics, anti-inflammatory compounds, minerals, and beneficial fatty acids. According to Michael Murray and Joseph Pizzorno in the *Encyclopedia of Natural Medicine,* aloe vera contains anthraquinones, which reduce the growth rate of urinary calcium crystals that contribute to the formation of kidney stones. Once kidney stones form, as reported by K. Riley in the 1981 edition of the *Journal of John Bastyr College of Natural Medicine,* aloe vera extracts can help reduce the size of stones and subsequently eliminate them.

Aloe vera is widely known as a skin moisturizer and healing agent, especially in treating cuts, burns, insect stings, bruises,

acne, poison ivy, welts, ulcerated skin lesions, eczema, and sunburns. It has also been used, according to James F. Balch and Phyllis Balch in *Prescription for Nutritional Healing,* to treat stomach disorders, ulcers, colitis, and many colon-related disorders. They suggest that aloe vera juice may be used to treat food allergies, varicose veins, skin cancer, and arthritis as well.

Aloe vera may help stop the spread of some viruses. Researchers at the University of Maryland in Baltimore tested the antiviral activity of a number of plant extracts, including aloe vera emodin. The results, according to R. Sydiskis writing in the December 1991 issue of *Antimicrobial Agents & Chemotherapy,* showed that aloe emodin inactivated herpes simplex virus type 1 and 2, varicella-zoster virus, pseudorabies virus, and the influenza virus.

Bitter Melon (Momordica Charantia)

Bitter melon, also known as balsam pear, is a tropical vegetable widely cultivated in Asia, Africa, and South America. According to Murray and Pizzorno, bitter melon is composed of several compounds, including charantin. Charantin, which acts as a hypoglycemic agent, is composed of mixed steroids that are more potent than the prescription drug Tolbutamide in treating some cases of diabetes. Bitter melon also contains polypeptide-P, which lowers blood sugar levels when injected in patients with Type 1 diabetes. Since it appears to have fewer side effects than insulin, Murray and Pizzorno suggest that it can be used as an insulin substitute for some patients.

S. Lee-Huang, writing in the October 15, 1990, issue of *FEBS Letter,* reports that an isolated, purified extract of bitter melon seeds and fruits (momordica charantia or MAP 30) formed an essential basic protein that inhibited cell-free HIV-1 infection and replications in animal experiments. No severe side effects have been identified. Lee-Huang concludes: "This data suggests that MAP 30 may be a useful therapeutic agent in the treatment of HIV-1 infections."

Chamomile

Chamomile, one of the best-selling herbs in the United States and often made into a tea, is actually two herbs with the same name: German or Hungarian chamomile (matricaria chamomilla) and Roman or English chamomile (anthemis nobilis). Both have flowers with yellow centers and white rays, and both produce a light blue oil that has medicinal properties.

Chamomile traditionally has been used as a digestive aid. According to Murray and Pizzorno, several chemicals in chamomile oil relax the smooth muscle tissue that lines the digestive tract. W. Mitchell, in his book *Naturopathic Applications of the Botanical Remedies,* claims that chamomile oil has been shown to relax the gastrointestinal tract as well as or better than the prescription drug Pavabid.

J. Duke, in the *Handbook of Medicinal Herbs,* states that German researchers have discovered that chamomile oil kills several bacteria including candida albicans, the fungus responsible for vaginal yeast infections. Chamomile is licensed in Germany as an over-the-counter drug for internal use against gastrointestinal spasms and inflammatory diseases of the gastrointestinal tract. It is also approved as a topical treatment for skin and mucous membrane inflammations, bacterial skin diseases of the mouth and gums, and inflammation of the throat and airways.

Chinese Skullcap (Scutellaria Baicalensis)

Chinese skullcap has confirmed antiarthritic and anti-inflammatory actions, similar in effect to the prescription drugs Phenylbutazone and Indomethacin. As reported by M. Kuba in a 1984 issue of *Chemical Pharmacology Bulletin,* Chinese skullcap does not appear to have any adverse side effects. Kuba hypothesizes that its effectiveness is due to its high content of flavonoid molecules.

Chinese skullcap also may prove useful in the treatment and prevention of HIV infections. Dr. B. Li, writing in a 1993 issue (Volume 39) of *Cellular & Molecular Biology Research,* states that baicalin, a purified extract of Chinese skullcap, inhibits infection and replication of HIV-1 in vitro. In addition, Li claims that Chinese skullcap shows no side effects. He concludes: "This data suggests that [baicalin] may serve as a useful drug for the treatment and prevention of HIV infections."

Dr. T. Nagai reported in the May 1990 issue of *Chemical & Pharmaceutical Bulletin* that of 103 species of flavonoids tested in Japan, Chinese skullcap was the most potent in inhibiting several influenza viruses.

Cranberries

Cranberries have long been used to treat bladder and urinary tract infections. In one study reported by Murray and Pizzorno, drinking 16 ounces of cranberry juice per day produced beneficial effects in 73 percent of the subjects (44 females and 16 males) with active urinary tract infections. Furthermore, withdrawing the cranberry juice from the people who benefited resulted in recurrence of bladder infection in 61 percent. Several components in cranberry juice appear to reduce the ability of bacteria to adhere to the lining of the bladder and urethra. In order for bacteria to infect they must first adhere to the mucosa, and by interfering with adherence, cranberry juice greatly reduces the likelihood of infection and helps the body fight off infection.

Significant variations of urinary pH now are known to cause urinary tract disorders and infections. Dr. B. Walsh suggests in the July–August 1992 issue of *Journal of Nursing* that urinary tract disorders are due to high alkaline levels in the urine. According to Walsh, ingesting cranberry juice and ascorbic acid is the "least risky method to promote the production of acidic, diluted urine."

Dandelion (Taraxacum Officinale)

Many Americans are familiar with dandelions, those stubborn weeds that often spoil a cultivated lawn. According to Murray and Pizzorno, dandelion contains more vitamins, iron, other minerals, protein, and nutrients than any other herb. Dandelion has been used in traditional medicine to treat anemia. It is extremely high in carotenoids, even higher than carrots (14,000 IU of vitamin A per 100 grams compared with 11,000 IU for carrots).

A. Leung, in the *Encyclopedia of Common Natural Ingredients Used in Food, Drugs, and Cosmetics,* reviews several studies conducted in China, Russia, and India in which dandelion was used to treat breast problems, liver diseases, appendicitis, and digestive ailments. According to Leung, dandelion enhances the flow of bile, alleviating liver congestion, bile duct inflammation, hepatitis, gallstones, and jaundice. Dandelion stimulates bile secretion by the liver (as opposed to expulsion of bile by the gallbladder). It has been clinically used to treat gall-stones, and may be a substitute for antacids in treating indigestion.

Dong Quai (Angelica Sinensis)

According to a medieval legend, the medicinal benefits of angelica were revealed to a monk by an angel during a terrible plague— and thus the plant's horticultural name became angelica, or "root of the Holy Ghost." Several varieties have been identified, including angelica norvegical in Scandinavia, angelica sativa in Holland and France, and angelica refracta and japonica in Japan. The botanical is popularly known in the United States as dong quai, and primarily acts as a regulator of female hormones, according to Dr. Andrew Weil.

Dong quai contains angelic acid, valeric acid, and a resin called angelicin. The Chinese have used it for many disorders, and herbalists consider it safe and nontoxic. However, its strong flavor can cause gastric acidity (gas) in some people, and as a result, it is usually mixed with other herbs. Dong quai is not recommended for use during menstruation or pregnancy.

According to Murray and Pizzorno, dong quai has been used to relieve osteoporosis, hay fever, asthma, and eczema. They suggest that dong quai selectively inhibits the production of allergic antibodies (IgE) that cause inflammation. Japanese researcher Y. Ozaki, writing in the April 1992 issue of *Chemical & Pharmaceutical Bulletin,* reports that angelica siensis contains tetramethylpyrazine (TMP) and ferulic acid (FA), both of which exert an anti-inflammatory effect during the early and late stages of inflammation.

Garlic (Allium Sativum)

Garlic has played an important medicinal role for centuries, according to Dr. J. Dausch of the National Cancer Institute. Writing in the May 1990 issue of *Preventive Medicine,* Dausch states: "It is now known that garlic contains chemical constituents with antibiotic, lipid-lowering, detoxification, and other medicinal effects in the body."

Steven Foster in a 1991 monograph entitled *Garlic,* published by American Botanical Council, reports that garlic has been used effectively to prevent common colds and flus, intestinal worms, dysentery, sinus congestion, gout, rheumatism, and some ulcers.

Alternative Medicine: The Definitive Guide reports that garlic also has important cardiovascular benefits, including lowering blood pressure levels, thinning the blood, and reducing platelet aggregations that cause blood clots. It has been shown to strengthen the immune system by increasing natural killer cells' activity.

Recently published studies in China and Italy, cited by Dr. E. Dorant in the March 1993 issue of *British Journal of Cancer,* suggest that consuming garlic also may help prevent certain types of tumors. Dorant emphasizes that the available evidence "warrants further research into the possible role of garlic in the prevention of cancer in humans."

Ginger (Zingiber Officinale)

Ginger is a tropical perennial herb that can grow to a height of two to three feet. It produces a yellow flower, and its underground roots (tubers) are used to make the familiar spice. Ginger is believed to have originated in India, and was one of the first spices to reach Europe from Asia.

Ginger has a very long history of use in the treatment of a wide variety of intestinal ailments, including many different types of flu. It promotes the elimination of intestinal gas and relaxes and soothes the intestinal tract. Ginger is also very effective in preventing the symptoms of motion sickness, and many consider it superior to Dramamine, a commonly used over-the-counter drug. Weil uses ginger as a general anti-inflammatory, especially for treating arthritis and bursitis. Dr. S. Phillips, writing in the August 1993 issue of *Anaesthesia,* cites a study that compared the effect of powdered ginger root with metoclopramide (a stomach and intestinal stimulatory drug) and a placebo in relieving nausea and vomiting in 120 women who had undergone elective laparoscopic gynecological surgery. Twenty-one percent of the women receiving ginger became nauseated, compared with 27 percent who took metoclopramide, and 41 percent who took the placebo. The ginger powder did not cause the usual side effects of prescription drugs such as abnormal movement, itching, or visual disturbance.

Michael Murray states in *The Healing Powers of Herbs* that ginger has been shown to lower cholesterol levels and inhibit platelet aggregation. Ginger (along with cinnamon, thyme, and rosemary) contains powerful candida killing substances as well.

Ginkgo Biloba

Ginkgo (or gingko) biloba is an ancient Chinese tree whose leaves contain flavonoids that appear to enhance functioning of the adrenal and thyroid glands and the central nervous system. Ginkgo flavonoids are extremely potent antioxidants that also are capable of improving the flow of blood to the brain. In one clinical trial, reported by Dr. G. Rai in a 1991 issue of *Current Medical*

Research & Opinion, 112 elderly patients with chronic cerebral insufficiency were given 120 milligrams daily of ginkgo biloba extract (GBE). The extract significantly regressed the major symptoms of vascular insufficiency. Rai believes that a reduced blood and oxygen supply to the brain may be the major causative factor of the so-called age-related cerebral disorders (including senility), rather than a true degenerative process of nerve tissue. Ginkgo biloba extract, by increasing blood flow to the brain and improving glucose utilization, offers relief from these presumed side effects of aging. Rai concludes that ginkgo biloba extract may be helpful in treating senility, including Alzheimer's disease.

Another extract of ginkgo biloba produced in Austria has been shown to be a free radical scavenger and to decrease platelet aggregation, protect against ischemia, inhibit cerebral edema, and enhance cerebral blood flow. Dr. G. Hitzenberger, writing in a 1992 issue of *Wiener Medizinische Wochenschrift,* states: "Clinically GBE has proven favorable effects on intellectual deficiency, equilibrium disturbances and peripheral artery occlusions."

Ginseng (Panax Ginseng)

Widely regarded as the "king of herbs," ginseng is perhaps the best known of all botanical medicines. There are at least five types of ginseng plants, each of which has different chemical properties. Panax ginseng has been grown in China for several thousand years. The genus name panax is derived from the Latin word panacea, meaning "cure all." American ginseng (panax quinquefolium) grows throughout the woods of eastern North America from Canada to the Carolinas. Ginseng root is now available as a whole root, powdered extract, liquid extract, tea granules, tinctures, tablets, and capsules.

Recent research in China, summarized by Dr. C. Liu in the February 1992 issue of the *Journal of Ethnopharmacology,* indicates that panax ginseng has 28 different ginsenosides that "act on the central nervous system, cardiovascular system and endocrine secretion, promote immune function, and have effects on anti-aging and relieving stress." Ginseng appears to help regulate the amount of adrenaline secreted by the adrenal glands. It also improves adrenal gland function and prevents the shrinkage of the adrenal gland due to aging, prolonged stress, or corticosteroid drugs.

Murray suggests in *The Healing Powers of Herbs* that ginsenosides increase nerve fiber growth and prevent nerve damage by radiation. They also protect the liver against damage by increasing the growth of cells in that organ. In addition, ginseng lowers total cholesterol, especially low density lipoproteins (LDL, or "bad," cholesterol) while increasing HDL ("good") cholesterol.

Goldenseal (Hydrastis Canadensis)

Goldenseal is a perennial herb native to eastern North America that was used by Native Americans to treat a wide variety of conditions, including infections. Goldenseal is considered a blood purifier and an antiseptic tonic for the digestive tract and mucous membrane.

According to *Alternative Medicine: The Definitive Guide,* the medicinal benefits of goldenseal are due to its high content of biologically active alkaloids—berberine, hydrastine, and canadine. Berberine has proven a potent activator of macrophages, cells that digest waste matter in the blood. Berberine has been used to effectively combat bacteria, protozoa, and fungi, including gardia lambia, candida albicans, and streptococcus.

According to Murray and Pizzorno, it is effective in treating many acute diarrheas, including those that are typical of patients with AIDS. Goldenseal is usually included in most detoxification formulas because it increases splenic blood flow, improves liver function, and increases white cell activity in patients with the Epstein-Barr virus.

Green Tea (Camellia Sinensis)

Green tea is made from the leaves of camellia sinensis, an evergreen plant. Both green and black teas are derived from camellia sinensis, but the black tea leaves are fermented before drying and lose their beneficial polyphenols. According to David Steinman, writing in the March/April 1994 issue of *Natural Health,* dietary surveys of the Japanese, the world's leading green tea drinkers, show that people who drink four to six cups daily have a much lower incidence of liver, pancreatic, breast, lung, esophageal, and skin cancers than do people who drink less green tea or none. Steinman hypothesizes that green tea prevents cancer (and possibly other diseases) by acting as an antioxidant.

Japanese researchers recently found the main physiologically active polyphenol in green tea extract, (-)epigallocatechin gallate (EGCG), appears to inhibit the growth of tumors. A. Komori, writing in the June 1993 issue of the *Japanese Journal of Clinical Oncology,* states that EGCG inhibits protein kinase C activation by teleocidin, a tumor promoter. Komori claims that EGCG prevents the growth of lung and breast cancer. Dr. N. Ito, in a 1992 issue of *Teratogenesis, Carcinogenesis, & Mutagenesis,* theorizes that green tea may have a sealing effect—it may block the interaction of tumor promoters, hormones, and growth factors with their receptors.

The Medical Benefits of Green Tea

- Drinking green tea lowers the risk of liver, pancreatic, breast, lung, esophageal, and skin cancers.
- Green tea lowers the risk of cardiovascular disease by inhibiting the production of platelets, which form atheromas (blockages) of the coronary arteries.
- Green tea reduces the risk of stroke.
- Green tea lowers blood sugars. Animal experiments have shown that animals who maintain moderate blood sugar levels live longer.
- Green tea and its active components combat viruses.

Hawthorn Berry (Crataegus Monogyna)

The leaves, berries, and blossoms of hawthorn contain many active flavonoid compounds, including anthocyanin-type pigments, cratagolic acid, glycosides, purines, and saponins.

Hawthorn berry and its flower extracts have been effective in clinical trials in reducing blood pressure and angina attacks, as well as in lowering serum cholesterol levels and preventing the deposition of cholesterol on arterial walls. C. Hobbs reviewed several studies in the 1990 issue of *HerbalGram* that document the wide use of hawthorn extracts by European physicians to lower blood pressure. The beneficial effects of hawthorn extracts in treating high blood pressure appear to be a result of dilating the larger blood vessels. In excessive amounts, however, hawthorn can be dangerous because it constricts the bronchial tubes and depresses respiration and heart rate. Hobbs also reports that studies show hawthorn berry increases blood flow to the coronary muscle, and decreases heart rate and oxygen use of the myocardium (the middle layer of the heart muscle). Hawthorn extracts are currently approved by the German Ministry of Health for declining heart performance and mild forms of bradyarrhythmia (slow heart beat).

Licorice (Glycyrrhiza Glabra)

Most Americans are familiar with licorice as the sweet black candy, but in the perennial temperate zones in Asia where it grows, licorice root has been used for its medicinal properties for several thousand years. It was originally used as an expectorant, or a medicine that helps moisten the mucous membranes when a person has a dry cough, bronchitis, or a sore throat.

Recent scientific evidence indicates that licorice is useful in combating bacteria and viruses. Its major components produce interferon, which binds to cell surfaces and stimulates the synthesis of proteins that have been shown to inhibit the growth of several human viruses in cell cultures, including herpes simplex type 1. W. Lu reports in the June 1993 issue of the Chinese journal *Chung-Kuo Chung Hsi i Chieh Ho Tas Chih* that a licorice extract inhibited HIV activity in 35 percent of 60 HIV-infected patients. Licorice apparently prevents the suppression of immunity by stress and cortisone, and has displayed antibiotic activity against staphylococcus, streptococcus, and candida albicans.

Double-blind clinical studies have shown that a licorice component (SNMC) is effective in treating viral hepatitis. Dr. S. Acharya, writing in the April 1993 issue of the *Indian Journal of Medical Research,* reports that 12 of 18 patients with the disease survived after being given SNMC. He cautions, however, that further studies are necessary to standardize the dosage and duration of SNMC therapy.

Ma Huang (Ephedra Sinica)

Commonly called ephedra in the West, ma huang is now included in many herbal formulas. It has been grown in China for more than 5,000 years and, according to Murray and Pizzorno, has been used to relieve allergies, asthma, hay fever, colds, and inflammatory conditions. The plant contains two primary alkaloids, ephedrine and pseudoephedrine. Ephedrine stimulates the circulatory system, increases cardiac contractions and pumping, and stimulates blood flow to the brain. It has similar effects as adrenaline, although it can be taken orally and is less toxic.

Ephedra's effect diminishes if used over a long period of time due to weakening of the adrenal glands caused by ephedrine. It is therefore often necessary to use ephedra in combination with adrenal gland supportive herbs such as licorice (glycyrrhiza glabra) and panax ginseng, as well as nutrients that support the adrenal glands such as vitamin C, magnesium, zinc, vitamin B6, and pantothenic acid.

Maitake Mushrooms (Grifola Frondosa)

The maitake mushroom is native to northeastern Japan and has been prized in Japanese herbology for hundreds of years because of its ability to strengthen the body and improve overall health. According to Anthony Cichoke, writing in the May 1994 *Townsend Letter for Doctors,* maitake mushrooms have inhibited some tumor formation in animal experiments. Currently, research is being conducted by Dr. Dennis Miller of the Cancer Treatment Centers of America on its effects in stabilizing stage IV colorectal cancer in human patients.

Cichoke also suggests that maitake mushrooms may help prevent the destruction of T-cells by HIV. Dr. Joan Priestley, a world-renowned AIDS specialist, has used the mushrooms to improve the condition of Kaposi's sarcoma patients, especially those who received radiation. Many symptoms of AIDS were generally improved after taking the mushrooms. Cichoke further reports that Dr. Ber, a homeopathic physician practicing in Phoenix, Arizona, has used maitake mushrooms to treat HIV/AIDS patients. Ber has been able to maintain T-cell counts and inhibit further infections characteristic of AIDS patients. Ber believes the mushrooms improve immune function and maintain CD-4 cell levels. Cichoke emphasizes that more comprehensive controlled studies are needed, however, to substantiate maitake's use in treating AIDS-related diseases.

Milk Thistle (Silybum Marianum)

Milk thistle is a biennial plant that grows in the Mediterranean region of southwest Europe and in parts of the eastern United States and California. It has been cultivated for centuries as a medicinal remedy. Milk thistle contains silymarin, which Murray and Pizzorno note has been used to treat cirrhosis, chronic hepatitis, and gallbladder inflammation. *Alternative Medicine: The Definitive Guide* states that milk thistle effectively shortens the course of viral hepatitis, minimizes

post-hepatitis complications, and protects the liver from complications resulting from liver surgery. Foster notes in the November/December 1993 issue of *Natural Healing* that silymarin also has been used to treat gallstones. Silymarin concentrations vary in milk thistle capsules, pills, and teas, and should be taken only upon the advice of an herbalist or physician.

Mistletoe (Viscum Album)

As N. Bloksma reports in a 1979 issue of *Immunobiology,* the mechanism underlying the long known antihypertensive action of mistletoe has not yet been clarified. Although mistletoe contains a large number of biologically active substances, it appears that the healing effect is not produced by any one of its components. Rather it is produced by the whole complex of biologically active substances contained in the plant.

Mistletoe is believed to function as a regulator of blood pressure, exerting a healing effect in both hypertension and hypotension. In Europe, mistletoe has often been combined with other herbs to treat hypertension. As Murray and Pizzorno emphasize, this potentially toxic herb should not be used in high dosages or for extended periods of time except under the supervision of a physician.

E. Mueller reports in a 1992 issue of *Cancer, Immunology, Immunotherapy* that mistletoe was first used to treat cancer in 1917. Mistletoe contains lectins, polysaccharides, and polypeptides that researchers believe may indirectly kill cancer cells by stimulating a nonspecific immune reaction. Unlike chemotherapy drugs, mistletoe kills only cancerous cells and does not damage healthy cells. Mistletoe extracts have low toxicity and no fatal side effects have been reported. More than 40 clinical studies have been carried out, mainly at the Lukas Klinik in, Switzerland, and the Ludvig Boltzmann Institute in Austria.

Mueller adds that European mistletoe has been used at the Lukas Klinik to boost the immune system and to transform cancer cells into normal cells when injected beneath the skin or taken orally. German researchers also have used a viscum album preparation called Helixor to prolong the survival rates of patients with colorectal and liver cancer, both of which are extremely difficult to treat with chemotherapy. Mueller reports that the average one-year survival rate for Helixor-treated patients is 40.3 percent, compared with 6.6 percent for untreated control patients.

Experiments at the University of Heidelberg substantiate the ability of mistletoe extracts (ABNOB Aviscum) and pure mistletoe lectins to prevent the growth of tumor cells. Dr. O. Janssen reports in the November 1993 issue of *Arzneimittel-Forschung* that ABNOB Aviscum and pure mistletoe lectins administered to human tumor cell lines in vitro inhibit tumor cell growth. The mechanisms of growth arrest were due to the induction of programmed cell death (apoptosis). Janssen argues that mistletoe extracts and lectins should be further studied for their possible cytogenic effects.

Pokeweed (Phytolacca Americana)

Pokeweed traditionally has been used to treat upper respiratory tract infections, pharyngitis, rheumatism, and lymphatic disease. The July–August 1993 issue of *European Cytokine Network* reports that pokeweed extracts are commonly used in research and laboratory investigations (as pokeweed mitogen or PWM). PWM is a nontoxic yet potent agent that stimulates the production of T lymphocytes. Pokeweed also

appears to stimulate antiviral activity against herpes simplex. It should be used with caution, however, since it can be toxic in high doses. Check with your holistic practitioner.

Purple Coneflower (Echinacea Angustifolia)

Purple coneflower, commonly known in the U.S. as echinacea, is a perennial plant native to the midwestern states. It was used by Native American tribes as a blood purifier, analgesic, antiseptic, and snake bite remedy. It contains several chemicals including betaine, echinacin, echinoside, fatty acids, inulin, resin, and sucrose.

According to Murray and Pizzorno, echinacea is "the most widely used herb for enhancement of the immune system." Echinacea has long been prescribed to treat infections and inflammation of the stomach and bowels. Its pain-relieving properties, along with its antibiotic, anti-inflammatory nature, also make it effective in treating wounds, poison bites, ulcers, infected sores, and other skin conditions including boils, eczema, and psoriasis. It has been used to treat bronchitis and pneumonia because it helps stimulate the immune system and supports respiratory tract drainage.

Recent research conducted in Germany suggests that echinacea has interferon-like properties that may protect some types of cells from viruses and cancer tumors. The 1989 German Ministry of Health monograph, *Echinacea Purpurea Leaf,* reports that echinacea contains inulin, which neutralizes some viruses and destroys bacteria. The resultant effect, according to the monograph, is enhanced T-cell mitogenesis (reproduction), macrophage phagocytosis (the engulfment and destruction of bacteria or viruses), antibody binding, natural killer cell activity, and increased levels of circulating neutrophils (white blood cells primarily responsible for defense against bacteria).

Shiitake Mushrooms (Lentinus Edodes)

The shiitake mushroom has been used in traditional Chinese medicine to strengthen immune resistance to disease. The Chinese regard shiitake mushrooms as one of the most beneficial botanical medicines. Chinese legends refer to it as a plant that gives eternal youth and longevity.

Shiitake mushrooms contain a polysaccharide complex, lentinan, which stimulates the production of T lymphocytes and macrophages, specifically interleukin. Interleukin (a compound that destroys cancer cells and viruses) and interferon are currently being tested as possible treatments for AIDS and other diseases of the immune system. Balch and Balch state in *Prescription for Nutritional Healing* that pokeweed extracts also have been used effectively to prevent high blood pressure and heart disease, and to lower blood cholesterol levels.

Nutritionist Donald Brown writes in the April 1994 *Townsend Letter for Doctors* that an extract of lentinus edodes has been shown to have marked antitumor activity and to suppress viral chemical and viral oncogenesis and prevent cancer recurrence (metastasis) after surgery. Results of clinical trials indicate that it prolongs the lifespan of patients with advanced and recurrent stomach, colorectal, and breast cancer with minimal side effects.

Lentinus edodes also increases resistance to several bacterial, viral, and parasitic infections. An extract of lentinus edodes has been used to block the development of herpes simplex. Dr. S. Sarkar, writing in the April 1993 issue of *Antiviral Research,* suggests that lentinus edodes mycelia (JLS-S001) may

Safety Tips for Using Botanical Herbs

Before using any botanical herb, first consult with a physician or an herbalist. Dr. Andrew Weil offers the following guidelines:

- Do not use medicinal herbs for infants or children without guidance from a doctor.
- Do not use medicinal herbs unless you know enough to use them safely.
- Discontinue use of any botanical product to which you have an adverse reaction.
- Do not take herbal medicines unless you need them.
- Experiment with herbal remedies conscientiously.
- Loose herbs sold in bulk are likely to be useless.

block the replication of the virus in late stages.

Summary

Various components of plants have been used for thousands of years by traditional healers as botanical medicines. Modern research has yielded a great deal of information about the complex chemical structure of plants and how certain plant chemicals can be used to treat or prevent human medical disorders. More than 370 botanicals, for example, are being investigated in China for their possible effect in delaying the aging process. Botanical medicines show great promise for offering low-cost and safe treatments for many disorders. Nevertheless, much more research must be conducted on the pharmaceutical and toxic effects of botanical medicines at the molecular level.

It is hoped that in the near future governments and research institutions around the world will establish common nomenclatures for botanical medicines and will coordinate research on the chemical and molecular structure of their many subspecies. P.D. Semt, writing in the March 1993 issue of the *Journal of Ethnopharmacology,* urges governments to improve the timely detection and quantification of adverse reactions to the many different botanical medicines, and to develop testing procedures to ensure their safety. He and others have advocated that biologists and chemists form international networks to document the effects of different botanicals. Their first task would be to develop an internationally accepted botanical drug classification system, or a special set of herbal classification codes.

Resources

References

Acharya, S. "A Preliminary Open Trial on Interferon Stimulator (SNMC) Derived from Glycyrrhiza Glabra in the Treatment of Subacute Hepatic Failure." *Indian Journal of Medical Research* (April 1993): 69–74.

Balch, James F., and Phyllis Balch. *Prescription for Nutritional Healing.* Garden City Park, NY: Avery Publishing Group, 1993.

Belch, J. "The Effects of Altering Dietary Essential Fatty Acids on Requirements for Non-Steroidal Anti-Inflammatory Drugs in Patients with Rheumatoid Arthritis: A Double-Blind Placebo Controlled Study."

Annals of the Rheumatic Diseases (1991, Volume 47): 94–104.

Bergner, Paul. "How to Use 12 Powerful Herbs." *Natural Health* (September/October 1993): 92–96.

Beuscher, N. "Stimulatin der Immunanwort durch Inhaltsstoffe aus Baptisia Tinctoria." *Planta Medica* (1985, Volume 5): 381–84.

Bloksma, N. "Cellular and Humoral Adjuvant Activity of a Mistletoe Extract." *Immunobiology* (1979, Volume 6): 309–19.

Bordia, A. "Effect of Garlic Oil on Fibrinolytic Activity in Patients with CHD." *Atherosclerosis* (1977, Volume 28): 155–59.

Boyd, M.R., et al. "AIDS Anti-Viral Sulforlipids from Cyanobacteria (Blue-Green Algae)." *Journal of National Cancer Institute* (1989, Volume 16): 1254.

Brown, Donald. "Phytotherapy Review & Commentary." *Townsend Letter for Doctors* (April 1994): 406–07.

Brown, J. "The Use of Botanicals for Health Purposes by Members of a Prepaid Health Plan." *Research in Nursing & Health* (October 1991): 339–50.

The Burton Goldberg Group. *Alternative Medicine: The Definitive Guide.* Puyallup, WA: Future Medicine Publishing, Inc., 1993.

Chang, H. *Pharmacology and Applications of Chinese Materia Medica.* Teaneck, NJ: World Scientific Publishing, 1987.

Cichoke, Anthony. "Maitake—The King of Mushrooms." *Townsend Letter for Doctors* (May 1994): 432–34.

Culbreth, D. *A Manual of Materia Medica and Pharmacology.* Portland, OR: Eclectic Medical Publications, 1983.

Dausch, J. "Garlic: A Review of Its Relationship to Malignant Disease." *Preventive Medicine* (May 1990): 346–61.

De Semt, P. "An Introduction to Herbal Pharmacoepidemiology." *Journal of Ethnopharmacology* (March 1993): 197–208.

Dorant, E. "Garlic and Its Significance for the Prevention of Cancer in Humans." *British Journal of Cancer* (March 1993): 424–29.

Duke, J. *Handbook of Medicinal Herbs.* Boca Raton, FL: CRC Press, 1985.

Duker, E. "Effects of Extracts from Cimicifuga Racemosa on Gonadotropin Release in Menopausal Women and Ovariectomized Rates." *Planta Medica* (October 1991): 420–24.

Foster, Steven. *Feverfew.* Botanical Series 310. Austin, TX: American Botanical Council, 1991.

———. *Garlic.* Botanical Series 310. Austin, TX: American Botanical Council, 1991.

———. "Herbal Antioxidants." *Herbal Renaissance* (November/December 1993): 67.

Furusawa, E. "Antileukemic Activity of Viva-Natural, a Dietary Seaweed Extract." *Cancer Letters* (March 1991): 197–205.

German Ministry of Health. *Echinacea Purpurea Leaf.* Monographs for Phytomedicines. Bonn, Germany, 1989.

Griffith, H. Winter. *Complete Guide to Vitamins, Minerals & Supplements.* Tucson, AZ: Fisher Books, 1988.

Heptinstall, S. "Extracts of Feverfew Inhibit Granule Secretion in Blood Platelets and Polymorphonuclear Leucocytes." *The Lancet* (1985): 1071–74.

Hitzenberger, G. *Wiener Medizinische Wochenschrift* (1992, Volume 17): 371–79.

Hobbs, C. "Hawthorn: A Literature Review."

HerbalGram (1990, Volume 21): 19–33.

Ito, N. "Strategy of Research for Cancer Chemoprevention." *Teratogenesis, Carcinogenesis, & Mutagenesis* (1992, Volume 12): 79–95.

Janssen, O. *Arzneimittel-Forschung* (November 1993): 1221–27.

Kast, A. "Helixor—Mistletoe Preparation for Cancer Therapy." *Schweizerische Rundschau fur Medizin Praxis.* (1990, Volume 10): 291–95.

———. "Iscucin—Mistletoe Preparations for the Pre- and Postoperative Treatment of Malignancies." *Schweizerische Rundschau fur Medizin Praxis* (1990, Volume 14): 427–29.

Komori, A. *Japanese Journal of Clinical Oncology* (June 1993): 186–90.

Kuba, M. "Studies on Scutellariae Radix." *Chemical Pharmaceutical Bulletin* (1984, Volume 32): 724–29.

Lee-Huang S. "MAP 30: A New Inhibitor of HIV-1 Infection Replication." *FEBS Letter* (October 15, 1990): 12–18.

Leung, A. *Encyclopedia of Common Natural Ingredients Used in Food, Drugs, and Cosmetics.* New York, NY: John Wiley & Sons, 1980.

Li, B. "Inhibition of HIV Infection by Baicalin—a Flavonoid Compound Purified from Chinese Herbal Medicine." *Cellular & Molecular Biology Research* (1993, Volume 39): 119–24.

Liu, C. "Recent Advances on Ginseng Research in China." *Journal of Ethnopharmacology* (February 1992): 27–38.

Louria, D. "Onion Extract in Treatment of Hypertension and Hyperlipidemia." *Current Therapeutic Research* (1985, Volume 37): 127–31.

Lu, W.B. "Treatment of 60 Cases of HIV-Infected Patients With Glyke." *Chung-Kuo*

Chung Hsi i Chieh Ho Tsa Chih. (June 1993): 340–42.

Mahajan, V. "Antimycotic Activity of Berberine Sulfate." *Sabouraudia* (1982, Volume 20): 79–81.

Morgan, Helen C., and Kelly J. Moorhead. *Spirulina: Nature's Superfood.* Kailua-Kona, HI: Nutrex Inc., 1993.

Mueller, E. "A Viscum Album Oigosaccharide Activating Human Natural Cytotoxicity Is an Interferon Gamma Inducer." *Cancer Immunology, Immunotherapy* (1990, Volume 4): 221–27.

Murray, Michael. *The Healing Powers of Herbs.* Rocklin, CA: Prima Publishing, 1992.

Murray, Michael, and Joseph Pizzorno. *Encyclopedia of Natural Medicine.* Rocklin, CA: Prima Publishing, 1991.

Nagai, T. "Inhibition of Influenza Virus Sialidase and Anti-Influenza Virus Activity by Plant Flavonoids." *Chemical & Pharmaceutical Bulletin* (May 1990): 207–17.

O'Brien, Jim. "The Herbal Cure for Migraine Pain." *Your Health* (October 19, 1993): 11–12.

Ozaki, Y. "Anti-inflammatory Effect of Tetramethypyrazine and Ferulic Acid." *Chemical & Pharmaceutical Bulletin* (April 1992): 124–28.

Petkov, V. "Plants with Hypotensive, Antiatheromatous and Coronary Dilating Action." *American Journal of Chinese Medicine* (1979, Volume 7): 197–236.

Phillips, S. "Zingiber Offinale (Ginger)—an Antiemetic for Day Case Surgery." *Anaesthesia* (August 1993): 96–99.

Rai, G. "A Soluble-Blind, Placebo Controlled Study of Ginkgo Biloba Extract ("Tanakan") in Elderly Outpatients with Mild to Moderate Memory Impairment." *Current Medical Research & Opinion* (1991, Volume 6): 350–55.

Riley, K. "The Biological Efficacy of Aloes." *Journal of John Bastyr College of Natural Medicine* (1981, Volume 2): 8–27.

Sarkar, S. "Antiviral Effect of the Extract of Culture Medium of Lentinus Edodes Mycelia on the Replication of Herpes Simplex Virus Type 1." *Antiviral Research* (April 1993): 293–303.

Steinman, David. "Why You Should Drink Green Tea." *Natural Health* (March/April 1994): 56.

Sydiskis, R. "Inactivation of Enveloped Viruses by Anthraquinones Extracted From Plants." *Antimicrobial Agents & Chemotherapy* (December 1991): 2463–66.

Walsh, B. "Urostomy and Urinary pH." *Journal of Nursing* (July–August 1992): 110–13.

Wlihinda, J. "The Insulin-Releasing Activity of the Tropic Plant Momordica Charantia." *Acta Biologische Medizine Germanische* (1982, Volume 41): 229–40.

Zhang, H. "Preliminary Study of Traditional Chinese Medicine Treatment of Minimal Brain Dysfunction: Analysis of 100 Cases." *Traditional & Western Medicine* (May 1990): 278–79.

Organizations

American Association of Acupuncture and Oriental Medicine
4101 Lake Boone Tr., Ste. 201, Raleigh, NC 27607.

American Association of Naturopathic Physicians
2366 Eastlake Ave., Ste. 322, Seattle, WA 98102.

American Botanical Council.

PO Box 201660, Austin TX 78720.

The American Herbalists Guild.

PO Box 1683, Sequel, CA 95073.

Additional Reading

Hoffman, David. *The New Holistic Herbal.* Rockport, MA: Element Books, 1992.

Tierra, Lesley. *The Herbs of Life.* Freedom, CA: Crossing Press, 1992.

RESOURCES

Chapter 6

EXERCISE

In 1991, public health specialists at the University of Michigan invited 75 men and women, most of whom were 75 years of age or older, to take part in an unusual experiment to test the effects of regular activity on older people. The majority of the participants were overweight and had never exercised regularly. Many of them also reported suffering from several chronic health problems such as arthritis, hypertension, heart disease, or diabetes.

Despite their particular infirmities, the men and women were asked to exercise for 30 minutes twice a week under the supervision of specialists at the university's School of Public Health. The exercises were not strenuous and included neck and shoulder rolls, spinal twists and side stretches, arm and leg extensions, and pelvic rotations. Slow deep-breathing exercises also were part of their routine.

At the end of the experiment, all the subjects reported that they felt better and had lost weight. Even minor physical improvements were noticeable. Participants said they could "get around and move faster" and "felt less stiff in the joints," or "had more energy and were able to walk longer distances," according to the 1991 publication *Aging* by the U.S. Department of Health and Human Services.

To the many Americans who exercise, these findings are not surprising. An increasing number of Americans of all ages make exercise a part of their daily routine and for a good reason. More and more studies show that by not exercising, people put their health at risk. The same studies show that, conversely, even moderate exercise can help people prevent many diseases. The

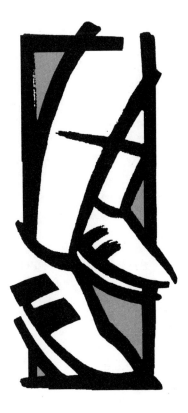

American Cancer Society, for example, has suggested that exercise alone can lower the risk of cancer for both men and women.

In one study of ten thousand men and three thousand women conducted by the Institute for Aerobics Research in Dallas, men who were most fit on a treadmill test had four times lower cancer rates over an eight-year period than nonexercisers. Women who were physically fit on the same treadmill test were sixteen times less likely to get cancer. Exercise, particularly in a woman's teenage and young adult years, directly lowers the rates of breast cancer and various hormone-related cancers of the reproductive tract. Nonathletes almost always have higher rates of cancers of the uterus, ovary, cervix, and vagina. The primary benefit of exercise in reducing cancer risk in women is believed to be a lower lifetime exposure to estrogen, which can stimulate growth of cells in the breasts and reproductive organs.

In a study at the Harvard School of Public Health, 5,400 women who had graduated from college between 1925 and 1991 were asked about their diet, health, and reproductive and exercise histories. Half the subjects were nonathletes; the other half had been college athletes, and 75 percent of this group reported that they had continued to exercise. After eliminating factors such as smoking and family history of cancer, "we found that the former athletes who continued to exercise had a significantly lower rate of breast cancer and cancers of the reproductive system," claims Dr. Rose Frisch, an associate professor who headed the research. Frisch also noted that with the exception of skin cancer, the athletes had markedly less of all types of cancer—including nonreproductive-tract cancers—than sedentary subjects, reports Michele Wolf in the October 1993 issue of *American Cancer.*

The Centers for Disease Control and Prevention (CDC) and the American College of Sports Medicine now recommend that every adult engage in at least 30 minutes of moderate physical activity throughout the day, at least five times a week, to prevent cardiovascular illness. This can be done by exercising through sports or walking or by adding physical activities, such as gardening and climbing up stairs, to a daily routine. The guidelines are aimed at increasing the proportion of adults who get enough exercise to achieve worthwhile health benefits. Currently, 54 percent of Americans over the age of 18 need more physical activity, according to an article in the December 1990 *University of California at Berkeley Wellness Letter.*

This chapter discusses the many physiological benefits of exercise. Clinical trials in which exercise has proven effective are analyzed, and general guidelines for measuring the effects and benefits of exercise are suggested. The major forms of exercise are then described, along with specific exercises for children, the elderly, and people with disabilities. Understandably, not everyone has the leisure time or inclination to exercise regularly out of doors or at a local health club. Yet anyone can find the time to do simple calisthenics at home that gently exercise the muscle and tissue systems of the body.

Starting an Exercise Program

Before starting an exercise program, it is important that people determine their current health status. Those who have been inactive for a number of years or who have an illness should consult their physician first. Individuals over age 30 who have been sedentary for a period of time should work up to higher levels of exercise very gradually. Some experts recommend that all potential exercisers undergo a complete physical examination before embarking on a regular training program.

Benefits of Exercise

As discussed by Kurt Butler and Lynn Rayner in *The Best Medicine: The Complete Health and Preventive Medicine Handbook,* various forms of exercise have different physiological effects. While not all of them have been studied comprehensively, definite benefits have been substantiated.

• *Exercise increases the functioning of the heart.* Exercise increases the size of the heart muscle and its chamber volume and greatly improves its efficiency.

• *Exercise improves oxygen circulation, especially in the heart muscle.* Oxygen-carrying blood is supplied to the heart muscle by two arteries arising from the aorta (which carries oxygenated blood out of the largest heart chamber, the left ventricle). These coronary arteries branch into smaller and smaller arteries, forming a network that can transport blood to any area of the heart muscle. Clinical observations indicate that regular aerobic exercise increases this network of tiny arteries as well as the size of the coronary arteries. If one of these arteries is impaired (coronary occlusion), a well-developed network can provide adequate blood to the entire heart until the blockage is cleared. Without this detour system, a region of heart muscle could go without blood long enough to damage it and possibly cause a heart attack.

• *Exercise lowers blood cholesterol.* Cholesterol is carried in the blood by different proteins, or lipoproteins: high-density (HDL), low-density (LDL), and very-low-density lipoproteins (VLDL). LDL cholesterol appears to be a significant factor in the formation of fatty plaques in the arteries, while HDL cholesterol appears to be protective. Exercise tends to decrease the LDL ("bad")

Choosing the Right Exercise Program

The components of a good exercise program are discussed and evaluated in this section. Before choosing an exercise program, every person should consider these basic questions:

• Current health status.

• Desired goals to be accomplished through exercise (such as living longer, losing weight, or increasing mental functioning).

• Maximum pulse rate and optimal exercise training range.

form if cholesterol and increase the HDL form, thereby reducing the formation of these plaques. Regular aerobic exercise, such as walking or cycling, has positive effects on blood fats, raises HDL ("good") cholesterol, and lowers triglycerides. In a recent study reported in the winter 1993 *Healthy Woman,* five months of resistance training (weight-lifting) alone—without any dietary changes—prompted a thirteen-point drop in total cholesterol in study participants. (Experts estimate that every one-point decrease in total cholesterol equals a two percent drop in a person's risk for heart disease.)

• *Exercise reduces high blood pressure to safe levels,* especially if aerobic exercise is accompanied by a proper diet. However, blood pressure may be increased dangerously in those with hypertension, so careful monitoring is essential.

• *Exercise improves glucose tolerance,* which is poor in diabetics and often in heart disease patients. Type 2 diabetes (the most common type) often can be prevented or kept under control without drugs by using exercise and good nutrition. Staying fit clearly helps prevent or delay blindness, loss of limbs, and other complications of diabetes.

• *Exercise promotes muscle and bone development* by increasing blood levels of anabolic hormones. The risk of developing osteoporosis is greatly reduced by regular exercise, especially activities like weight training that increase bone mass.

• *Exercise reduces stressful emotions and depression,* associated with coronary artery disease and heart attacks. Studies have shown that regular exercise increases endorphins, reduces muscle tension and anxiety levels, and increases self-confidence and emotional stability. This effect is due to improved cerebral circulation resulting from general cardiovascular improvement. As a result, many psychiatrists now prescribe moderate aerobic exercise such as jogging to help patients suffering from depression and anxiety. Beneficial effects on the mind may include improved concentration, memory, creativity, and mental speed and stamina.

• *Exercise helps people resist stress and injuries.* People who are fit, with strong muscles, are more capable of withstanding sudden illness, injury, surgery, and serious emotional stress such as grief than are physically weak and unfit people. In life-threatening emergencies requiring prolonged swimming, running, or walking for safety or help, people who are fit have a clear advantage.

• *Exercise helps reduce body weight.* As noted in Chapter 2, diet is the most important element in weight loss, although regular exercise can be the deciding factor in losing weight and keeping it off. While a meager diet may help a person lose weight, most of what is lost—besides some fat—is water and protein. The body tends to maintain its level of fat when drastic weight loss occurs. According to the Harvard School of Public Health, 30 minutes of exercise every day can take off (and keep off) as many as 25 pounds a year.

• *Exercise helps lose weight while maintaining muscle tissue.* People who reduce their body weight without exercising lose up to 30 percent of their muscle tissue. A 1988 Stanford University study found that exercise promotes fat loss while preserving muscle. Dieters in the study lost total body weight (fat weight and lean weight), while the exercisers lost fat weight but not lean weight. Therefore, the optimal way for overweight or obese people to lose weight is to eat less fat and to exercise more.

• *Exercise reduces back pain.* Many doctors believe that exercise not only prevents most back problems, but is also the most effective treatment once they occur. In a 1991 clinical trial performed at the University of Copenhagen in Denmark, 105 patients with chronic low-back pain were divided into three groups. One group performed 30 intense workouts over the course of the three-month trial. A second group performed only a fraction of these exercises. The third group did mild exercise but spent more time receiving heat treatments and massage. The patients who performed the intense exercises were found to have the best backs during the follow-up year. All of the patients with sciatic back problems significantly reduced the amount of pain they experienced, according to an article by Joel Posner in the March 15, 1992, issue of *Patient Care*.

Back pain is almost always associated with muscular weakness. Regardless of whether this weakness is a cause or an effect of pain, exercise usually can increase the strength and functioning of the back and decrease the pain. Dr. Richard A. Deyo, professor of medicine and health services at the University of Washington School of Medicine, uses exercise to reduce the number of days back pain patients spend in the hospital. He prescribes a minimum bed rest period for back-pain patients, normally no more than two days if necessary (most doctors recommend two weeks in bed). Deyo suggests that prolonged bed rest may increase future back pain because it contributes to bone loss, general weakness, and blood clots in the legs, Posner reports.

Exercise Goals

While people of all ages should exercise to maintain good health, the type of exercise varies for different age groups. Not all forms of exercise are equally beneficial for any individual's specific goals. In general, exercises are either aerobic or isometric. In aerobic exercises such as walking, running, swimming, and cycling, rhythmic contraction and relaxation of flexor and extensor muscle groups occurs, promoting blood flow through the blood vessels to and from the heart. At the right pace, such activities can be continued for long periods. In isometric exercises where muscles are held in contraction for prolonged periods, on the other hand, the sustained contraction limits blood flow by compressing the small arteries, and fails to help pump blood back to the heart. Moreover, the acute increase of blood pressure associated with isometrics can be very hazardous to people with heart disease or high blood pressure.

Maximum Pulse Rate and Optimal Exercise Training Range

The safety and effectiveness of any exercise is partially determined by measuring heart rate (number of heartbeats per minute). Exercise physiologists recommend training at a level of between 70 and 80 percent of maximum heart rate; under no circumstances should the rate exceed 85 percent.

To determine maximum heart rate, simply subtract a person's age from 220. To determine the training range, multiply this number by 70 to 80 percent. A 50-year-old individual, for example, would have a maximum heart rate of 170, and a training range of 119 to 136. The heart rate should never exceed 145 beats per minute. To gain significant benefits from exercise, a person must exercise at least 30 minutes at a time, 3 days a week, at the proper training heart rate.

Taking Precautions

People should never exceed their capacity for exercise, or serious injury can result. Exercising at a level that makes the heart beat at or near its maximum capacity forces the muscles into more anaerobic metabolism, which quickly uses up available glucose and increases the breakdown of muscle tissue. Normally, the lost tissue from exercise is more than replaced during the recommended rest period of approximately 20 hours after exercise. If exercise is resumed before full recovery, a net loss of muscle tissue—rather than a gain—may occur.

Overexercise can result in significant loss of muscle mass and fat-burning capacity. The older a person is, the more likely this is to occur, because tissue repair rate slows down with age. People who consistently overexercise can become sore and tired, and end up in worse condition than before they started.

Many experts now warn that overexercise can precipitate a heart attack, even in apparently healthy individuals. Exercisers should monitor their heart rates while exercising and should not ignore symptoms such as tightness or pain in the chest, dizziness, light-headedness, stomach pain, or breathing difficulties. Exercises that cause pain also can lead to severe injuries. In moderate-to-intensive aerobic training programs, which are more beneficial to cardiovascular fitness and general health, there is no reason to experience pain in order to gain fitness.

Another precaution to keep in mind is to drink water or other nonsugar liquids while exercising, particularly during hot weather when the body loses fluids most rapidly. Perspiring excessively can lead to dehydration (with symptoms including increased body temperature, dizziness, and weakness), which in turn can cause heat stroke. Most experts suggest drinking a glass of water or a noncarbonated sports beverage which also provides small amounts of sodium and potassium. Carbonated or sugary drinks can upset the stomach if people are dehydrated. Check the label for serving sizes and calorie counts. Drink 8 to 12 ounces of fluid at least 15 minutes before exercising and replenish the body's supply of liquids before thirst occurs.

According to *Food Insight,* the bulletin of the International Food Information Council, "drinking enough fluid is certainly key to maximum athletic performance. But it is even more basic than that. It can make the difference between feeling great or drained after exercise." *Food Insight* says that the average adult needs 64 ounces (8 cups) of fluid a day. The fluid can come from water, milk, meat, or vegetables. Even dry cereal or bread contains from 8 to 35 percent water.

Approximately 12 to 15 percent of Americans suffer from exercise-induced asthma (EIA). Some may have this problem without being aware of it, since EIA typically occurs in people who have no history of asthma or allergies. Early signs of difficulty include a drop in performance or post-exercise fatigue. During heavy exercise, an athlete normally breathes in 18 to 20 times more air than when he or she is at rest. If the body cannot consume and humidify this large volume of air, spasms or constriction of the airways may result. Colds, pollution, and recent upper respiratory tract infection (like bronchitis) also can trigger this reaction.

During exercises such as running, swimming, and cycling, people can monitor for

EIA by noting their breathing response and lowering the intensity of the workout, if necessary. Swimming is an ideal sport for athletes with EIA, because the warm, moist air decreases the incidence of spasms or constriction of the airways. Sports that involve intermittent exertion, such as baseball and volleyball, are usually low risk as well. People with EIA who exercise regularly should use medication, if prescribed, 30 to 60 minutes before starting, and warm up at 50 percent of maximum heart rate for 10 to 15 minutes. They should also cool down by walking or stretching for 10 to 20 minutes after exercising and should, in all cases, stay well hydrated.

Proper exercise can be beneficial even for people with a number of illnesses, including hypertension and diabetes, but a vigorous exercise program should not be undertaken without consulting a physician or health practitioner. Individuals susceptible to EIA should talk with their physician as well. There may be reasons why any individual, due to genetic factors, age, gender, and prior activity levels, should not perform a certain exercise.

Aerobic Exercises

Aerobic exercise is defined as any form of movement that conditions the heart and lungs to work more efficiently. When the body works harder than it is accustomed to working, the muscles demand more oxygen. The capacity of the lungs increases and the heart becomes stronger and larger as it works to pump oxygen-rich blood through the arteries.

Exercising aerobically less than three times a week does not increase aerobic capacity or help in achieving or maintaining weight loss. At the same time, exercising aerobically more than five times per week does not provide a significant increase in fitness and may result in injury if the exercise is too strenuous.

Aerobic exercise includes any activity that uses large muscle groups in a rhythmic, continual motion that increases oxygen consumption. A three-mile daily walk is the simplest aerobic exercise. Hiking, bicycling, swimming, dancing, rowing, skating, and cross-country skiing are other good aerobic exercises. Indoor exercises include cross-country ski machines, aerobic dance and step aerobics, weight training, and indoor climbing.

Aerobic Dancing

Aerobic dancing is a special type of exercise that is scientifically designed to maximize aerobic respiration. Programs vary in length and degree of difficulty. A session should include at least 10 minutes of stretching and warming-up exercises, followed by 15 to 30 minutes of nonstop aerobic movements at a pace determined by a person's fitness level (beginner, intermediate, advanced). At least 5 minutes of cooling-down activities such as walking and stretching should conclude the program.

Aerobic dancing has proven effective in improving fitness and reducing weight. The workouts popularized on television videos provide significant benefits, but exercisers should remember that to be of real value, any aerobic dance workout should increase heartbeat up to 75 percent of its maximum rate for at least 15 minutes. Many aerobic dance injuries can result from prior foot, leg, or back injuries, and good shoes and a resilient surface should always be used.

Bicycling

Bicycling provides an excellent aerobic workout. Today an increasing number of Americans bicycle to work, school, or to go shopping, or use a stationary cycle at home or at the gym.

In bicycling, the peak oxygen load is not as great as with running or cross-country skiing. It is also much less physically stressful than running or aerobic dancing. To produce exertions, a person must bicycle hard enough to increase heart rate for at least 15 consecutive minutes. In order to burn 300 to 360 calories, it is necessary to cycle at least 8 miles per hour. To burn 350 to 420 calories, a person must cycle at least 10 miles per hour. According to Dr. Roger Kennedy, internist and bioethicist at Kaiser Permanente Medical Center in Santa Clara, California, stationary bicycling is especially beneficial for people with knee problems.

Brisk Walking

In the last 10 years, brisk walking has become one of America's favorite exercises, particularly for women. Research indicates that brisk walking may offer virtually the same health and fitness benefits as running or jogging, but without stress to the joints and risk of injury. Physicians recommend brisk walking as an efficient and safe form of exercise for almost everyone. Many participants achieve a level of fitness in which they are able to easily walk a 13-minute mile or ascend a two-thousand-foot hill.

Cross-Country Skiing

Butler and Rayner recommend cross-country skiing as one of the best aerobic exercises, because it provides all the benefits of running without the jarring stresses that accompany it. The large leg muscles are used more than in swimming, and very high levels of oxygen consumption can be reached by the fit cross-country skier. Unfortunately, the sport is not accessible or affordable for all people, although it is much less expensive than downhill skiing. Some exercise devices now mimic cross-country skiing very well and are excellent for skiers and nonskiers alike.

There are two different techniques involved in cross-country skiing, both of which provide excellent exercise for the legs and heart. In the skating technique, the skier pushes off from the rear ski in a motion similar to ice skating. The pushing portion is known as the propulsive phase and occurs between pole plant and toe off. The remainder of the cycle is the stride phase. The skating technique is a slightly more effective form of aerobic exercise.

Rowing

Rowing is both an intensely demanding physical activity and a competitive sport. Noncompetitive rowing is an excellent aerobic exercise, although it is normally used in combination with running or bicycling as part of a total fitness program. Adaptive rowing is a popular exercise in the U.S., and many different types of boats have been marketed to appeal to different age groups. Many homes now also have a rowing machine. Rowing is an ideal form of exercise for many disabled persons (see Exercise and the Disabled, later in this chapter). One variant of the rowing machine is the landrower, a rowing bicycle that propels the upper body forward as the rower pulls on the oars.

Running (Jogging)

Running is a high-impact sport and should be undertaken only by people in good health who have no ankle, knee, or back problems. Individuals who can comfortably walk two miles in 30 minutes without dangerously increasing their heart rate are good candidates for running. Sports physicians normally advise beginning runners to alternate between walking and jogging for 20 minutes, doing two- to three-minute stretches of each, and

then to slowly build up to 30 uninterrupted minutes of running.

As a high-risk aerobic exercise, running can be quite stressful to the body and lead to injuries. Butler and Rayner cite one survey of a thousand runners that found "60 percent had been injured for considerable periods of time. The most common injuries are of the knee, shin, Achilles' tendon, forefoot, hip, thigh, heel, ankle, arch, and groin. Almost one-fourth of those surveyed suffered knee injuries, while only two percent had groin injuries." As with any form of exercise, injury can be avoided by choosing appropriate shoes, running surfaces, and running habits, and by consulting a trainer or sports physician.

An increasing number of women are taking up jogging, although more seem to prefer brisk walking. At one time, it was thought that the stress of jogging could weaken the connective tissue supporting the uterus and drive it down, causing it to protrude into the vagina. Recent surveys of women runners, however, seem to suggest that this is unlikely. However, women with prolapsed uteruses should be cautioned that running and lifting heavy weights can aggravate the condition. Jogging also can cause breast sagging and pain. This problem usually is prevented by wearing a sports bra that prevents lateral and spiraling motions of the breast.

Step Aerobics

Step aerobics (or bench aerobics) is an increasingly popular form of aerobics that utilizes a small platform approximately the height of a stair-step. Working to music, aerobicizers step on and off the bench in routines that give them a cardiovascular workout while toning legs and buttocks. This form of aerobics is low in impact, because one foot is always on the floor or on the step, and is less

Safe Running Tips

Dr. R. James Gregg of the International Chiropractors Association recommends the following injury-prevention guidelines for people who jog:

- Wear a running shoe with ample heel padding. Each heel hits the ground about fifteen hundred times per mile, and pressure on the lower back increases an average of three times an individual's body weight every time it strikes down. Air-cushioned shoe inserts help absorb shock.

- Run on surfaces that "give," such as grass, pathways, and dirt roads.

- Run on alternate sides of the road. Running continually in the same direction on the same side of the road may cause a muscle imbalance in the lower back because the grade of the road surface may slope toward the sides of drainage.

- Stretch at least five minutes before and after the jog; stretch both leg and back muscles.

- Avoid running downhill frequently. With the pull of gravity on a downgrade, a normal three-foot stride can become five feet long. To compensate for a longer gait, the body leans backwards, which increases the curve of the lumbar spine and may tighten back muscles.

- Measure heart rate and do not exceed the proper training range.

---

likely to result in the exercise-related injuries typically associated with dance aerobics.

Researchers at San Diego State University found that working at a rate of 120 steps per minute while pumping the arms was as exerting as running at seven miles per hour. However, impact forces were similar to those created by walking at only three miles per hour. In a second study at the University of Pittsburgh, subjects working at a rate of 80 steps per minute burned almost 300 calories in 30 minutes. The calorie expenditure increased 19 percent when one-pound hand weights and a pumping arm motion were added.

As with any aerobic exercise, it is important to warm up and stretch before the cardiovascular session and cool down after the exercise is concluded.

Swimming

Swimming is considered by many experts to be the safest form of exercise. It also uses more muscles than most other aerobic alternatives. Swimming is an excellent choice for people of all age groups and physical fitness levels because swimmers can pace themselves, both in terms of duration and intensity (speed) of the workout. Swimming has been shown to help relieve varicose veins by increasing circulation in the legs. And, as discussed later in this chapter, it is ideal for people with physical disabilities. In order to derive the benefits of aerobic exercise, a person must swim for at least 15 minutes nonstop. Because swimming entirely immerses the individual in water, all of the cells of the skin are stimulated, and relaxation is induced.

Walking

Walking is the fastest growing form of exercise among Americans and also the most popular. More than 68 million Americans walk regularly to satisfy their exercise needs. According to a study in the *British Medical Journal,* reported in the *San Jose Mercury News* on December 23, 1992, those who participate in moderate physical activity such as walking have a 40 percent lower risk of stroke than inactive people. Walking also has been shown to bolster human defense against colds. Tests at Appalachian State University in Boone, North Carolina, revealed that walking strengthens the specific components of the immune system that fight cold viruses. Test subjects who walked did not always avoid colds, but when they got them, the colds were less severe and lasted only half as long as those suffered by physically inactive people, according to Posner in *Patient Care.*

According to the American College of Sports Medicine, as reported by the Associated Press on October 31, 1993, regular, moderate-intensity endurance exercises, such as 30 minutes of walking every other day, can reduce mild to moderate hypertension and help people avoid developing high blood pressure.

Walking requires no special skills or equipment and can be stopped at any time without danger. A good pair of walking shoes is essential, and any comfortable, well-cushioned athletic shoe that fully supports the sole of the foot is adequate.

Susan Johnson, author of *The Walking Handbook,* suggests that beginners start with a simple 10-minute walk at any speed, 5 minutes out and 5 minutes back. During the second week, build up to 15 minutes a day. In the third week, increase to 20 minutes a day. And by the fourth week, continue to walk 20 minutes a day, warming up with a slow stroll for 5 minutes and then increasing to a brisk pace. End the exercise by slowing down to a stroll; then cool down with passive stretching, and drink an 8- to 12-ounce glass of water.

Johnson says that walkers will see more strength and firmness in their legs in three to four weeks. By the end of eight weeks, they will begin to lose body fat. At that time, walkers can concentrate on strengthening calf and hamstring muscles by pushing off their back foot rather than reaching with the front, or by developing a long, even, rhythmic stride that will tone the buttocks.

Other Sports

Sports such as tennis, basketball, and volleyball can be very tiring, although they often consist largely of standing around between short bursts of action, and are not as aerobically valuable as sports with nonstop movements. It has been estimated that jogging at a rate of at least three miles per hour for 15 minutes is equivalent to an hour or more of most other sports, including tennis, racquetball, and Ping-Pong. This, of course, depends on how fast and vigorously the latter games are played.

Although these sports tend to be less aerobically effective, an exception is two-on-two volleyball, which can be extremely demanding, especially between players good enough to keep long volleys in play. Baseball and football players often keep in shape by jogging, sprinting, and other exercises that combine nonstop smooth movements of all major muscle groups.

Calisthenics

Virtually everyone, despite their age or physical condition, should exercise regularly each day. And it is not necessary to belong to a sports gym, exercise facility, or sports team to do so. The Centers for Disease Control and Prevention has, in fact, stated that most

Americans can achieve the physiological benefits of exercise by doing simple tasks around the house, such as walking up and down stairs and doing yardwork.

One of the easiest and most systematic methods of gently exercising all parts of the body is calisthenics, or a variety of gymnastic exercises that move all parts of the body. Calisthenics are familiar to many who have attended a public school, competed in athletics, or served in the Armed Forces. The purpose of calisthenics is to gently exercise all the muscle groups of the body and increase aerobic breathing. People suffering from stress tend to take shorter breaths and, as a result, not enough oxygen reaches their lungs. Physical exercises such as calisthenics or yoga can be an excellent way of coping with stress. Calisthenics are not physically difficult or dangerous and people of all ages, including those with disabilities, can perform them.

Calisthenics are practiced in most societies of the world, as virtually all cultures recognize the importance of regularly moving all parts of the body. In India, exercise includes practices such as yoga, which combines movement with deep breathing and mental exercises. In China, exercise has been practiced for twenty-five hundred years using martial arts such as tai chi, and a series of 108 slow, fluid movements intended to increase the body's agility and calm the mind. People who have visited China or cities in America with large Chinese populations have seen young and old Chinese alike practicing tai chi every morning in front of their homes or in the parks. To the Chinese, exercise is as important as eating or sleeping.

The Chinese maintain that exercises such as tai chi not only tone the muscles and tissues, but also supply energy that must be kept circulating in the body. One important purpose of tai chi is, through movement and concentration, to find your center or "chi," which the Chinese believe is health itself. Elderly

Door Stretch Exercise

1. Find a narrow doorway.
2. Lay the forearms up against each side of the doorway, with one foot behind the other and begin to lean forward.
3. As the body leans forward, the shoulders should be pulled back.
4. Done correctly, this exercise will fully stretch the chest muscles as well as the muscles around the shoulders. The force of the stretch can be controlled by moving the front leg farther forward.
5. As the leg is moved forward, there should be a strong stretch along the calves and hamstrings. The hip flexors, the muscles surrounding the hipbone, also are being stretched.
6. Now turn to one side and lean forward. This helps to stretch the serratus interior, the rippled muscles above the rib cage.
7. Put the other foot forward and repeat the exercise.

proponents maintain that through tai chi they can recapture the energy of their youth.

Exercising at Work

Americans spend an average of eleven to twelve hours a day working and commuting to and from work, which often results in a lack of time or inclination to exercise. For people who cannot exercise before, during, or after work, the following gentle exercise is recommended to effectively stretch various body muscles.

Exercise and Children

One of the most valuable gifts parents can give their children is the motivation to stay physically fit. If children's early years are physically active, they will lay a solid foundation for a healthier adult life. Unfortunately, an estimated 25 million American children are not fit, and more than half of the children who participate in organized athletics cannot pass a basic fitness test, according to the American Physical Therapy Association (APTA).

The National Exercise for Life Institute in Excelsior, Minnesota, further claims that 50 percent of all American children are not getting enough exercise to develop healthy cardiorespiratory systems; 67 percent of children have at least 3 heart risk factors; and obesity figures are 54 percent higher than in the 1960s. One study found that typical gym classes give children only 1 to 3 minutes of vigorous exercise per class. However, the U.S. Public Health Service recommends that children ages 6 through 17 exercise vigorously for 20 minutes 3 times a week. For a free pamphlet on children's health and fitness, contact the National Exercise for Life Institute at 1-800-358-3636.

APTA publishes an activity booklet for children in grades one through four that encourages fitness through illustrations, games, and puzzles. (For a copy of the booklet, write to "Fit Kids," PO Box 37257, Washington, DC 20013.) Several of the exercises that APTA recommends for children appear in the following pages. Children should be advised to undergo flexibility screening before exercising. The exercises should be done slowly and rhythmically, and children should hold the positions steady, without jerking or bouncing.

Exercise and the Disabled

Many people with physical or emotional disabilities are nevertheless able to exercise parts of their bodies and even take part in athletic competition. Physically challenged people now regularly participate in events such as the Special Olympics that recognize their physical abilities. Many people with disabilities keep their bodies in shape and try to be the best they can be in their chosen sport. For these athletes, exercise is not only good for their health, but it is part of the recovery process that in some cases allows them to live independently.

Many disabled people swim, ski, bicycle, and lift weights. With recent advances in equipment and techniques, new exercise programs are available for people who are physically challenged, including senior citizens who use wheelchairs. The Idaho State University's Senior Enhancing Lifelong Fitness program, for example, has been very successful in tailoring chair aerobic exercise programs for wheelchair users who wish to remain physically active, outgoing, and independent. Adaptive rowing is especially helpful for people who move about in wheelchairs or on crutches. Water-based exercise is probably the most beneficial for the disabled because it allows them a great range of movement and physical exertion without fighting the forces of gravity. People with disabilities now water walk, play water polo, snorkel, and scuba dive. Rowing has become one of the most popular sports for the disabled, who now hold their own regattas each year in the U.S. and Europe.

Exercise and the Elderly

Only one of four elderly persons exercises regularly or maintains the level of physical activity recommended by medical specialists. Yet research has conclusively demonstrated both the conditioning and rehabilitative effectiveness of physical activity for this age group.

Calf Muscle Stretch Exercise

1. Stand facing a wall with the arms stretched out straight. The palms of the hands should be touching the wall.

2. Keep the knees straight and heels flat on the floor.

3. Point the toes toward each other.

4. Bend the elbows and lean in toward the wall until there is a stretch in the back of the legs. Stay like this for a count of 10.

Fit Kids, Vol. 1, 1993. Reprinted by permission.

Vigorous physical activity, especially if it is recreational, has been linked to longevity. According to a 1986 report in the *New England Journal of Medicine,* formerly sedentary middle-aged men who take up a moderately vigorous activity such as swimming, brisk walking, or tennis live an average of 10 months longer than men who never work out. (Although women were not included in the study, the researchers believe that exercise has a positive impact on their longevity as well.) The findings, based on questionnaires filled out by 10,269 Harvard University alumni who were followed between 1962 and 1985, suggest that it is never too late to begin an exercise regimen. The study also confirmed that the earlier in life a person begins a program—including at least 30 minutes of exercise 3 times a week— the greater the chances of extending lifespan.

Exercise also has been proven to enhance cardiovascular fitness. At a given level of

Back Thigh (Hamstrings) Stretch Exercise

1. Sit flat with legs out in front, knees slightly bent.
2. Stretch down the legs and try to hold the ankles for a count of 10. Don't bounce.
3. Come back up slowly.

Fit Kids, Vol. 1, 1993. Reprinted by permission.

Front Thigh Stretch Exercise

1. Lie on the stomach.
2. Bend the right knee and grab the ankle with the right hand.
3. Pull the foot in as far as you comfortably can.
4. Hold for a count of 10.
5. Slowly unbend the leg and return it to a straight position on the floor.
6. Do the same thing with the left leg and left hand.
7. Be sure to hold again for a count of 10.

Fit Kids, Vol. 1, 1993. Reprinted by permission.

exertion, physical training results in decreased oxygen requirements of the heart as well as decreased blood pressure. Physicians therefore often recommend exercise for elderly patients with moderate hypertension, risk of coronary heart disease, or angina pectoris.

Regular exercise increases muscle mass in the elderly and maintains muscular strength, both essential in the prevention and rehabilitation of many musculoskeletal problems. For example, osteoporosis (the loss of mineral bone mass) causes approximately 700,000 fractures annually, one-third of which occur in the hip joint. Physical activity may prevent or delay the onset of osteoporosis by stimulating bone mineralization. Finally, moderate exercise training has been associated with a 20 percent increase in serum immunoglobulins, thereby helping to strengthen the immune system.

Water exercise programs are an option for people who prefer not to participate in traditional walking or low-impact aerobic programs. Water-based programs allow these people to gain the full benefits of aerobic exercise without strain or pressure on their joints. With the aid of water walkers (buoyancy devices which attach easily around the waist), exercisers have total freedom of move-

ment and can participate at their own pace.

The cardiovascular and musculoskeletal benefits of water exercise for older people are similar to those of "on the ground" aerobic exercise. The American College of Sports Medicine now recommends aquatic aerobic activity involving large muscle groups for elderly patients with rheumatoid arthritis (RA), because of the soothing effects of warm water. Water-based workouts cause less exercise-induced asthma than other forms of exertion. Traditional low-impact and chair aerobic programs geared for seniors also have proven popular.

In this article in the March 15, 1992, issue of *Patient Care,* Posner describes the Optimal Aging Program at the Medical College of Pennsylvania, which uses a variety of exercises to help elderly patients stay physically fit. The most important part of the program is lifting weights 3 times a week for 40 minutes. The sessions are individually tailored, and the smallest weights are only 2 pounds. One set of 10 repetitions may be enough for the beginning exerciser. When 3 sets of 10 repetitions can be done easily, the weight loads are increased. Lower body work includes exercising the quadriceps, hamstrings, and legs. Exercises for the hip are important, especially for women, in preventing falls and hip fractures. A weight-stack machine or ankle weights gently tones the knee joints.

Upper body weight lifts, including shoulder work (overhead presses and/or lateral raises on the weight-stack machine), pectoral work, upper and lower back exercises, abdominal work, and trunk exercises also are included in the Optimal Aging Program. People in their seventies can increase upper body strength by approximately 20 percent after six months. In addition to these benefits, those who play golf or tennis will find the power of their swing or serve considerably enhanced. In addition, lower back pain is often alleviated by strengthening the lower back and abdominal muscles. The fitness program amounts to a total commitment of one and one-half hours three times a week.

Summary

In both Eastern and Western cultures, exercise is a vital component of maintaining good health. Studies consistently show that exercise improves circulation, increases energy, stimulates digestion, strengthens bones, helps regulate hormones, and provides increased stamina for responding to both physical demands and emotional stress. Regular activity also is essential for maintaining a healthy body weight and increasing longevity.

Perhaps the well-known Chinese adage best sums up the importance of exercise: "The body is like a hinge on a door. If it is not swung open, it will rust." Dr. Ralph Paffenbarger, a professor of epidemiology at the Stanford University School of Medicine, also puts it well: "Exercise seems to improve quality of life, as well as longevity. People who exercise regularly and live healthy lifestyles consistently look and feel younger than their years."

Resources

References

Butler, Kurt, and Lynn Rayner. *The Best Medicine: The Complete Health and Preventive Medicine Handbook.* New York, NY: Harper & Row Publishers, Inc., 1985.

"Health Worries? Take a Hike." *San Jose Mercury News* (December 23, 1992).

"Let Your Feet Do Walking to Lower Blood Pressure." Associated Press (October 31, 1993).

Posner, Joel. "Optimal Aging: The Role of Exercise." *Patient Care* (March 15, 1992): 35–39.

"The Next Step in Aerobics." *The University of California at Berkeley Wellness Letter* (December 1990): 6.

U.S. Department of Health and Human Services. *Aging.* No. 362. Washington, DC: U.S. Department of Health and Human Services, 1991. Reprinted in: "Exercise Isn't Just for Fun." *Public Citizen Health Research Group Health Letter* (August 1991): 8–9.

Wolf, Michele. "Can Exercise Ward Off Cancer?" *American Cancer* (October 1993): 77.

"You Can Prevent Many of the So-called By-Products of Aging—or Even Reverse Them by Doing One Thing: Weight Lifting." *Healthy Woman* (winter 1993): pp. 42–45.

Organizations

American Heart Association.
7320 Greenville Ave., Dallas, TX 75231.

American Physical Therapy Association (APTA).
PO Box 37257, Washington, DC 20013.

International Chiropractors Association.
1901 L St. NW, Ste. 800, Washington, DC 20036.

President's Council on Physical Fitness and Health.
450 5th St. NW, Washington, DC 20001.

Additional Reading

Adams, G. "Physiological Effects of Exercise Training Regimen Upon Women Aged 51 to 79." *Journal of Gerontology* (1973): 50–55.

American Heart Association. *Statement on Exercise.* Dallas, TX: American Heart Association, 1990.

Awbrey, B. "Chronic Exercise Induced Pressure." *American Journal of Sports Medicine* (1988): 391–97.

Challis, S. "Treating Arthritis the Holistic Way." *Professional Nurse* (May 1991): 448–51.

Cumming, M. *Rowing Beyond Handicaps.* U.S. Rowing Association, 1989.

Dorsen, P. "Overuse Injuries from Nordic Ski Skating." *Physician Sports Medicine* (1986): 34.

Doyne, E. "Running Versus Weight Lifting in the Treatment of Depression." *Journal of Consultative Clinical Psychology* (1987): 748–55.

"Exercise During Pregnancy." *Health Tips Index.* California Medical Association, June 1990.

"Exercise and Heart Disease." *Health Tips Index.* California Medical Association, April 1989.

Fletcher, G. *Exercise Standards: A Statement for Health Professionals from the American Heart Association.* Dallas, TX: American Heart Association, 1990.

Guiton, Arthur, M.D. *Textbook of Medical Physiology.* Philadelphia, PA: Harcourt Brace Jovanovich, 1991.

Harkcom. T. "Therapeutic Value of Graded Aerobic Exercise Training in Rheumatoid Arthritis." *Arthritis Rheumatism* (1985): 32–39.

Hausman, Patricia, and Judith Been Hurley. *The Healing Foods.* Emmaus, PA: Rodale Press, Inc., 1989.

Hoeger, W. "Effect of Low-Impact Aerobic Dance on the Functional Fitness of Elderly Women." *Gerontologist* (1990): 189–92.

Nehlsen-Cannarella, S. "The Effects of Moderate Exercise on Immune Response." *Medical Science Sports Exercise* (1991): 64–70.

Norris, R. "The Effects of Aerobic and Anaerobic Training on Fitness, Blood Pressure and Psychological Stress and Well-Being." *Journal of Psychosomatic Research* (1990): 367–75.

Simon, Harvey B., and Steven R. Levisohn. *The Athlete Within: A Personal Guide to Total Fitness.* Boston, MA: Little, Brown, 1987.

Stevenson, J. "A Comparison of Land and Water Exercise Programs for Older Individuals." *Medical Science Sports Exercise* (1988): 537.

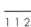

RESOURCES

Chapter 7

STRENGTHENING THE IMMUNE SYSTEM

In the course of a single day, the average American may be exposed to a multitude of potentially harmful toxins while driving to and from work, working at the office or factory, eating meals or shopping, and carrying out simple household chores. In the home alone, there are hundreds of toxins in the walls, floors, building materials, carpets, paints, cleaning materials, drinking water, and even in the food.

Some people are exposed to high levels of these toxins and rarely get sick, yet their friends or neighbors may be exposed to the same toxins at much lower levels and become ill far more frequently. What accounts for the difference in the way people fight off the toxins that can cause infection and illness?

The answer has a great deal to do with how each person's immune system eliminates toxins. It is the immune system that prevents infectious and chronic diseases and is most responsible for guaranteeing optimal holistic health. However, a balanced natural diet and adequate amounts of vitamins, minerals, herb supplements, and exercise—which all play a critical part in maintaining the health of the immune system—may not protect everyone from dangerous toxins in the air, food, and water. And, depending on the amount of toxins absorbed, it may be necessary for some people to regularly eliminate dangerous toxins from their bodies. This chapter discusses the major toxins and the body's immune system attempts to eliminate them and outlines the components of a basic gentle detoxification program.

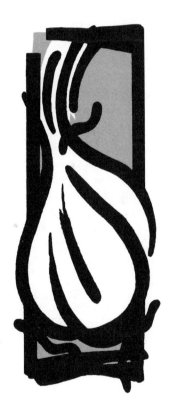

Types of Toxins

Chemical and Metal Toxins

What are environmental toxins? Basically, they are substances in the environment that can cause physiological or psychological disorders and even death. These toxins can be in the air, the water, foods, and even inside homes and offices.

Polluted air contains the most potentially dangerous toxins. Gordon Edlin and Eric Golanty, in *Health and Wellness: A Holistic Approach,* explain that clean air, which is essential for all living things to function normally and maintain health, consists of approximately 21 percent oxygen, 78 percent nitrogen, and trace elements of seven other gases. The human body must have a constant source of pure oxygen. If the oxygen content of air drops below 16 percent, body and brain functions are adversely affected.

The air in many industrialized countries is now severely polluted. Air pollution limits the amount of pure oxygen available and forces the body to breathe in hundreds of chemical toxins that are harmful to the lungs, blood, and body tissues. This can be particularly disastrous for people who already suffer from cardiovascular or respiratory diseases. Edlin and Golanty report that the American Lung Association estimates one out of every five Americans suffers from some kind of pulmonary disease, including asthma, emphysema, bronchitis, and chronic coughing. Equally ominous is the association's survey revealing that 66 percent of the U.S. population lives in counties and cities that violate the federal clean air standards for ozone, carbon monoxide, and lead, according to an article in the September/October 1993 issue of *Natural Health.*

Unfortunately, virtually everyone is familiar with smog, the grey or yellow haze produced when gases from automobiles, electricity generating plants, furnaces, or oil refineries mix with sunlight. According to the Natural Resources Defense Council, long exposure to smog may cause irreversible cell damage, reduced lung functioning, higher susceptibility to respiratory illness, and accelerated lung aging. Children are particularly vulnerable to the effects of air pollution because their bodies are still growing and much of their day is spent outdoors. The council claims, as reported by the Associated Press on October 28, 1993, that in southern California, 90 percent of children under the age of 14 live in areas that do not meet U.S. air-quality standards.

Almost every day, a person in a modern industrialized nation can be exposed to any of an estimated 100,000 new chemicals or by-products that have been invented in the past 50 years. Many have not been studied to determine if they are toxic or dangerous. Several, however, already have been proven to cause disease. For example, asbestos and cigarette smoke have been shown to cause cancer. Lead and pesticides such as DDT have been linked to birth defects and mental retardation. Other toxins have been linked to mood changes, allergies, visual and mental disturbances, rashes, flu-like symptoms, nervous system disorders, and respiratory diseases.

Soot, the tiny particles emitted from industrial plants and the exhaust of diesel vehicles, is another dangerous toxin. Several studies have concluded that as many as 60,000 deaths are caused by soot in the U.S. each year, a figure that rivals the death toll from some cancers. Deaths due to soot occur mostly among children with respiratory problems, people of all ages suffering from asthma, and elderly Americans who have bronchitis, emphysema, or pneumonia. While soot particles do not create heart or lung disease, nevertheless, long-term exposure to the particles worsens existing cases, and short-term

Natural Ways to Combat Heavy-Metal Poisoning

People can effectively combat heavy-metal poisoning by including certain foods and nutritional supplements in their diet. These include:

- A high potency multiple vitamin and mineral supplement.

- Minerals such as calcium, magnesium, zinc, iron, copper, and chromium.

- Vitamin C and B-complex vitamins.

- Sulfur-containing amino acids (methionine, cysteine, and taurine).

- High sulfur-content foods such as garlic, beans, onions, and eggs.

- Water-soluble fibers such as oat bran, pectin, and psyllium seeds.

exposure may reduce the odds of surviving medical crises brought on by the diseases, according to a report in the July 19, 1993, *New York Times.*

Most new heavy metals result from environmental contamination. Common sources include lead from the solder in tin cans, pesticide sprays, cadmium and lead from cigarette smoke, mercury from dental fillings, contaminated fish, cosmetics, and aluminum from antacids and cookware. In the *Encyclopedia of Natural Medicine,* Michael Murray and Joseph Pizzorno say that these heavy metals tend to accumulate within humans in the brain, kidneys, and immune system, where they can severely disrupt normal functioning.

Lead, for example, is now linked to high blood pressure, strokes, heart attacks, and kidney disease. Since the 1920s, millions of tons of lead have been added to gasoline to improve engine performance. Lead also has been used extensively in paints, although some countries now limit its use. Studies show that adults who suffer from acute lead poisoning may become alcoholics and suffer mental depression. According the U.S. Centers for Disease Control (CDC), "children are particularly susceptible to lead toxic effects." It is now estimated that from three to four million American children under six years of age have high enough levels of lead in their blood to suffer neurological damage or a reduced Intelligence Quotient (IQ). Studies have documented that women who work with lead in factories suffer higher rates of sterility, miscarriage, premature birth, and birth defects. Brain damage, comas, and convulsion can result in severe cases of lead poisoning, states Dr. R. Wedeen, in *Poison in the Pot: The Legacy of Lead.*

Food Toxins

The foods purchased at the local grocery store probably contain some toxins. For example, fruits and vegetables that are not grown organically often contain chemical residues from pesticides, insecticides, larvicides, and herbicides. These substances kill rodents, insects, molds, and weeds that interfere with crop production, but they also bury themselves in the soil and water and remain in food products which, once eaten, enter the human body. Human tolerance levels for insecticides and pesticides are extremely low. The U.S. National Academy of Sciences estimates that one million cases of cancer over the next decade will result from pesticide poisoning in food alone, not taking into account

Natural Protectors Against Lead

Dr. Steven Schecter, author of *Fighting Radiation and Chemical Pollutants with Foods, Herbs and Vitamins* and a leading authority on allergies, suggests that supplementing diets with the following vitamin and mineral supplements can help the body combat daily lead exposure.

- Optimal amounts of zinc, iron, and copper protect against the absorption of lead in the body.
- Optimal levels of calcium prevent the absorption of lead into the intestinal tract. Deficiencies of calcium can result in higher lead levels in the blood, bones, and soft tissues.
- Megadoses of vitamin B1 (thiamin), along with a high potency whole B-complex, may counteract lead poisoning.
- Vitamin C neutralizes the toxic effects of lead, increases its elimination, and specifically protects muscle tissue from lead damage.
- Several forms of fiber (particularly algin and pectin) are natural chelating agents—they attack the lead in the intestinal tract and eliminate it quickly from the body.

---

pesticide risk from water and atmospheric contamination, states Leon Chaitow in *The Body/Mind Purification Program,* published in 1990.

Meat and fish are increasingly doused with chemical insecticides and toxic artificial hormones. In fact, today's meat contains as much as thirty times more saturated fats and artificial hormones than it did forty years ago. Meats from animals raised on hormones can cause infertility, impotence, behavioral disorders, and cancer, according to Chaitow.

Many people assume that meat, fish, and dairy product toxins are not dangerous to human health. Recent studies indicate, however, that 95 to 99 percent of all food poisoning comes from meat, fish, dairy products, and eggs. Furthermore, most of the poisons found in meat and dairy products are carcinogenic at the lowest levels tested in laboratory animals. They have been shown to suppress the human immune system and cause birth defects, sterility, and neurological disorders, Chaitow states.

Immunotoxins

Some newer chemicals that are being released into the environment are immunotoxic—that is, poisonous to the human immune system. Young children, whose immune systems are still in development, and persons with chronic illnesses such as asthma are especially vulnerable. One problem with these new immunotoxins is that their long-term effects are unknown.

Scientists studying the immune system have identified more than two dozen immune-damaging chemicals, including sulfur dioxide and nitrogen dioxide emitted from power plants and automobiles. The most dangerous immunotoxic chemicals are industrial gases that many people breathe every day. Inhaled gases readily find their way into the bloodstream. Although the lungs are coated with cells that normally eliminate toxic particles, some pollutants, such as asbestos and silica, cannot be eliminated by the human body.

Microbial Toxins

Toxins also can be produced by the bacteria and yeast in the intestines. Examples include endotoxins, exotoxins, toxic amines, toxic derivatives of bile, and various carcinogenic substances. Intestinal toxins have been linked to a wide variety of diseases including liver disease, Crohn's disease, ulcerative colitis, thyroid disease, psoriasis, allergies, asthma, and many immune disorders, according to Murray and Pizzorno. One danger of these internal toxins is that they prevent the development of natural antibodies that normally fight infections. In effect, microbial toxins form antigens that cross-react with the body's own tissues, thereby causing autoimmunity— that is, the body's immune system cannot protect itself. Murray and Pizzorno state that autoimmune diseases that have been associated with cross-reacting antibodies include rheumatoid arthritis, diabetes, and autoimmune thyroiditis.

Office Toxins

A typical office building is likely to contain at least 50 (possibly as many as 500) volatile organic compounds and gases, emitted by everything from caulking to carpeting. The EPA ranks indoor pollution in offices as one of the five most urgent environmental issues in the U.S. Thirty to 75 million workers are estimated to be at risk of developing an illness due to office pollution, say Edlin and Golanty. Harmful gases usually are greatest in newly constructed or recently renovated buildings. Some gases, however, cannot be detected by odor, and many gases and chemicals combine to form even more dangerous toxins. For example, Edlin and Golanty cite the work of Danish researcher Lars Molhave, who found that more than 40 common office chemicals irritate the eyes, nose, and throat. Some forms of indoor air pollution are known to cause asthma and a severe lung inflammation called hypersensitivity pneumonitis. A

Natural Ways to Protect Against Toxic Chemicals in Food

People can strengthen their liver's ability to detoxify itself after exposure to toxic chemicals (including food additives, solvents, pesticides, and herbicides) by consuming the following:

- The amino acid methionine.
- Antioxidants such as vitamins A, C, and E, and beta-carotene.
- Choline.
- Botanicals such as dandelion root, milk thistle, artichoke leaves, and curcuma root.

small percentage of office workers develop "multiple chemical sensitivity," crippling their immune system. People who suffer from indoor toxicity may experience dizziness, headaches, nausea, burning eyes, and nosebleeds. In addition, they may find themselves unusually tired, suffer from coughing and sneezing, or have itchy skin and throats. Contact lens wearers may suffer eye irritation. Some building-borne pollutants can be fatal, as demonstrated in 1991 when an outbreak of Legionnaire's disease at the Social Security Administration building in Richmond, California, killed two workers.

Radioactive Gases

Exposure to high concentrations of radioactive gases also can cause cancer. The most dangerous radioactive gas in the U.S. is radon, a naturally occurring gas contained in certain rocks (especially granite) and building materials such as concrete, bricks, and tiles.

Radon is believed to be the second leading cause of lung cancer, resulting in 7,000 to 30,000 deaths annually, according to the Environmental Protection Agency (EPA). Because several cities in the U.S. recently had radon scares, the EPA now advises people to contact their local authorities or ecological groups to determine if they live in a radon area. Since approximately 6 percent of American dwellings have elevated radon levels, people who live in a radon area may wish to buy a radon detector to assess the toxicity in their home.

Sunlight

Sunlight also contains harmful radiation, and too much exposure to the sun's rays over time can cause squamous-cell carcinoma, a skin cancer developed by more than 100,000 people in the U.S. each year. While only about 2 percent of patients die from the disease, which is the second most common skin cancer after basal-cell carcinoma, it can prove lethal if allowed to spread. The cancer is often preceded by actinic keratoses—a condition in which red, rough, and scaly spots appear on the face, the top of the hands, or other locations frequently exposed to the sun.

Once the skin is burned by high levels of the sun's radiation, the body becomes more susceptible to immunotoxic chemicals. Relatively small doses of ultraviolet light—for example, the amount received from a mild sunburn—can suppress the immune response against bacteria and yeast infections. Sunscreen lotions containing the B vitamin PABA and the antioxidant vitamins A, C, and E provide the best protection.

Toxins in the Home

The home may also be full of toxins—even from seemingly innocuous sources. Ordinary building materials used for house walls, floors, insulation, roofing treatments, paints, and plastic tiles often are toxic. New carpeting has been linked to a variety of respiratory and nervous ailments. According to the federal Consumer Products Safety Commission, these ailments have flu-like symptoms such as weakness, aching joints, congestion, nosebleeds, and even dementia, the Associated Press reported on November 3, 1993. Many people now have their homes

Indoor Toxins

- Some textiles are potential sources of pollutants.

- Padded partitions, curtains, and carpets may be toxic.

- Office machinery contributes to indoor pollution. Some photocopying machines give off ozone—detectable by its metallic odor—that may cause nosebleeds, irritate the eyes and throat, and make life difficult for contact lens wearers.

- Machines that duplicate an executive's signature emit butyl methacrylate, which can trigger allergic reactions.

- Blueprint copiers give off ammonia and acetic acid vapors, causing the eyes, nose, and throat to burn.

- Shredders release irritating particles of paper into the air. Proper ventilation minimizes such hazards.

- Ventilation systems harbor molds, fungi, and bacteria, which collect moisture that condenses when air is cooled. If the systems are not kept clean, the biological agents proliferate, traveling through the building in the air currents.

- Water leaks may cause mold or fungus to build up in carpets and ceiling tiles.

professionally examined for toxins and replace hazardous materials with nontoxic substitutes where possible.

Water Toxins

More than 100 potentially toxic chemicals have been introduced in drinking water supplies in the U.S. Some are compounds that seep into underground water supplies adjacent to industrial complexes or toxic waste dumps. Several are carcinogenic (cancer-causing), including benzene, carbon tetrachloride, dioxin, ethylene dibromide (EDB), polychlorinated biphenyls (PCBs), and vinyl chloride. Studies show that children are especially vulnerable to these toxins.

Tap water in some areas of the U.S. also may carry toxins. Ordinary drinking water stored in wells may be contaminated by wastes, pesticides, or other toxins. Well water can carry heavy metals from copper or lead pipes, which can result in mental retardation in children and nervous system illnesses. Some American cities control bacteria in drinking water by using small amounts of chlorine, which may be toxic if it exceeds recommended levels. A recent National Cancer Institute survey showed that in ten areas of the U.S., regular consumption of chlorinated tap water was responsible for between 12 and 27 percent of bladder cancers, according to Edlin and Golanty. People who are worried about water contamination should drink only pure spring or filtered water, or buy a water purifier.

Measuring Toxicity Levels

With so many toxins in the air, water, home, and office, how can people prevent infections and diseases caused by these substances? The answer is regular elimination of toxins from the body. The first step is to be alert to the symptoms of toxicity and, if nec-

Common Sources of Toxins in the Home

Kitchens

- Paper towels fortified with formaldehyde can cause skin rashes, nausea, and menstrual irregularities.
- Avoid using bleached paper containing dioxin.
- Air fresheners (carbolic acid or formaldehyde) can cause nausea and eye and lung irritation.
- Oven cleaner formulas contain lye, phenols, formaldehyde, benzene, or ammonia, which can cause blisters and rashes.
- Some deep frying oils are carcinogenic. Ventilators should be used when cooking with these oils.

Bathrooms

- Antiperspirants contain aluminum chlorohydrate which blocks skin pores.
- Commercial toothpastes contain ammonia, ethanol, formaldehyde, mineral oil, or saccharin.
- Furniture and tile polish contain sodium phosphate or turpentine, which can burn the skin and is dangerous when inhaled.
- Toilet cleaners contain cresol which is easily absorbed through the skin and can damage major organs.

Clothing

- Spot removers often contain benzene, sulfuric acid or toluene, which can cause skin rashes and nervous system complications.
- Leather dyes in shoes contain nitro-benzene, which can turn skin blue, affect breathing, and induce vomiting.

Recommendations

- Use all natural non-toxic products: i.e., corn flour or arrowroot instead of talc, bicarbonate of soda instead of antiperspirant, peppermint oil instead of deodorant, or natural herb toothpastes instead of commercial brands.
- Avoid using plastic products and containers when possible.
- Use deodorants made of essential oils instead of strong chemical deodorants.
- Avoid drain cleaners that contain lye or sulfuric acid.
- Avoid using paper towels that contain formaldehyde, air fresheners that contain carbolic acid, and oven cleaners that contain lye.
- Use natural, nontoxic, antidandruff shampoos.

essary, to measure toxicity levels. Special laboratory techniques are useful in detecting toxins in the body. A detailed medical examination by an experienced physician may be necessary, or a laboratory analysis that involves measuring blood and fatty tissue for suspected chemicals. It is extremely important to test the liver, because it is responsible for eliminating most toxins from the body. The serum bile acid assay test measures liver toxicity, along with other tests for liver function, including serum bilirubin and liver enzymes.

Natural Ways to Strengthen the Immune System

Toxins are in the air, soil, water, and many foods, and it is virtually impossible for people to seal themselves off from these substances. Once toxins enter the body, they must be eliminated. The rest of this chapter describes how the immune system eliminates toxins and how it can be strengthened through detoxification programs. The most important components of the immune system are discussed, as are vitamin, mineral, and herbal supplements that have proven effective in detoxifying them.

The skin, the body's largest organ, is the first line of defense against external toxins. It can prevent the entry of most microorganisms, while the mildly acid surface of the skin neutralizes harmful bacteria. A number of toxins are eliminated through the skin, principally through sweat. The skin needs to be strong, supple, and moist. Natural supplements that detoxify the skin include PABA (ointment) and beta-carotenes. The herb dandelion root is used in Europe as a skin detoxicant and to treat various skin problems.

The mucous membranes of the eyes, nose, throat, and lungs also protect against toxic substances by secreting enzymes that degrade toxins and eliminate them naturally from the body. Tears wash away toxins from the eye, and ear wax protects the ear canal.

As Murray and Pizzorno explain, "the spleen is the largest mass of lymphatic tissue in the body. In addition to producing lymphocytes which engulf and destroy bacteria and cellular debris, the spleen is responsible for destroying worn-out blood cells and platelets. The spleen also serves as a blood reservoir." During emergencies such as hemorrhage, the spleen releases stored blood to prevent shock. Goldenseal, an herb, improves spleen function by enhancing the blood flow through this important organ.

The liver performs more than fifteen hundred different functions, many of which directly maintain the body's immune system. Except for some fats, the liver processes all foods absorbed by the intestines before they are released into the bloodstream. It filters the blood by removing, deactivating, or reprocessing wastes, toxins, and bacteria. The liver also helps eliminate the by-products of alcohol and pesticides. Perhaps most importantly, it helps produce interferon, the special chemical agent that activates white blood cells to destroy and eliminate disease-causing microbes and toxins. Several nutrients are known to enhance the liver's production, including zinc, manganese, and vitamin C. Lipotropic formulas or silymarin from silyhum marianum and vitamin C help detoxify the liver, as do echinacea and goldenseal.

The kidneys remove toxins from the blood for elimination in the urine and also reabsorb valuable nutrients that are recycled for further use in the body. The kidneys gradually decline in efficiency with age and excessive toxicity due to diet, drugs, or pollutants that place stress on them. Cranberry juice has been used to treat bladder infections by toning the kidneys. Several compounds isolated from rubia, cassia, and aloe vera also help maintain healthy kidneys. Murray and Pizzorno, in the *Encyclopedia of Natural Medicine,* recommend the following nutritional supplements to detoxify the kidneys: vitamin B6 and K supplements, glutamate, magnesium citrate, and potassium citrate.

A healthy, intact intestinal lining allows properly broken down particles of fats, proteins, and starches to be assimilated into the blood. When the intestinal lining becomes disturbed, it loses its effectiveness as a filter, and allergies and food sensitivities can develop, along with chronic infections and inflammation. Shortages of beneficial bacteria can

Fighting Can Make You Sick

Harsh words and name-calling between men and women not only result in hurt feelings, but also weaken the immune system. A study conducted by Janice Kiecolt-Glaser, an Ohio psychologist, and her immunologist husband, Ronald Glaser, found that the immune systems of married couples who became hostile toward one another were weakened more dramatically than those of couples whose disagreements were milder. Although exploding with anger can significantly weaken the immune system, not dealing with important conflicts can damage a marriage as well, the researchers claimed.

damage the intestinal lining. Caprylic acid, a naturally occurring fatty acid, has been reported to be an effective intestinal compound. Lactobacillus acidophilus, the type of bacteria found in natural yogurt, also strengthens the intestine's natural microflora and retards the growth of candida, a bacteria linked to AIDS. Garlic has proven effective in preventing fungi from growing in the intestine. The common barberry plant has been used to prevent a wide range of harmful bacteria in the intestines, including candida albicans.

The colon probably contains most of the dangerous toxins in the body, many of which lead to the production of free radicals that may be responsible for systemic degenerative autoimmune conditions such as cancer, arthritis, arteriosclerosis, and possibly AIDS. Many of these diseases can be prevented by continually eliminating toxins that collect in the colon. Herbs that help eliminate toxins from the colon include alfalfa, bentonite, goldenseal, and echinacea. Buckthorn has long been used as a laxative to increase peristalsis,

the muscular activity of the colon. Cassia senna leaves are commonly used for their laxative properties, as is psyllium seed powder mixed with a full glass of water.

When toxic bacteria, viruses, pollen, microorganisms, or certain chemicals enter the body, the organs discussed here attempt to neutralize them. This process produces specific protein molecules called antibodies and special blood cells called lymphocytes. In a strong immune system, antibodies and lymphocytes inactivate the toxins, which are removed by macrophages and phagocytic cells in the blood. Macrophages and phagocytic cells are transported throughout the body by lymphatic vessels that run parallel to arteries and veins and drain waste products from tissues. Important nutrients that detoxify the lymph are vitamins A, B6, and C, and the trace mineral zinc. Herbs which enhance lymphatic function include goldenseal, echinacea, Korean ginseng, Siberian ginseng, and licorice, according to Murray and Pizzorno.

Basic Detoxification Programs

The body's immune system can naturally eliminate most external toxins. However, if people are exposed to high levels of certain toxins, or lower levels of other toxins over a protracted period of time, their immune system may be weakened. Given that more than 100,000 new, potentially toxic chemicals have been released into the environment during the past 50 years, regular detoxification of the body should be considered.

The most important components of any detoxification program are the organs they specifically detoxify; the diet, vitamins, minerals, herb supplements, and botanical medicinal formulas they prescribe; and the exercise regimen (aerobics, meditation, yoga, visualizations) they incorporate. Comprehensive one-day detoxification programs are designed to detoxify each organ system through careful diet or fasting; vitamin, mineral, and botanical supplements; and stretching, relaxation, visualization, and biofeedback. People should contact a holistic physician for recommendations about a specific diet for their program, whether to fast, and which vitamins, minerals, and botanical supplements will most efficiently and gently detoxify their bodies.

Before starting a detoxification program, be aware of the possible side effects. These are not dangerous but may cause slight discomfort. Before taking any vitamins, herbs, or supplements, it is important to consult with a physician.

Summary

Many people today have less than optimal health because their bodies contain potentially dangerous toxins. While a normal immune system can eliminate most toxins, if the body has an excess of these substances the immune system may become depressed and unable to function effectively. The best protection against the adverse effects of toxins is to regularly eliminate toxic debris through gentle detoxification programs that rejuvenate the immune system. Given the right proportions of nutrients; vitamin, mineral, and botanical supplements; exercise; and meditation and relaxation, the body has the miraculous ability to maintain the health of all its systems. This ability of the body to detoxify, to eliminate toxins, largely determines an individual's life energy ("chi" or elan vital) and health.

Resources

References

"Carpet Industry Will Adopt Cautionary Label." Associated Press (November 3, 1993).

Possible Side Effects of Detoxification Programs

- Headaches may occur during the first forty-eight hours. To alleviate a headache, use the acupressure points or self-massage.
- Nausea, especially if fasting. Nausea can be relieved by drinking a light herbal tea such as chamomile.
- Loss of body heat.
- Inability to focus.
- Constipation due to fluid loss.
- Diarrhea.
- Weight loss due to reduced food intake.
- Rashes and blemishes.
- Loss of amino acids.

Chaitow, Leon, M.D. *The Body/Mind Purification Program.* New York, NY: Simon & Schuster, Inc., 1990.

Edlin, Gordon, and Eric Golanty. *Health and Wellness: A Holistic Approach.* Boston, MA: Jones and Bartlett Publishers, Inc., 1992.

Hilts, P. "Studies Say Soot Kills Up to 60,000 in U.S. Each Year." *New York Times* (July 19, 1993).

"Indoor Air Pollution." *Mayo Clinic Health Letter* (November 1993): 4.

Murray, Michael, and Joseph Pizzorno. *Encyclopedia of Natural Medicine.* Rocklin, CA: Prima Publishing, 1991.

"Report Tells How Smog Affects Kids." Associated Press (October 28, 1993).

"Two-thirds of the U.S. Population Breathes Polluted Air." *Natural Health* (September/October 1993).

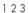

Wedeen, R., M.D. *Poison in the Pot: The Legacy of Lead.* Carbondale, IL: Southern Illinois University Press, 1984.

Organizations

Consumer Product Safety Commission. 5401 Westbard Ave., Bethesda, MD 20207.

Environmental Protection Agency (EPA). 401 M St. SW, Washington, DC 20460.

Food and Drug Administration (FDA). 5600 Fishers Ln., Rockville, MD 20857.

National Institute for Occupational Safety and Health (NIOSH). 1600 Clifton Rd. NE, Atlanta, GA 30333.

Occupational Safety and Health Administration (OSHA). 200 Constitution Ave., Washington, DC 20210.

Additional Reading

Agency for Toxic Substance and Disease Registry. *The Nature and Extent of Lead Poisoning in Children in the United States: A Report to Congress.* Agency for Toxic Substance and Disease Registry, 1988.

Brown, Lester, et al. *State of the World.* New York, NY: W.W. Norton & Co., Inc., 1988.

Bunyard, Peter. *Health Guide for the Nuclear Age.* London, England: Macmillan, 1988.

————. *The Radiation Protection Plan.* London, England: Thorstens, 1989.

Cook, Judith. *Dirty Water.* London, England: Unwin Hyman, 1989.

Dudley, Nigel. *The Poisoned Earth.* London, England: Piatkus Publishers, 1987.

Greeley, Alexandra. "Getting the Lead Out of Just about Everything." *FDA Consumer Reports* (July/August 1991): 26–31.

Haddy, R.I. "Aging, Infections, and the Immune System." *The Journal of Family Practice* (October 1988): 409–13.

Jaroff, Leon. "Controlling a Childhood Menace: Lead Poisoning Poses the Biggest Environmental Threat to the Young." *Time* (February 25, 1991): 68–69.

Marwick, C. "As Immune System Yields Its Secrets, New Strategies Against Disease Emerge." *JAMA* (November 24, 1989): 2786–87.

Nossal, G.J.V. "The Basic Components of the Immune System." *New England Journal of Medicine* (May 21, 1987): 1320–25.

Office of Air and Radiation. *The Inside Story: A Guide to Indoor Air Quality.* Washington DC: Office of Air and Radiation, Environmental Protection Agency, September 1988.

Pearson, David. *The Natural House Book.* New York, NY: Simon & Schuster, Inc., 1989.

Schecter, Steven. *Fighting Radiation and Chemical Pollutants with Foods, Herbs and Vitamins.* Berkeley, CA: Vitality, Inc., 1990.

Stanway, Andrew, M.D. *The Natural Family Doctor.* New York, NY: Simon & Schuster, Inc., 1987.

Chapter 8

COPING WITH STRESS

In one study, as reported by Gurney Williams III in the October 1990 issue of *Longevity,* the London School of Hygiene and Tropical Medicine invited 192 men and woman between the ages of 35 and 64 to experiment with managing their stress levels. Each of the participants had at least two of the following risk factors: high blood pressure, high cholesterol, and a smoking habit of 10 or more cigarettes a day. The volunteers were divided into two groups: some took eight one-hour lessons in relaxation, meditation, stress management, and breathing exercises, while the rest received no instruction.

After eight weeks, the doctors discovered that blood pressures were significantly lower for participants in the group taught to relax and breathe correctly, compared with those in the other group. Four years later, they still showed lower blood pressure readings. Compared with those who had no instruction, they were less likely to be in treatment for hypertension and less apt to show symptoms of heart disease, or to have died of a heart attack.

Virtually everyone has experienced "stress" to some degree. The December 1993 issue of *New Body* magazine, for example, states that a 1993 U.S. Public Health survey estimates that 70 to 80 percent of Americans who visit a physician suffer from a stress-related disorder. Job-related stress costs U.S. businesses $60 million a year, and stress-related disability cases have doubled since 1981.

This chapter discusses how the body responds to stress and describes alternative therapies for reducing stress and its effects, including nutritional, vitamin, and mineral therapies; exercise; guided imagery; yoga; meditation; biofeedback; massage; and group support.

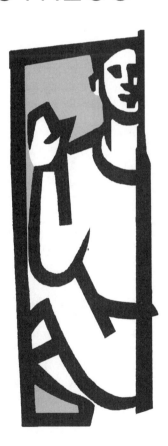

What Is Stress?

In 1925, Hans Selye, a European physician trained at the German University in Prague, noticed that most of his patients displayed the same symptoms, including fatigue, aching bones and joints, fever, and loss of appetite and weight. He subsequently developed the concept of "stress"—and the body's adaptive reactions to any demand, or "the rate of wear-and-tear caused by life." In his book *Stress Without Distress*, Selye explains how a number of agents can cause stress, including intoxication, trauma, nervous strain, heat, cold, muscular fatigue, polluted air, and radiation.

According to Selye, the body reacts to stress in the same way it reacts to danger by going through a series of biochemical changes that he called the General Adaptation Syndrome (GAS). In the first stage, which he termed "the alarm reaction," the body mobilizes its defenses against the stressor agent. Nerve impulses from the brain stimulate the adrenal medulla to secrete adrenalin and other stress-related hormones such as cortisol. This is known as the "fight or flight" response: the heartbeat is accelerated, blood pressure levels are elevated, an increased amount blood flows to the muscles, and the lungs dilate to increase respiratory effort.

Selye called the second stage of the General Adaptation Syndrome the "resistance" phase—the phase during which the body continues to fight the stressor long after the effects of the "fight or flight" response have worn off. If the stress is induced by infective agents, the body's immune system activity increases. If the stress is physical, the neuroendocrine system converts protein to energy. If the stress is psychological, a combination of responses may occur, such as anxiety and shortness of breath.

Prolongation of the resistance reaction or continued stress can lead to "exhaustion," the

The Fight or Flight Response

- The rate of breathing increases to supply necessary oxygen to the heart.
- The heart rate and force of contraction of the heart increase to provide more blood to the muscles and brain.
- The liver dumps more stored glucose into the bloodstream to energize the body to begin physical activity.
- Sweat production increases to eliminate toxic compounds produced by the body and to lower body temperature.

third stage of the General Adaptation Syndrome. During this stage, glucocorticoid reserves become depleted and some body cells do not receive a sufficient amount of glucose or other nutrients.

Exhaustion may manifest itself in a total collapse of body functions or a collapse of specific organs. Prolonged stress can overwork many organ systems, especially the heart, blood vessels, adrenals, and immune system. When stress is overwhelming, the response is general depression, low blood pressure and heart rate, increased cortisol (natural steroid hormone), and low sex steroid hormone secretions. Failure to cope with stress can lead to disorders such as headaches, hypertension, heart disease, stroke, and ulcers.

Measuring Stress Levels

Many people may not be aware they are undergoing stress. To help people assess their own stress levels, Dr. Thomas Holmes and Dr. Richard Rahe developed a list of potential stressors that have been linked to medical dis-

The Social Readjustment Rating Scale

Read the list of life events below and enter the score for each event that has occurred in the past year. If any event occurred more than once, multiply the point value by the number of times the event occurred. Then total the score.

Life Event	Point Value	Score
1. Death of spouse	100	___
2. Divorce	78	___
3. Marital separation	65	___
4. Detention in jail or other institution	63	___
5. Death of a close family member (other than spouse)	63	___
6. Major personal injury or illness	53	___
7. Marriage	50	___
8. Dismissal from job	47	___
9. Marital reconciliation	45	___
10. Retirement	45	___
11. Major change in health or behavior of family member	44	___
12. Pregnancy	40	___
13. Sexual difficulties	39	___
14. Gain of a new family member (through birth, adoption, parent moving in)	39	___
15. Major business readjustment (merger, reorganization, bankruptcy)	39	___
16. Major change in financial status	38	___
17. Death of a close friend	37	___
18. Change to a different line of work	36	___
19. Major change in number of arguments with spouse	35	___
20. Taking out a mortgage or loan for a major purchase (home, business)	31	___
21. Foreclosure of mortgage or loan	30	___

→

The Social Readjustment Rating Scale (continued)

Life Event	Point Value	Score
22. Major change in responsibilities at work	29	——
23. Son or daughter leaving home (college, marriage)	29	——
24. Trouble with in-laws	29	——
25. Outstanding personal achievement	28	——
26. Spouse begins or ceases work outside the home	26	——
27. Beginning or ceasing formal schooling	26	——
28. Major change in living conditions (new home, remodeling, moving)	25	——
29. Revision of personal habits (dress, manners)	24	——
30. Trouble with boss	23	——
31. Major change in working hours/conditions	20	——
32. Change in residence	20	——
33. Change in schools	20	——
34. Major change in usual type/amount of recreation	19	——
35. Major change in church activities	19	——
36. Major change in social activities	18	——
37. Taking out a loan for a lesser purchase (car, TV)	17	——
38. Major change in sleeping habits	16	——
39. Major change in family get-togethers	15	——
40. Major change in eating habits	15	——
41. Vacation	13	——
42. Christmas/holiday season	12	——
43. Minor legal violations (traffic or jaywalking ticket)	11	——
TOTAL		——

→

The Social Readjustment Rating Scale (continued)

What the Score Means

The higher the score (i.e., the more changes occurring in the past year), the more likely a person is to develop a stress-related illness.

Below 150 Points: Statistically, there is a 30 percent chance a significant health problem will develop in the near future.

Between 150 and 300 Points: There is a 50 percent chance that a significant health problem will occur in the near future.

More than 300 Points: There is an 80 percent chance that a significant health problem will develop in the near future.

orders. The Social Readjustment Rating Scale (see above) ranks stressful life events. The highest value, 100 points, is attached to the most grievous loss, the death of one's spouse. The scale demonstrates that stress is cumulative. A few significant events, or a number of smaller events, may overload the adaptive system of the body.

Methods for Coping with Stress

Successfully coping with stress involves using therapies that are designed to counteract the effects of the "fight or flight" response by inducing its opposite reaction—the "relaxation response." The term was coined by Dr. Herbert Benson of Harvard Medical School, who found that people undergoing stress could control their reaction to it by relaxing. In his book, *The Relaxation Response,* Benson suggests that a variety of techniques can induce the relaxation response, including yoga, meditation, progressive relaxation, autogenic training, self-hypnosis, and biofeedback.

Acupuncture and Acupressure. Acupuncture and acupressure also are effective in relieving stress. Acupuncture, as noted in Chapter 1, is based on the theory that the body contains chi. Acupuncture treatments rebalance the chi force, and the physical symptoms associated with stress are alleviated and usually disappear.

Practitioners of acupressure (also known as shiatsu) use their thumbs, fingers, and elbows to stimulate the body's 361 tsubos, or acupuncture points. The technique involves repetitively pressing the tsubos for three to five seconds, and then releasing pressure. Acupressure is most useful for rebalancing energy blockages associated with stress, rather than for curing specific diseases.

Massage is another useful stress-relieving therapy. A Chinese form of massage called tui na uses a combination of gentle hand pats and stretches to redistribute the chi flow throughout the body. Tui na is based on the same model of the body as acupuncture and acupressure, although it is less forceful and focuses on broader areas rather than specific points.

Botanical Medicines. Many people experiencing mild stress symptoms treat themselves with sedatives and sleeping pills. These can result in chemical addictions, however, and

The Relaxation Response

- Heart rate and blood pressure are reduced.
- The rate of breathing decreases, because oxygen demand is reduced when a person becomes relaxed.
- The stomach produces more hydrochloric acid, which aids digestion.
- The liver secretes less glucose, and blood sugar levels are reduced.

alternative physicians emphasize that natural medicinal herbs also can be effective in reducing stress.

Michael Murray and Joseph Pizzorno in the *Encyclopedia of Natural Medicine* claim that a number of botanical medicines have proven effective in calming nerves, reducing tension, and relieving stress-related symptoms. These herbs typically are used in conjunction with recommended changes in nutrition and lifestyle. Although herbs can be effective in treating stress and anxiety, Dr. Roger Kennedy, internist and bioethicist at Kaiser Permanente Medical Center in Santa Clara, California, strongly suggests that people consult a physician or herbalist and only take those botanical or herbal stress relievers that are recommended by them.

Ginseng (especially Korean or Chinese ginseng) has been shown to enhance adrenal gland function and to improve reactions against a variety of stresses. Ginseng is regarded as an "adaptogen," or an herb that protects against both mental and physical fatigue and helps the body maintain its natural equilibrium. Murray and Pizzorno cite 10 studies that document how ginseng improves adrenal functions and helps the body withstand extremely stressful conditions. They also state that hops assists digestion and is especially effective in treating digestive complaints related to stress. Chamomile, a sedative that aids digestion, also is a botanical stress reducer. Lemon balm is used in many parts of the world to relax the nervous system, reduce heart palpitations, and relieve headaches.

Exercise. Exercise is one of best techniques for reducing stress because physical activity allows the body to "throw off" tension. Anyone who runs, walks, or swims regularly knows how the body feels after exercising—tired, even drained, but relaxed. A growing body of evidence suggests that regular exercise boosts the body's ability to withstand stress. Exercise also can help to protect the cardiovascular and immune systems from the consequences of stressful events.

Physical exercise appears to be effective in reducing stress for a variety of reasons. For example, many types of physical exercise take people outdoors and expose them to fresh air and sunshine, which are vital to the functioning of the immune system. Most exercise is also social and provides a natural and enjoyable way of being with other people, while helping to put aside stressful problems for a time. From a physiological point of view, exercise relieves muscle tension and helps dissipate the hormones that can build up in response to stress. The primary psychological benefit of exercise is that it helps people maintain control of their health. One aspect of stress is the sense of feeling out of control, or of not being able to respond to a stressor. When people are afraid and lose their sense of control, their heart races and their blood pressure increases. But exercise, along with relaxation, helps to reverse this process.

Mindful Exercise (Exercise Plus Meditation). A University of Massachusetts Medical School study recently showed that mindful exercise (exercise combined with meditation) elicits immediate, positive psychological states such as enthusiasm, alertness, and greater self-esteem. The research, reported by Suzanne Hildreth in the January/February 1994 issue of *Natural Health,* was done in collaboration with the Center for Balance and Fitness and Dr. Benson's Mind/Body Medical Institute at the New England Deaconess Hospital in Boston. During the course of the study, one group followed a low-intensity walking program; the second group did the walking while listening to a relaxation tape developed by Benson. The third group practiced a combination of visualization and tai chi movements, while the fourth walked at a higher intensity than the others. Those who walked while listening to the tape, participated in the tai chi and visualization class, or exercised more briskly reported less irritability, guilt, fear, and hostility, along with increased feelings of excitement and strength, than did the low-intensity walking group, according to Hildreth.

Nutritional Therapies. According to Dr. Serafina Corsello, executive medical director of the Corsello Centers for Nutritional Medicine in New York, the link between stress and diet is indisputable. She states in the March 1994 issue of *Delicious:* "Stress depletes the body's energy reserves while food supplies the body with fuel it needs to produce energy. How much energy you have also depends on the quality of the food you ingest and the distribution of food in the digestive system that works properly. If you're under stress, you can't properly digest food. Therefore, you are not getting all the nutritional benefits of the food you eat."

Corsello recommends a diet high in complex carbohydrates (which provide a steady supply of slow-burning fuel as well as protective antioxidants) and low in animal fat. "The best diet includes raw or steamed fresh veg-

Stress Reduction Exercise Hints

- Start slowly, progress gradually, and do not overexercise.

- Work out with friends or as part of an exercise class. Social support makes exercise more fun and decreases the tendency to stop exercising.

- If possible, start with an activity involving repetitive motion, such as running or brisk walking. Running and brisk walking prompt a meditative effect from the sound of feet hitting the pavement or ground.

- Exercise regularly.

- Don't rush back to a normal routine. Take at least a few minutes after exercising to enjoy feeling relaxed.

etables, whole-grain foods such as brown rice, oatmeal and whole wheat pasta, and a small amount of oily fish such as salmon, which contains essential fatty acids," she counsels. Corsello also suggests avoiding coffee and other caffeine-containing substances that "in the long run contribute to adrenal fatigue."

Comprehensive vitamin, mineral, and nutritional therapies that curb the effects of stress are discussed in Chapters 2, 3, and 4.

Progressive Relaxation. Progressive relaxation, according to Benson, is an effective therapy for inducing the relaxation response. People are taught to contract to and relax their face and neck muscles. These muscles are tensed for one to two seconds and then relaxed. This simple procedure helps patients experience the difference in blood flow **to** a muscle when it is stressed—and **away** from the muscle when it is relaxed. The procedure is repeated progressively from the face and neck to the upper chest and arms, the abdomen, hips, buttocks, thighs, knees, calves, and feet. The process is repeated two or three times, producing a deep state of relaxation.

Qi Gong. Qi gong, a Chinese meditative exercise, also effectively relieves stress. There are several variations of the exercise. In one form, practitioners sit in a relaxed pose and use their mental concentration to channel chi to specific parts of the body. Chi is a vital energy force that circulates freely in a healthy body. Chi is altered when a body is undergoing stress, and an unbalanced chi force can cause disease. In the movement form of qi gong, practitioners combine graceful, rhythmic movements while meditating on the movement of chi throughout their bodies. According to an article by R. Jahnke in the January–February 1991 issue of the *Townsend Letter for Doctors,* qi gong initiates the "relaxation response," which reduces stress, decreases the heart rate, lowers blood pressure, and increases tissue regeneration.

Social Support and Stress Reduction. Psychosocial processes often mediate the relationship between stressful events and how the body reacts to stressors. A 1993 Swedish study reported by Daniel Goleman in the December 7, 1993 issue of the *New York Times* suggests that stress is easier for individuals to cope with if they have the support of close friends or family. In the study, a random sample of 50-year-old men living in Göteborg were given a physical examination and psychological evaluation in 1986. Seven years later, researchers analyzed official records and found that the death rate from stressful events for those men who were socially isolated and who had identified themselves as lacking

emotional support was three times higher than that of men who were not socially isolated.

Research on the effects of social isolation, stressful events, and death rates began in the 1970s when Dr. Lisa Berkman, an epidemiologist at the Yale University School of Medicine, and Leonard Syme, an epidemiologist at the University of California at Berkeley, first conducted a study of more than 7,000 men and women in Alameda County, California. They reported in a 1979 issue of the *American Journal of Epidemiology* that between 1970 and 1979, people with the fewest social ties were twice as likely to die as those with the strongest ties. Scientists still are uncertain as to precisely how social support decreases a person's likelihood of dying from a stress-related experience. In Goleman's article in the *New York Times,* Berkman is quoted as saying that in the Swedish study "there's ample evidence now that having a rich social network protects health somehow." She suggests that people with social ties may have healthier habits in general—or that such ties may help strengthen a person's neuroendocrine and immune systems.

Dean Ornish, M.D., in his book *Dr. Dean Ornish's Program for Reversing Heart Disease,* states that scientists at the Ohio State University College of Medicine have found "that patients who scored above the average in loneliness had significantly poorer immune functioning." Ornish also notes that research conducted by Dr. James Goodwin and colleagues at the Medical College of Wisconsin suggests that social support may strengthen the immune system. Studying 256 healthy elderly adults, Goodwin found that individuals with strong support systems tended to have higher indices of immune function and lower blood cholesterol levels.

Spiral Relaxation. Spiral relaxation is a variation of progressive relaxation. To begin the procedure, a person lies comfortably on a bed with the palms of the hands facing up. With the eyes closed, the person imagines a point of light or heat that begins a series of three clockwise spirals around the top of the head and moves down around the face, neck, upper chest, each arm, the abdomen, waist, hips, thighs, knees, calves, and feet. Each part of the body relaxes as the series of three spirals encircles it.

Another variation can be done alone or with a partner. Lying comfortably on a bed on their back, participants imagine their body being filled from the top of the head to the tip of the toes with healing energy. The energy enters through an opening at the top of the head and moves through the frontal lobes to the lower brain stem. Relaxees feel the back of the brain sink into the bed. The cranium, skull, ears, eyes, mouth, cheeks, throat, nose, and ears progressively relax. This is repeated, moving down the body. The arms, chest, abdomen, hips, buttocks, thighs, knees, calves, and feet fill with heavy healing energy that "melts" into the bed.

Visualization. Another way of inducing the relaxation response is to use a visualization exercise or guided imagery. In these therapies, summarized by Gerald Epstein in *Healing Visualizations,* people imagine themselves in an environment they associate with relaxing—a peaceful beach, for example, or a lake or favorite mountain. Closing their eyes and taking a few deep, easy breaths, they remember the details of the setting—the sights, smells, and sounds—and focus on feeling peaceful and relaxed.

Vitamin and Mineral Therapies. The adrenal glands play a critical role in how most people respond to stress. Murray and Pizzorno in the *Encyclopedia of Natural Medicine* suggest that vitamin C, vitamin B6, zinc, magnesium, potassium, and pantothenic acid are nutrients needed for the normal functioning of

the adrenal glands. Supplementation of all these nutrients may be appropriate during periods of extreme stress for people who need adrenal support. However, appropriate supplementation should be discussed with a physician or a nutritionist.

Yoga and Meditation. Goleman, in his book *The Meditative Mind,* states that more than a thousand studies since the 1970s have proven that yoga and meditation effectively reduce stress and anxiety, lower blood pressure, relieve addictions, and improve metabolic and respiratory functioning. He notes that because meditation has proven highly effective in reducing stress and tension, the National Institutes of Health has recommended that it replace prescription drugs as the first treatment for mild hypertension.

Yoga schools can be found in many parts of the United States. Although there are many variations, all forms of yoga involve gentle movements and regular breathing exercises. Some yoga practices also include visualization, progressive relaxation exercises, and meditation.

There are several different forms of meditation, but all share the goal of quieting the mind. In some traditions, such as Buddhism, meditators sit comfortably in silence and think no thoughts. In transcendental meditation, practitioners silence their minds by internally reciting a mantra—or holy sound. In qi gong, tai chi, and other Chinese disciplines, practitioners perform gentle dancelike movements while meditating on the flow of chi energy through their bodies. In *The Relaxation Response,* Benson details a number of studies showing that meditation helps slow the breathing rate. It also increases oxygen consumption and blood flow to the brain, producing a more relaxed brain wave rhythm.

Dr. Jon Kabat-Zinn, founder of the Stress Reduction Clinic at the University of Massachusetts, has used meditation to help

Summary of Stress Relieving Therapies

- Biofeedback: Use biofeedback to voluntarily relax specific muscles, reduce blood pressure and heart rate, and improve digestion.

- Botanical Medicines: Ask a physician, nutritionist, or herbalist about adding ginseng, hops, chamomile, or lemon balm as supplements

- Exercise: Start a moderate exercise program, such as brisk walking or running, that combines aerobic exercise, repetitive motion, and social interaction.

- Nutritional Therapies: Eat a diet high in complex carbohydrates, raw or steamed fresh vegetables, whole-grain foods, and fish such as salmon, which contains essential fatty acids.

- Relaxation Exercises: Practice progressive relaxation, spiral relaxation, or guided imagery and visualization exercises.

- Vitamin and Mineral Therapies: Ask a physician or nutritionist about adding vitamin C, vitamin B6, zinc, magnesium, potassium, and pantothenic acid supplements to a nutritional program.

- Yoga and Meditation: Practice yoga and meditation to reduce stress and anxiety, lower blood pressure, and improve metabolic and respiratory functioning.

people suffering from chronic diseases and stress-related disorders such as abdominal pain, ulcers, and chronic diarrhea. In his book, *Full Catastrophic Living: Using the Wisdom of Your Body and Mind to Face Stress, Pain, and Illness,* he details how a majority of his clinic's patients reduced their pains associated with stress and improved their health by meditating.

Summary

Stress is unavoidable in normal living, and, when utilized efficiently, can provide an opportunity for growth and development. Excessive, prolonged stress is harmful, however, and increases the risk of medical disorders such as atherosclerosis, headaches, hypertension, and ulcers. More important than the stress level itself is how efficiently a person converts the stress into useful energy, and how successfully he or she manages it, rather than being managed by it. Recognizing the early signs of stress and doing something positive to handle stress through exercise, relaxation, and other techniques—rather letting the stress become destructive—can make an important difference in a person's quality of life and sense of well-being.

Resources

References

Arnold, Kathryn. "Energy!" *Delicious* (March 1994): 18–20.

Benson, Herbert. *The Relaxation Response.* New York, NY: William Morrow, 1975.

Berkman, L.F., and S.L. Syme. "Social Networks, Host Resistance, and Mortality: A Nine-Year Follow Up Study of Alameda County Residents." *American Journal of Epidemiology* (1979, Volume 2): 186–204.

Epstein, Gerald. *Healing Visualizations.* New York, NY: Bantam Books, 1989.

Goleman, Daniel. *The Meditative Mind.* Los Angeles, CA: Jeremy P. Tarcher, Inc., 1988.

———. "Stress and Isolation Tied to a Reduced Life Span." *New York Times* (December 7, 1993): B8.

Hildreth, Suzanne. "The New Body/Mind Workout." *Natural Health* (January/February 1994): 54–56.

Jahnke, R. "The Most Profound Medicine— Part II and Part III: Physiological Mechanisms Operating in the Human System During the Practice of Qi gong and Yoga Pranayama." *Townsend Letter for Doctors* (January–February 1991): 124–30, 281–85.

Kabat-Sinn, J. *Full Catastrophic Living: Using the Wisdom of Your Body and Mind to Face Stress, Pain, and Illness.* New York, NY: Delacorte Press, 1990.

Murray, Michael, and Joseph Pizzorno. *Encyclopedia of Natural Medicine.* Rocklin, CA: Prima Publishing, 1991.

Ornish, Dean, M.D. *Dr. Dean Ornish's Program for Reversing Heart Disease.* New York, NY: Ballantine Books, 1990.

Scofield, M. *Work Site Health Promotion.* Philadelphia, PA: Hanley & Belfus, Inc., 1990.

Selye, Hans. *Stress Without Distress.* New York, NY: New American Library, 1975.

"Stress is Sickening." *New Body* (December 1993).

Williams, Gurney, III. "Don't Let Stress Number Your Days." *Longevity* (October 1990): 58–59.

Organizations

American Heart Association
7320 Greenville Ave., Dallas, TX 75231.

The American Institute of Stress
Dept. U, 124 Park Ave., Yonkers, NY 10703.

National High Blood Pressure Education Program, 120/80
4733 Bethesda Ave., Bethesda, MD 20814.

The National Institute of Mental Health
Parklawn Bldg. 15C-05, 5600 Fishers Ln., Rockville MD 20857.

Additional Reading

Benson, Herbert, and William Proctor. *Beyond the Relaxation Response.* New York, NY: Berkeley Publishing Group, 1987.

Girdano, Daniel, and George Everly. *Controlling Stress and Tension: A Holistic Approach.* Englewood Cliffs, NJ: Prentice-Hall, 1986.

"How to Fend Off Stress." *Good Housekeeping* (February 1991): 106, 130.

Kirsta, Alix. *The Book of Stress Survival.* New York, NY : Simon & Schuster, Inc., 1986.

Mason, L. *Guide to Stress Reeducation.* Berkeley, CA: Celestial Arts, 1985.

Murphy, Michael. *The Future of the Body.* Los Angeles, CA: Jeremy P. Tarcher, Inc., 1992.

Shimer, Porter, and Sharon Ferguson. "Unwind and Destress (Part 1)." *Prevention* 42 (July 1990): 75–92.

———. "Unwind and Destress (Part 2)." *Prevention* 42 (August 1990): 99–117.

"Stress Can Make You Sick, But Can Managing Stress Make You Well?" *Consumer Reports Health Letter 2* (January 1990): 1–3.

Wilkinson, Greg. "Stress: Another Chimera." *British Medical Journal* (January 26, 1991): 191–92.

Chapter 9

STRESS-RELATED DISORDERS

As discussed in the previous chapter, certain experiences are so physically or emotionally stressful that they can severely compromise the immune system's ability to ward off disease. Prolongation of stress can exhaust specific organ systems, especially the heart, blood vessels, and adrenal glands. This chapter discusses the alternative prevention and treatment of medical disorders associated with chronic stress: headaches, hypertension (high blood pressure), irritable bowel syndrome (IBS), ulcers, and atherosclerosis.

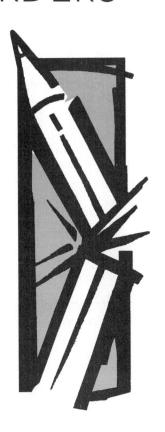

Atherosclerosis

Arteriosclerosis is the general term for the thickening and hardening of the arteries that occurs as part of the aging process. Atherosclerosis, one form of arteriosclerosis, is caused by hypertension and other risk factors including high cholesterol levels, a rich diet (with large amounts of meat, butter, whole milk, eggs, and calories), genetics, diabetes, poor physical fitness, and cigarette smoking. Atherosclerosis, according to Kurt Butler and Lynn Rayner in *The Best Medicine: The Complete Health and Preventive Handbook,* causes or contributes to more deaths in the U.S. than all other diseases or accidents combined.

People with atherosclerosis have deposits of fatty substances of cholesterol, cellular waste products, calcium, or fibrin (a clotting material) on the inner linings of their arteries. These substances combine to form arterial blockages called plaque. Plaque may partially or totally block the blood's flow through an artery and cause bleeding (hemorrhaging) in the plaque, or blood clots (thrombi) on the plaque's surface. If a coronary artery becomes blocked, less blood is supplied to the heart, and a heart attack can occur. If the arteries supplying blood to the brain are occluded, a stroke can occur. The clogging of arteries feeding the kidneys can lead to kidney failure.

Treatments for atherosclerosis include removal of the fatty substances or plaque by surgery or laser, widening of affected arteries using small balloons (angioplasty), and the use of various drugs. Therapies also include diet, treating hypertension, and not smoking.

Alternative Treatments for Atherosclerosis

Ayurvedic Medicine. Ayurvedic physicians use herbal food supplements, detoxification, and purification techniques to reduce free radicals and lipid peroxides that are believed to contribute to atherosclerosis. Sodhi states in *Alternative Medicine: The Definitive Guide* that one hospital in Bombay, India, has treated more than 3,000 cases of coronary heart disease using herbals and detoxification and purification therapies that eliminate toxins from the blood and reduce stress. The hospital's stress reduction program combines yoga and meditation.

Botanical Medicines. Michael Murray and Joseph Pizzorno cite several studies in the *Encyclopedia of Natural Medicine* that indicate garlic oil, alfalfa leaf, and hawthorn berry may help lower cholesterol levels and inhibit the formation of plaque. Garlic oil increases the breakdown of fibrin and inhibits atherosclerotic platelets from forming. Alfalfa leaf appears to exert a "shrinkage" effect on atherosclerotic plaque. Hawthorn berry and its flower extracts have been widely used in Europe in clinical trials to lower serum cholesterol levels and to prevent the deposition of

cholesterol in arterial walls. Hawthorn berry can be toxic in excessive amounts, however, and should be taken only under the supervision of a physician or nutritionist.

Chinese physicians have used an herbal extract from the plant mao-tung-ching (ilex puibeceus) to treat coronary atherosclerosis. The extract, according to Chung San Yuan in an article that appeared in the 1973 *Chinese Medical Journal*, helps dilate blocked blood vessels and increase blood flow to the heart. Of a total of 103 cases, 101 patients showed significant improvement.

Exercise. Regular aerobic exercise such as walking or cycling raises HDL ("good") cholesterol blood levels and lowers triglycerides. A study reported in the April 1993 issue of *Archives of Internal Medicine* suggests that resistance exercise helps lower both total cholesterol and LDL ("bad") cholesterol levels, at least in premenopausal women. In the study, inactive women with normal cholesterol levels were assigned to either an exercise group or a control group. The participants were told to continue their usual eating patterns. Those in the exercise group were placed on a supervised program of strength-training—12 resistance exercises for one hour three times a week. At the end of the five-month period, the exercise group showed significant declines in cholesterol levels. As a group, the women who trained with weights lowered their total cholesterol by 13 percent and their LDL cholesterol by 14 points.

Nutritional Therapies. In his best-selling book *Dr. Dean Ornish's Program for Reversing Heart Disease,* Ornish outlines a combination of alternative treatments he has used successfully to reverse coronary atherosclerosis. A diet of vegetables, fruits, and dietary fiber (including flax seed, oat bran, and pectin) is a key component. Ornish suggests that patients with coronary atherosclerosis must totally avoid saturated fats, cholesterol, sugar, and animal proteins. To prevent atherosclerosis and heart disease, he recommends that people limit their fat consumption to 20 percent of calories consumed. To reverse heart disease caused by coronary atherosclerosis, he counsels his patients to limit their fat intake to 10 percent of calories.

Butler and Rayner claim that dietary fibers such as cellulose, pectin, lignin, and other indigestible components of whole grains, legumes, fruits, and vegetables appear to reduce cholesterol (a key risk factor in atherosclerosis). They report one study in which participants who ate a quarter-pound of raw carrots for breakfast for three weeks reduced serum cholesterol levels by an average of 11 percent. The effect lasted for three weeks after patients stopped eating the carrots. Butler and Rayner theorize that the fiber may decrease intestinal absorption of cholesterol.

They also note that vegetarians are known to be less susceptible to atherosclerosis, which traditionally was linked to their lower fat and cholesterol intake. However, as Butler and Rayner suggest, it also could be the result of their higher consumption of vitamin B6 (pyridoxine), which is abundant in plant foods. By comparison, meat eaters (especially those who also eat a lot of processed and sugary foods and little fresh produce) usually consume very little vitamin B6.

Vitamin and Mineral Therapies. Several studies summarized in Chapter 3 have shown that vitamins C, E, and B help prevent atherosclerosis. Vitamin C dissolves cholesterol, aids in fat metabolism, and helps restore the integrity of the arterial walls. Supplemental vitamin E helps prevent atherosclerosis by inhibiting platelet aggregation and elevating HDL cholesterol levels. Niacin also has been used to lower cholesterol levels, although its use should be supervised by a physician, because it can lead to liver damage and glu-

cose intolerance. Pantetheine lowers LDL cholesterol levels and increases HDL cholesterol levels.

Magnesium and calcium supplementation (see Chapter 4) also increases HDL cholesterol levels, decreases platelet aggregation, and prolongs the time it takes plaque and blood clots to form. According to Murray and Pizzorno, carnitine, a vitamin-like compound, stimulates the breakdown of long-chain fatty acids and can help prevent fatty plaques from forming in the blood. Lecithin increases the solubility of cholesterol and helps remove cholesterol from tissue deposits. Onions and bromelain, an enzyme found in pineapples, also decrease platelet aggregation, they claim.

Butler and Rayner report that studies have confirmed the ability of lecithin to increase HDL cholesterol and inhibit platelet clumping or aggregation. It is found in unbleached soy flour, seeds, nuts, whole grains, and cold-pressed vegetable oils, all of which contain other important nutrients as well.

Headaches

Nine out of ten people in the U.S. experience at least one headache a year, while as many as 45 million Americans suffer from chronic or severe headaches that seriously interfere with their lives, according to studies cited in a November 1990 article in *The University of California, Berkeley Wellness Letter.* Headaches now account for 150 million lost work days and 80 million visit to doctors' offices each year in the U.S. More than $400 million is spent annually on over-the-counter pain relievers.

Headaches almost always are due to dilation, constriction, spasm, irritation, or inflammation of arteries or muscles of the head and neck. Sometimes more than one factor is involved. There are several types of

Types of Headaches

Tension headaches are caused by sustained constriction of scalp, neck, and face muscles, with symptoms of tightness and pressure in the forehead and the back of the head and neck.

Migraine headaches are caused by constriction of the arteries with symptoms that include flashing lights, extreme pain in one side of the head, and numbness.

Cluster headaches are characterized by piercing pain around and behind one eye, and may occur in clusters of several a day with recurrences every few weeks.

Food sensitivity headaches are caused by chocolate, red wines, cheeses, excessive salt, preservatives such as monosodium glutamate (MSG), and other foodstuffs.

Alcohol headaches occur hours after drinking and often are the main aspect of a hangover.

Smoking headaches are caused by inhaling nicotine.

Toxic headaches are caused by exposure to chemicals such as benzene, gasoline, formaldehyde, paints, glue, or carbon dioxide.

High blood pressure headaches (which occur in 10 percent of hypertension cases) resemble migraines and usually necessitate antihypertensive drug therapy.

Bruxism headaches are caused by excessive clenching and grinding of the teeth, excessive gum chewing, or jaw disorders.

TMJ headaches are caused by abnormal temporomandibular joints (where the jaws meet the skull) due to arthritis, biting on hard objects, excessive gum chewing, or malocclusion (bad bite).

---

headaches, each overlapping in symptoms and response to treatment. The triggering factors and modes of relief vary from person to person. The majority of primary headaches (those caused by stress and lifestyle factors such as smoking or drinking, and not by other diseases) fall into three categories: tension headaches, migraine headaches, and cluster headaches.

Nine out of ten headaches are tension-related, caused by the sustained constriction of scalp, neck, and face muscles and characterized by tightness and pressure in the forehead and the back of the head and neck. Poor posture on the job, with prolonged flexing of the neck, can trigger such a headache. Depression, fatigue, mental tension, and emotional distress also can be factors. Tension

headaches affect men and women in equal numbers.

According to Butler and Rayner, migraines affect approximately 8 percent of the U.S. population and tend to run in families. In migraine headaches the pain usually is limited to one side of the head and is pounding and often incapacitating. It often is accompanied by nausea and vomiting. Certain neurological symptoms may occur 10 to 30 minutes before an attack, such as flashing lights, blind spots, blurred vision, or a tingling, numbing sensation on one side of the body. Other vague symptoms beforehand include mental fuzziness, mood changes, fatigue, and unusual retention of fluids. Migraines, which affect three times as many women as men, are believed to be caused by several factors including emotional stress, depression, unstable levels of the brain chemical serotonin, alcohol, allergies, nitrates, excessive sun, motion sickness, fluctuating levels of female hormones, and genetics. Migraine pain can last several hours to several days. These headaches strike as often as several times a week or as rarely as once every few years.

Cluster headaches occur when the blood vessels on the surface of the brain widen excessively; they usually last between 30 and 45 minutes. Although some specialists consider them migraine variants, cluster headaches are distinguished by a knifelike, piercing pain around and behind one eye, which is tearing and red, and by a runny nose and accelerated heartbeat. The pain is very severe but non-throbbing, and both the onset and cessation are sudden. These headaches tend to occur in clusters of several a day, with recurrences every few weeks. They are much less common than migraines (only 1 percent of the U.S. population suffers from them), affect men much more often than women (especially those who are heavy smokers and heavy drinkers), and do not run in families. They seem to be linked to seasonal changes in the amount of daylight, according to the October 1993 issue of the *Mayo Clinic Health Letter*.

Treatments for Headaches

Acupuncture. In the last 20 years, acupuncture has become a respected therapy in many American hospitals. It is widely used to reduce pain in patients with migraine headaches. A New Zealand study, reported by L. Lenhard and P. Waite in a 1983 issue of the *New Zealand Medical Journal* (Volume 96), found that 40 percent of the subjects experienced a 50 to 100 percent reduction in the severity and frequency of migraine headaches after acupuncture treatment.

Acupuncture may be useful in relieving other types of headaches as well, although few clinical double-blind trials have been conducted.

Bodywork Therapies. Many stress-related headaches occur when the muscles that run between the base of the skull and along the top of the shoulders become tight or go into spasm. Massage therapy, rolfing, or other techniques such as the Feldenkrais method, the Alexander technique, the Trager approach, or polarity therapy help relax these tensed muscles as well as the neck and can relieve some headaches.

Botanical Medicines. Feverfew, a perennial composite herb, has a long folk history in the treatment of fever, arthritis, and migraine headaches. Steven Foster, in a 1991 pamphlet entitled *Feverfew* published by the American Botanical Council, states that feverfew's effectiveness in relieving migraines apparently is due to its ability to inhibit the secretion of serotonin and to reduce the size of inflamed blood vessels in the brain that cause throbbing pain in sufferers. Canada's Health and Welfare Department has approved the sale of feverfew for migraine prevention. Approval was based on two clinical trials conducted in the United Kingdom in 1985 and 1988, as reported by Jim O'Brien in the October 19, 1993 issue of *Your Health*. He quotes Dr. D. Awang, head of the Natural Products Bureau of Drug Research, as saying that feverfew "effectively reduced the incidence and severity of migraine attacks." Approximately 70 percent of patients in the 1988 study had fewer migraines after they took the equivalent of two medium-sized feverfew leaves daily. By comparison, only 50 percent of a group of control patients derived benefits from prescription migraine drugs. Canadian health officials currently advise consumers not to take feverfew continuously for more than four months without the advice of a physician.

Chiropractic Therapy. Headaches caused by a misalignment of the neck sometimes can be relieved with chiropractic therapy. In a six-month clinical trial conducted in Australia, as reported by G. Parker in a 1978 issue of the *Australian/New Zealand Journal of Medicine* (Volume 8), 85 patients reduced the severity of their migraine headaches through cervical spine manipulation by a chiropractor. Another study found that five treatments every month, given over a period of six months, decreased recurrences of headaches in 45 percent of patients.

Exercise. Dr. Joseph Primavera, co-director of the Comprehensive Headache Center at Germantown Hospital and Medical Center in Philadelphia, uses moderate exercise to treat patients suffering from headaches. According to Primavera, as quoted in the January 1994 issue of *American Health,* 20 minutes of aerobic exercise three times a week—running, brisk walking, bicycling, or swimming—can help prevent headaches. Primavera suggests that exercise improves cardiovascular functioning, reduces stress, and produces endorphins, the body's natural pain relievers.

Regular sexual activity also may relieve tension and migraine headaches. According to Kristin Von Kreisler, writing in the January 11, 1994 issue of *Your Health,* researchers at Southern Illinois School of Medicine studied the effect of regular sexual activity in 52 female migraine sufferers. Eight patients who made love during the headache reported that their headaches were eliminated, while 16 experienced some relief.

Homeopathic Remedies. According to Maesimund Panos and Jane Heimlich in *Homeopathic Remedies for Everyday Ailments and Minor Injuries,* homeopathic therapies have successfully treated many types of headaches. Homeopaths prescribe individualized remedies based on the patient's symptoms and overall mental and physical condition. The most frequently used homeopathic remedies include aconitum nappellus, arnica montana, belladonna, bryonia, gelsenium, iris versicolor, kali bichronicum, nux vomica, and sanguinaria canadensis.

In *Everybody's Guide to Homeopathic Medicine,* Dr. Stephen Cummings and Dana Ullman cite 107 controlled studies in which homeopathic therapies effectively treated a variety of medical disorders, including headaches. They list several homeopathic remedies such as belladonna, bryonia, nux vomica, pulsatilla, gelsenium, and sanguinaria.

Nutritional Therapies. James F. Balch and Phyllis Balch suggest in *Prescription for Nutritional Healing* that most stress-related headaches can be relieved by avoiding salt and acid-producing foods. They recommend that people who suffer frequent headaches consult a nutritionist who can design a customized rotation diet that will eliminate fried, fatty, and greasy foods. Some people may benefit from eliminating dairy products, yellow cheese, and cherries. The nitrate preservatives found in hot dogs and luncheon meats should be avoided as well.

Murray and Pizzorno claim that food allergies are a major cause of migraine headaches. They suggest that migraine sufferers adopt a food elimination diet that avoids alcoholic beverages, cheese, chocolate, citrus fruits, and shellfish. The diet should be low in animal fats and high in foods that inhibit platelet aggregation, including fish oils, vegetable oils, garlic, and onion. Butler and Rayner also identify certain foods as possible precipitating factors for migraine headaches. These include cheeses, wine, beer, chocolate, vinegar, pickles, organ meats, preserved fish and meat, soy beans, lima beans, onions, spinach, and foods with MSG or nitrates.

Stress Reduction Therapies. Biofeedback, yoga, meditation, and hypnosis help prevent migraines, although they are not effective in all cases. Simeon Margolis and Hamilton Moses III report in *The Johns Hopkins Medical Handbook* that biofeedback therapy teaches patients how to consciously raise their hand temperature, which can reduce the number and intensity of headaches including migraines. In this therapy, while the patient tries to warm his or her hands, a computer monitor provides a reading as the temperature increases. In another type of biofeedback, called electromyographic or EMG training, patients learn to control muscle tension in the face, neck, and shoulders. Both types of biofeedback sometimes are combined with relaxation training techniques that help patients mentally reduce their tension levels without the use of biofeedback machines. Dr. Andrew Weil, quoted in the October 19, 1993, issue of *Your Health,* recommends that people who get frequent headaches combine biofeedback with other relaxation methods such as yoga, meditation, visualization, and guided imagery.

Vitamin and Mineral Therapies. Several vitamins, minerals, and amino acids improve brain oxygenation and relieve migraine headaches. Murray and Pizzorno recommend that people who suffer recurring migraine headaches consult a physician who may recommend vitamin B3 (niacin), magnesium, or quercetin supplements. Niacin dilates blood vessels and helps prevent premenstrual headaches. Niacinamide is generally used in treatment because, unlike niacin, it does not cause burning, flushing, or itching of the skin. Evening primrose oil capsules and MaxEPAS, a form of fish oil, are sources of essential fatty acids that supply the body with anti-inflammatory agents and help prevent constriction of cerebral blood vessels.

Hypertension (High Blood Pressure)

Hypertension (excessive and sustained blood pressure against the walls of the arteries) is the most common stress-related disorder in the U.S. and a major cause of death. According to a September 1989 article in the *Johns Hopkins Medical Letter,* approximately 60 million Americans (or one in four) have blood pressure that is high enough to require treatment. Only half of the 60 million know they have the condition, however, and only 25 percent of those 30 million receive adequate medical care. Chronic hypertension (called a "silent killer" because of its lack of symptoms) can damage the kidneys, heart, brain, and retinas if left untreated. The article goes on to claim that hypertension is a factor in 75 percent of strokes and 68 percent of first heart attacks in the U.S. Butler and Rayner point out that because hypertension is so harmful, blood pressure is the most important factor life insurance companies use to predict life expectancy and to determine premiums.

There are two main types of hypertension: that resulting from other medical disorders such as diabetes; and essential hypertension, for which the cause has not been fully established. Factors that have been tentatively linked to essential hypertension include obesity and inactivity; excess salt, sugar, and licorice intake; heredity; smoking; coffee; alcohol; prolonged stress; and drugs, including estrogens, indomethacin, phenylpropanolamine (the appetite suppressant), amphetamines, and cocaine. Long-term studies have shown that chronic high blood pressure typical of essential hypertension increases the risk of heart disease, stroke, atherosclerosis, and kidney disease. Anxiety, heart palpitations, increased pulse rates, or feeling "all wound up" are not necessarily reliable indicators of high blood pressure. The only way to detect abnormal pressure and to minimize the

Dangerous Headache Symptoms

While headaches generally are not life threatening, they can signal a serious medical disorder such as a blood clot, brain tumor, or weakened blood vessel that could burst (aneurysm). People experiencing any of the following symptoms should consult a physician immediately:

- Abrupt, severe headache, often like a thunderclap.

- Headache with fever, stiff neck, rash, mental confusion, seizures, double vision, weakness, numbness, or speaking difficulties.

- Headache after a recent sore throat or respiratory infection.

- Headache after a head injury, even if it is a minor fall or bump, especially if the pain gets worse.

- Chronic, progressive headache that worsens after coughing, exertion, straining, or a sudden movement.

- New headache pain after age 55 (which could signal temporal arteritis, an inflammation that affects arteries in the scalp, brain, and eyes).

risk of hypertension is to have an annual blood pressure examination.

Treatments for Hypertension

Ayurvedic Medicine. Dr. Virender Sodhi, director of the American School of Ayurvedic Sciences in Bellevue, Washington, states in *Alternative Medicine: The Definitive Guide* that Ayurvedic medicine has helped patients suffering from hypertension. Patients are treated with diets low in sodium, cholesterol, and triglycerides; yogic breathing; relaxation, and Ayurvedic herbs. According to Sodhi, Ayurvedic herbs such as cas onvolvulus pluricaulis, ashwaganda, and rauwolfia help lower blood pressure levels. Herbs often are used in combination, depending on the patient's individual needs, along with calcium, magnesium, silicon, and zinc.

Bodywork Therapies. *Alternative Medicine: The Definitive Guide* suggests that one or several of the following bodywork therapies may be appropriate for treating hypertension: acupressure, reflexology, shiatsu, massage, rolfing, the Feldenkrais method, the Alexander technique, the Trager approach, and polarity therapy. Although these techniques are popular in the U.S. and have been used for 20 years to treat a variety of medical problems, their effectiveness has not been proven conclusively in clinical trials.

Botanical Medicines. Seaweed preparations have been shown to lower blood pressure more effectively than prescription medicines. Dr. M. Krotkiewski, writing in the June 1991 issue of the *American Journal of Hypertension*, reports that Swedish scientists reduced the blood pressure of 62 middle-aged patients suffering from mild hypertension by giving them seaweed fiber. This decrease, according to Krotkiewski, "was dependent on the decreased intestinal absorption of sodium and increased absorption of potassium released from the seaweed preparation." He concluded that seaweed fiber is a useful treatment for mild hypertension.

Murray and Pizzorno report that hawthorn berry extracts are widely used in Europe to lower blood pressure. The extracts appear to work by dilating the larger blood vessels, increasing intracellular vitamin C levels, and decreasing capillary permeability and fragility. The extracts also may help ward off angina attacks by lowering serum cholesterol levels and preventing the deposition of cholesterol on arterial walls.

Mistletoe is used by European physicians (combined with crataegus) to treat hypertension. The berries, leaves, and stems of the plant contain beta phenyethylamine and tyramine, which help regulate blood pressure. However, as mistletoe is toxic, it should not be used in high doses or for extended periods of time except under the supervision of a physician. Balch and Balch report that alfalfa, barley, spirulina, and wheatgrass, all of which are sources of concentrated chlorophyll, help lower blood pressure as well.

Exercise. Moderate exercise has been shown to directly reduce both stress and blood pressure. However, people with hypertension should consult a physician before starting any form of exercise, because even mild exercise can temporarily raise blood pressure. The best exercises, according to clinical trials, reduce the level of stress hormones in the bloodstream that constrict the arteries and veins. For example, a Johns Hopkins University Medical Center study cited by Margolis and Moses in *The Johns Hopkins Medical Handbook* found that progressive weightlifting reduced blood pressure 13 to 14 points in a group of 52 men, while intensive heavy lifting raised systolic blood pressure by 5 to 7 points. To lower blood pressure, a person should lift light weights three times a week at 40 percent of maximum strength in conjunction with aerobic exercise. The same study also found that walking or jogging three times a week for 20 minutes reduced blood pressure by approximately 6 points. Researchers are not certain how weightlifting reduces blood pressure, but researchers suggest that exercise

Alternative Therapies for Hypertension

- **Lose excess weight.** An estimated 20 to 30 percent of hypertension cases result from excess body weight, which, if lost, results in a commensurate drop in blood pressure.

- **Reduce sodium intake.** Recent studies show that approximately half of those people who have hypertension can lower their blood pressure by making a moderate reduction in dietary sodium consumption.

- **Reduce dietary fats** to 20 percent of caloric intake. Dr. Ornish's research proves that hypertension can be greatly reduced through a totally vegetarian diet that has less than 20 percent of its calories from fats.

- **Increase calcium.** Increased calcium intake may slightly lower blood pressure.

- **Increase potassium.** Potassium lowers blood pressure, although the benefit is modest.

- **Reduce alcohol intake.** Curtailing alcohol consumption has corresponded to decreases in blood pressure in limited trials.

- **Exercise.** Exercise helps to lower blood pressure.

- **Relaxation.** Relaxation routines such as deep breathing, meditation, and progressive muscle relaxation relieve muscular tension and lower blood pressure.

- **Stop smoking.** Nicotine constricts the arteries and increases blood pressure.

relaxes the blood vessels so blood flows through them more efficiently.

Nutritional Therapies. Many nutritional factors, according to Murray and Pizzorno, have been linked with high blood pressure, including sodium to potassium ratios, high cholesterol, and low fiber consumption. People who consume large quantities of salt are at risk of developing hypertension, and reducing dietary sodium directly lowers high blood pressure in some patients. The chloride present in table salt, along with sodium, may affect hormonal regulation of fluid and salt retention and contribute to hypertension. A calcium deficiency also may contribute to hypertension, because people who decrease their calcium intake usually experience increased blood pressure. A high-calcium diet helps counteract the harmful effects of a high-sodium diet, and sodium may be indirectly related to hypertension by its direct effect on calcium metabolism. For maximum benefits, Murray and Pizzorno recommend that people with high blood pressure adopt a diet that is low in sodium and high in potassium and calcium.

Ornish notes in *Dr. Dean Ornish's Program for Reversing Heart Disease* that people with hypertension often have low levels of magnesium. Elevated blood pressure returns to normal levels when magnesium-rich foods are added to the diet, and magnesium is believed to help the heart and blood vessels contract and relax. People who think they might have hypertension should also reduce their dietary fats. When dietary fats are reduced to 20 percent of total calories, blood pressure declines by as much as 10 percent. Ornish notes that vegetarians generally have lower blood pressure, and lower incidences of hypertension and other cardiovascular diseases, than do nonvegetarians. Vegetarian diets typically contain more potassium, complex carbohydrates, polyunsaturated fat, fiber,

calcium, magnesium, vitamin C, and vitamin A, all of which lower blood pressure.

According to both Ornish and Murray and Pizzorno, high-fiber diets effectively prevent and treat hypertension. The best fiber diet includes oat bran, apple pectin, psyllium seeds, guar gum, and gum karaya. This diet reduces cholesterol and promotes weight loss, which helps lower blood pressure. Ornish further recommends that table sugar be eliminated because it elevates blood pressure, and claims that garlic and onions decrease both systolic and diastolic blood pressure levels.

Stress Reduction Therapies. Elmer and Alyce Green of the Menninger Foundation claimed in a 1980 issue (Volume 6) of *Primary Cardiology* that four out of five people with essential hypertension can restore and maintain normal blood pressure without drugs, through biofeedback and stress reduction ("psychophysiological") training. W.S. Agras reported in the May 1983 issue of *Hospital Practice* that biofeedback, yoga, meditation, visualization, and hypnosis are clinically proven, effective therapies for lowering blood pressure in hypertensive patients.

In one study of 20 hypertensives using yoga relaxation and biofeedback, reported by Butler and Rayner, 16 improved greatly. The average blood pressure dropped from 160/102 to 134/86, and most of the group were able to reduce or eliminate the drugs they had been taking for hypertension. Butler and Rayner go on to say that other studies of those using meditation regularly, and attaining a deep relaxation one to four times a day, showed significant blood pressure reductions. These reductions lasted over a period of weeks, not just for the duration of the session, as long as the sessions continued.

Traditional Chinese Medicine (TCM). Hypertension is viewed in TCM as a problem in the circulation of energy (chi) in the body.

According to *Alternative Medicine: The Definitive Guide,* Chinese physicians have treated it successfully with acupuncture, herbs, exercises such as qi gong, meditation, and a diet high in vegetables and low in fat, sugar, and alcohol.

Vitamin, Mineral, and Botanical Therapies. Dr. Robert Atkins, director of the Atkins Center in New York City, claims in the May/June 1994 issue of *Well Being Journal* to have helped thousands of patients lower their blood pressure by using nutrient combinations. Atkins recommends pantetheine, chromium picolinate, GLA, hexanicotinate, calcium, lecithin, magnesium, garlic, olive oil, avocado, gum guggulu, DHEA, fenugreek seed powder, psyllium husks, guar gum, and vitamin C.

Irritable Bowel Syndrome (IBS)

Irritable bowel syndrome is a chronic disorder in which the muscle of the lower portion of the colon functions abnormally and produces exaggerated contractions. Put another way, IBS is a disorder of the natural conveyer-belt mechanism of the bowels, the mechanism that helps move waste products through the body. Approximately 15 percent of Americans suffer from IBS, and twice as many women as men have the disorder. While doctors have been unable to pinpoint its organic cause, IBS often is linked to emotional conflict or stress. Patients usually complain of lower abdominal pain, gas, bloating, constipation, or diarrhea, or alternating constipation and diarrhea. Although IBS can cause a great deal of discomfort, it is not serious, nor does it lead to any serious disease such as ulcerative colitis or cancer. With attention to proper diet, stress management, and, in some

cases, medications, most people with IBS can keep their symptoms under control.

Treatments for Irritable Bowel Syndrome

Botanical Therapies. Murray and Pizzorno recommend peppermint oil capsules, ginger, and herbal antispasmodics as botanical medicines that reduce the overgrowth of candida albicans, a common yeast, and sometimes offer relief for IBS sufferers. Ginger has a long history of use in relieving digestive complaints. Other herbs that have proven effective include chamomile, valerian, rosemary, and balm. David Hoffman recommends in *Alternative Medicine: The Definitive Guide* a combination mix of tinctures of bayberry, gentian, peppermint, and wild yam.

Colonic Therapy. IBS disorders sometimes are characterized by the inability of the colon to effectively eliminate wastes, which can then be passed into the lymph glands, bloodstream, and intestines. Colonic therapy, which irrigates the colon with water, helps dislodge fecal material and restores normal bacteria flora. A single session normally lasts 30 to 45 minutes. Another option suggested by Balch and Balch is to take regular enemas to keep the colon clean.

Nutritional Therapies. Because of the variable nature of the disorder, IBS patients must be treated on a case-by-case basis. In general, however, consuming a diet rich in complex carbohydrates and dietary fiber (present in whole grain breads and cereals, fruits, and vegetables) often is curative. Fiber supplements such as guar, pectin, psyllium seed, or oat bran also help eliminate waste from the colon.

The National Institute of Diabetes and Digestive and Kidney Diseases further counsels IBS sufferers to eat smaller meals more frequently, or to eat smaller portions of foods, especially if they are low in fat and rich in carbohydrates and proteins. Foods high in carbohydrates and low in fat include pastas, rice, breads, cereals, fruits, and vegetables. Those high in protein and low in fat include chicken and turkey without the skin, lean meats, most fish, and low-fat dairy products such as skim milk and low-fat cheeses.

Murray and Pizzorno cite a study in which approximately two-thirds of the patients with IBS had at least one food intolerance, and some had multiple intolerances. When IBS symptoms were caused by food sensitivities, sufferers who used a food elimination diet normally experienced improvement within five or six days. For this reason, IBS sufferers should first determine whether or not they have any food intolerances and, if so, begin to follow a diet that eliminates these foods.

Stress Reduction Therapies. Many patients with IBS complain of psychological symptoms such as anxiety, fatigue, hostile feelings, depression, and sleep disturbances. It is not known whether these are a cause or a result of bowel disturbances. According to Murray and Pizzorno, psychological stress reduction techniques such as biofeedback, progressive relaxation, deep breathing, massage and hypnosis are often quite helpful in alleviating IBS symptoms.

Peptic Ulcers

According to the National Digestive Disease Information Clearinghouse, one out of every ten Americans develops a peptic ulcer, although many—too minor to cause pain—will go unnoticed. Butler and Rayner warn, however, that even ulcers that have been treated tend to recur. Care and watchfulness are required throughout life to avoid hemorrhage, surgery, and even—in extreme cases—removal of the stomach.

Peptic ulcers are sores, usually one-quarter to three-quarters of an inch in diameter, that form in the lining (mucosa) of the stomach or the first part of the small intestine below the stomach, called the duodenum. Peptic ulcers that occur in the lining of the stomach are called gastric ulcers, and those in the lining of the duodenum are called duodenal ulcers. As Margolis and Moses point out in *The Johns Hopkins Medical Handbook,* duodenal ulcers are more common than gastric ulcers in the U.S., while the reverse is true in Japan.

Both the stomach and the duodenum secrete hydrochloric acid and the digestive enzyme pepsin, which help break down foods. If too much hydrochloric acid or pepsin is secreted, it begins to erode the mucosa of the stomach or duodenum and causes an ulcer—hence the name "peptic" ulcer. The linings of the stomach and duodenum also lose their ability to resist erosion as people age, and peptic ulcers sometimes occur in older people with low acid levels. Butler and Rayner and others claim that sustained emotional stress—such as anxiety, anger, and fear—can contribute to excessive acid production and sometimes is the main factor; even noise can be a problem. In some cases, there are no identifiable causes.

The most common symptom of a gastric ulcer is a burning pain in the stomach, which may be temporarily relieved by food or antacids. The most common symptom of a duodenal ulcer is a burning pain in the abdomen between the navel and the lower end of the breastbone. Other symptoms include lower back pain, headaches, choking sensations, and itching. A physician should be consulted if these pains persist, because serious complications may develop. If they are not treated, ulcers can erode blood vessels and cause bleeding into the digestive tract. If the damaged blood vessels are small, the blood may seep out slowly and the patient can become anemic. If the damaged blood vessels are large, the patient may vomit blood or collapse suddenly. If the ulcer erodes through the wall of the stomach or duodenum, partially digested food and bacteria from the digestive tract can inflame the abdominal cavity. This condition, called a "perforated ulcer," produces sudden, severe pain and usually requires hospitalization and corrective surgery.

Treatments for Ulcers

Acupuncture. William Cargile, chairman of research for the American Association of Acupuncture and Oriental Medicine, reports in *Alternative Medicine: The Definitive Guide* that acupuncture can aid some patients with ulcers. He suggests that ulcers be treated by using acupuncture points associated with stress, anxiety, and stomach gastrointestinal problems (especially the stomach meridian). Some patients who receive acupuncture treatments for ulcers no longer need to use prescription drugs such as Tagamet.

Antacids. As Butler and Rayner note, antacids—best taken between meals and at bedtime—have long been standard medication for ulcers. They relieve the burning pain, and studies have shown that they speed healing. Since antacids can be harmful, however, if taken in large doses or over a prolonged period of time, they should be used with caution and awareness of side effects such as constipation or diarrhea.

Anti-Inflammatory Medications. The December 1990 issue of the *Johns Hopkins Medical Letter* suggests that elderly people who take nonsteroidal anti-inflammatory drugs (NSAIDs) for arthritis—such as aspirin, ibuprofen (Motrin, Advil, Nuprin), naproxen (Naprosyn, Anaprox), or piroxicam (Feldene)—are especially susceptible to stomach ulcers. Therefore, one of the first steps in

alternative treatment of ulcers is to help patients reduce or eliminate their need for these drugs.

Botanical Medicines. Paul Bergner, editor of *Medical Herbalism: A Clinical Newsletter for the Herbal Practitioner,* states in the September/October 1993 issue of *Natural Health* that licorice may be helpful in treating ulcers. He cites several studies that found licorice to be "as effective in preventing recurrence of ulcers as anti-ulcer drugs like Tagamet."

Murray and Pizzorno confirm that licorice can prevent and heal both gastric and duodenal ulcers. As noted earlier, however, licorice can be toxic and should be taken under the supervision of a physician. Other botanicals recommended in *Alternative Medicine: The Definitive Guide* to relieve ulcer symptoms include marshmallow, calendula, chamomile, goldenseal, meadowsweet, and cayenne pepper.

Balch and Balch suggest bayberry, catnip tea, myrrh, sage, slippery elm, and cayenne (also known as capsicum). Soothing herbal teas such as chamomile, anise, fennel, and flax seed are recommended by Butler and Rayner. However, they warn against certain herbs that are likely to irritate the stomach lining, such as peppermint, spearmint, and such stimulating herbs as gotu kola (which contains caffeine), desert tea, and damiana.

Nutritional Therapies. Alternative treatments for ulcers focus on neutralizing acid and pepsin levels while regenerating the integrity of the lining of the stomach and gastrointestinal tract. The first stage of treatment usually involves eliminating foods that cause allergies, quitting cigarette smoking, and reducing stress. Allergies are a primary factor in peptic ulcers, according to Murray and Pizzorno, and food elimination diets often are effective. People who develop ulcers are advised to stop smoking, because smoking slows the healing of ulcers and makes them more likely to recur. It may also be necessary to reduce consumption of alcohol; alcoholic cirrhosis has been linked to an increased risk of ulcers, and heavy drinking has been shown to delay the healing of ulcers.

Butler and Rayner warn that alcohol, caffeine (coffee, tea, and cola), and cigarettes can provoke and aggravate ulcers. They point out that while decaffeinated coffee can be easier on the stomach, it sometimes stimulates as much acid flow as regular coffee, either by a conditioned reflex association with the flavor or by the action of oils or other substances in the coffee.

Diets rich in fiber help prevent duodenal ulcers because they promote mucus secretion and delay gastric emptying, counteracting the rapid movement of food into the duodenum that normally occurs in ulcer patients. Raw cabbage juice also has been documented to help heal peptic ulcers. Murray and Pizzorno claim that one liter per day of fresh cabbage juice, taken in divided doses, can heal an ulcer in an average of 10 days. Not only do fiber-rich foods such as fruits, vegetables, and whole grain breads protect against the formation of ulcers and promote healing, but they also prevent relapses once ulcers develop. It is believed that the fiber somehow slows down or buffers stomach acid.

Balch and Balch recommend a diet of easy-to-digest, nutritious, and chemical-free foods, which they claim has produced excellent results after 30 days. It includes well-cooked millet, cooked white rice, raw goat's milk, and soured milk products such as yogurt, cottage cheese, and kefir. If symptoms are severe, soft foods such as avocados, bananas, potatoes, squash, and yams should be eaten daily. They advise putting all vegetables through a blender or processor, and consuming well-steamed vegetables such as broccoli and carrots occasionally. Balch and Balch

counsel those with bleeding ulcers to eat baby foods, and to add nonirritating fiber such as guar gum and psyllium seed.

Stress Reduction Therapies. Some nutritionists, including Murray and Pizzorno, believe there may a link between stress and peptic ulcers. However, the chemical mechanisms by which stress promotes the development of ulcers have not been identified. It seems likely that a stressful lifestyle works in combination with food allergies, diets high in animal fat, cigarette smoking, alcohol, and NSAIDS to cause the growth of ulcers. Stress reduction therapies that are effective in relieving hypertension, such as yoga, meditation, biofeedback, and hypnosis, also may help with the symptoms of ulcers.

Vitamin and Mineral Therapies. Butler and Rayner recommend that certain vitamins and minerals may be especially useful in treating ulcers. Supplementary vitamin A seems to help by maintaining the healthy functioning of the mucus-producing cells that line the stomach and protect it from the powerful pepsin acid. Zinc and vitamin E also may be beneficial, they advise, but large doses (more than three times the RDA) should not be used without consulting a physician or health practitioner.

Summary

Everyone experiences some stress in the course of daily living. Over the last few years, many studies have documented that stress is a major factor in the development of atherosclerosis, headaches, hypertension, irritable bowel syndrome, and ulcers. Repeated incidences of stress can interfere with digestion, increase heart rates and blood pressure, alter brain chemistry, and affect metabolic immune functioning. The holistic treatment for stress-related disorders emphasizes a whole-body approach that includes nutritional therapies; vitamin, mineral, and botanical therapies; and stress-reduction techniques such as exercise, massage, yoga, meditation, hypnosis, biofeedback, and relaxation. While some stress cannot be avoided, it can be managed using alternative biological and psychoimmunological therapies that induce the "relaxation response."

Resources

References

Agras, W.S. "Relaxation Therapy in Hypertension." *Hospital Practice* (May 1983): 129–37.

Atkins, Robert C. "Lower Cholesterol: Seventeen Natural Ways to Bring Cholesterol Under Control." *Well Being Journal* (May/June 1994): 1, 5.

Balch, James F., and Phyllis Balch. *Prescription for Nutritional Healing.* Garden City Park, NY: Avery Publishing Group, 1993.

Benson, Herbert. *The Relaxation Response.* New York, NY: William Morrow, 1975.

Beverly, Cal, ed. *Natural Health Secrets Encyclopedia.* Peachtree City, GA: FC&A Publishing, 1991.

Butler, Kurt, and Lynn Rayner. *The Best Medicine: The Complete Health and Preventive Medicine Handbook.* New York, NY: Harper & Row Publishers, Inc., 1985.

Chaitlow, Leon, M.D. *The Body/Mind Purification Program.* New York, NY: Simon & Schuster, Inc., 1990.

Cummings, Stephen, M.D., and Dana Ullman. *Everybody's Guide to Homeopathic Medicine.* New York, NY: St. Martin's Press, 1991.

Feinstein, Alice. *Symptoms: Their Causes & Cures.* Emmaus, PA; Rodale Press, Inc., 1993.

Foster, Steven. *Feverfew.* Botanical Series 310. Austin, TX: American Botanical Council, 1991.

Green, Elmer, and Alyce Green. "The Ins and Outs of Mind–Body Energy." *Science Year* (1974): 137–47.

———."Self-Regulation Training for Control of Hypertension." *Primary Cardiology* (1980, Volume 6): 126–37.

"Headache." *Mayo Clinic Health Letter* (October 1993): 1–8.

"Heading Off Headaches." *The University of California, Berkeley Wellness Letter* 7 (November 1990): 4–5.

"Irritable Bowel Syndrome—Can Medication Help?" *Harvard Medical School Health Letter* (January 1989).

Kirchheimer, Sid. *The Doctor's Book of Home Remedies.* Emmaus, PA: Rodale Press, Inc., 1993.

Krotkiewski, M. "Effects of a Sodium-Potassium Ion-Exchanging Seaweed Preparation in Mild Hypertension." *American Journal of Hypertension* (June 1991): 483–88.

Lenhard, L., and P. Waite. "Acupuncture on the Prophylactic Treatment of Migraine Headache: Pilot Study." *New Zealand Medical Journal* (1983, Volume 96): 663–66.

Malagelada, Juan. "About Stomach Ulcers." *National Digestive Disease Information Clearinghouse Fact Sheet.* NIH Pub. No. 87–676 (January 1987): 1–3.

Margolis, Simeon, and Hamilton Moses III. *The Johns Hopkins Medical Handbook.* New York, NY: Medletter Associates, Inc., 1992.

Murray, Michael, and Joseph Pizzorno. *Encyclopedia of Natural Medicine.* Rocklin, CA: Prima Publishing, 1991.

National Digestive Disease Information Clearinghouse. *Fact Sheet About Stomach Ulcers.* Bethesda, MD: National Digestive Disease Information Clearinghouse, 1993.

O'Brien, Jim. "The Herbal Cure for Migraine Pain." *Your Health* (October 19, 1993): 11–12.

Ody, Penelope. *Complete Medicinal Herbal.* London, England: Dorling Kindersley, 1993.

Ornish, Dean, M.D. *Dr. Dean Ornish's Program for Reversing Heart Disease.* New York, NY: Ballantine Books, 1990.

Panos, Maesimund B., and Jane Heimlich. *Homeopathic Medicine At Home.* Los Angeles, CA: Jeremy P. Tarcher, Inc., 1980.

Parker, G. "A Controlled Trial of Cervial Manipulation for Migraine." *Australian/New Zealand Journal of Medicine* (1978, Volume 8): 589–93.

Petkov, V. "Plants with Hypotensive, Antiatheromatous and Coronary Dilating Action." *American Journal of Chinese Medicine* (1979, Volume 7): 197–236.

Radetsky, Peter. "You Don't Have to Suffer Anymore: How to Handle Headaches." *Your Health* (January 11, 1994): 64–69.

"Ulcers: New Thinking on Causes and Cures." *Johns Hopkins Medical Letter: Health after 50* (December 1990): 4.

Von Kreisler, Kristen. "Sexual Healing." *Your Health* (January 11, 1994): 30–31.

Weil, Andrew, M.D. *Natural Health, Natural Medicine.* Boston, MA: Houghton Mifflin, 1990.

Yuan, Chung San. "Treatment of 103 Cases of Coronary Disease with Ilex pubescens." *Chinese Medical Journal* (1973, Volume 6): 6–7.

Organizations

American Heart Association
7320 Greenville Ave., Dallas, TX 75231.

Chronic Fatigue Immune Dysfunction Society
PO Box 230108, Portland, OR 97223.

Chronic Fatigue and Immune Dysfunction Syndrome Association
PO Box 220398, Charlotte, NC 28222-0398.

National Chronic Fatigue Syndrome Association
919 Scott Ave., Kansas City, MO 66105.

National Digestive Disease Information Clearinghouse
Box NDDIC, Bethesda, MD 20892.

National Foundation for Colitis
444 Park Ave. S., New York, NY 10016.

National High Blood Pressure Information Center
4733 Bethesda Ave., Bethesda, MD 20814.

Additional Reading

Altman, Nathaniel. *Everybody's Guide to Chiropractic Health Care.* Los Angeles, CA: Jeremy P. Tarcher, Inc., 1989.

American Heart Association. *About High Blood Pressure.* Dallas, TX: American Heart Association, 1986.

Chopra, Deepak, M.D. *Perfect Health: The Complete Mind/Body Guide.* New York, NY: Harmony Books, 1991.

"Hypertension: Lower Your Blood Pressure Without Drugs." *Mayo Clinic Nutrition Letter* (May 1990): 2–3.

Moser, M. "Controversies in the Management of Hypertension." *American Family Physician* (May 1990): 1449–60.

National High Blood Pressure Information Center. *High Blood Pressure and What You Can Do about It.* Bethesda, MD:

National High Blood Pressure Information Center, 1987.

Newberry, Benjamin H., Janet Madden, and Thomas Gertsenberger. *A Holistic Conceptualization of Stress & Disease.* New York, NY: AMS Press, Inc., 1991.

Porkett, Manfred, M.D. *Chinese Medicine.* New York, NY: Henry Holt & Co., 1992.

Reid, Daniel. *Chinese Herbal Medicine.* Boston, MA: Shambhala Publications Inc., 1993.

Santillo, Humbart. *Natural Healing with Herbs.* Prescott, AZ: Hohm Press, 1991.

Schwartz, Harry. "Initial Therapy for Hypertension—Individualizing Care." *Mayo Clinic Proceedings* (January 1990): 73–87.

Chapter 10

DRUG ABUSE AND ADDICTION

Most people at one time or another have taken drugs to relieve headaches, indigestion, tension, cramps, fatigue, or anxiety. Many types of drugs exist, each differentiated by the effect they have on the body. Medical (pharmaceutical) drugs, for example, contain chemicals that can prevent, cure, or aid in the recovery from certain diseases and help protect against viral infections and antibiotics that can destroy pathogenic microorganisms.

This chapter discusses another class of drugs that people take not to prevent an illness or eradicate symptoms, but to stimulate pleasurable feelings. They sometimes are referred to as "psychoactive drugs" because they psychologically alter a person's thoughts, feelings, perceptions, or moods. Some of these drugs can become addictive, and alternative treatments are described.

Many people tend to associate psychoactive drugs with illegal substances such as marijuana, LSD, and cocaine. However, alcohol, nicotine, amphetamines, and tranquilizers, which are all psychoactive drugs, are legal in the United States and in many other countries. In fact, according to Gordon Edlin and Eric Golanty in *Health and Wellness: A Holistic Approach,* more than 25 percent of all legal drugs sold in the U.S.—and virtually all illegal drugs—are psychoactive drugs.

According to Edlin and Golanty, many psychological factors contribute to a person initially taking a psychoactive drug. Using a drug infrequently usually is not dangerous or habit forming. In fact, most people are able to tolerate and eliminate small quantities of most drugs without harmful side effects.

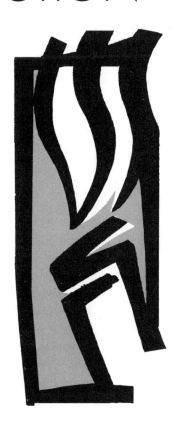

Edlin and Golanty go on to suggest that some individuals, however, for a variety of reasons, become habituated or addicted to a drug. Habituation is defined as the use of a drug to the point that a person becomes psychologically dependent on it. Addiction, on the other hand, is defined as a condition in which the removal of a drug can cause a severe or even fatal physiological reaction.

In the early stages of habituation, each use of the drug increases a person's feelings of pleasure and reduces anxiety, fear, or stress. Eventually, however, habituation can lead to subtle changes in people's rational judgment and their ability to perceive how the drug is affecting their behavior. Personality may become altered under the influence of the drug and, as a consequence, people may put their relationships, jobs, or families at risk.

Drug addiction is more dangerous than habituation because it creates a physiological dependency. Many legal drugs, including barbituates, tranquilizers, analgesics, opiates, alcohol, and tobacco, can be addictive. As discussed below, physical dependency varies with each drug and which parts of the body are affected. When people who are physically addicted to a drug are denied access to it, they go through withdrawal. This process can be extremely painful and difficult because a number of physiological effects occur before the body no longer needs the drug. Even those who take small amounts of heroin can easily become physically dependent on it—and curing this particular addiction is extremely hard. Sometimes, however, people can partly alleviate their physical need for heroin by using another drug, methadone, which is less damaging. The following sections describe the major types of psychoactive drugs, their withdrawal symptoms, and alternative therapies for treating habituation and addiction.

Alcohol

Alcoholism is a leading cause of disease, physical disorders, and death throughout the world. Current estimates indicate that alcoholism affects at least 22 million people in the United States and causes 200,000 deaths each year, making it one of America's most serious health problems. As many as 88 million people in the U.S. are adversely affected by an alcoholic parent, family member, friend, or associate. A 1992 Gallup poll, reported in the October 24, 1993, *New York Times,* found that approximately 81 million Americans have been directly or indirectly hurt by someone else's drinking problem.

Alcoholism, which is partially a genetic disease, involves progressive stages, and is complicated by the fact that drinking, even to excess, is still socially acceptable. In the first stage, people develop a tolerance for alcohol and are able to drink it in great quantities without appearing to be drunk. In the second stage, tolerance increases and people require more alcohol to achieve the desired effect. During this stage, they often become sick from alcohol but deny that they have an illness. In the third stage, people may experience severe withdrawal symptoms if they go without alcohol, and they are at risk of developing several severe physiological disorders. Third-stage alcoholics often black out (alcoholic amnesia) for several minutes to several days during a prolonged drinking binge.

Physiological Effects of Alcohol

The alcohol that humans drink contains a chemical called ethyl alcohol. Most alcohols, including ethyl alcohol, are toxic in small amounts. The human liver metabolizes ethyl alcohol into carbon dioxide and water, which can be eliminated, but alcohol does considerable damage to many parts of the body before it exits. The specific damage varies with each

Physiological Consequences of Alcohol Abuse

Cell Damage. Alcohol causes some metabolic damage to every cell.

Birth Defects. Birth defects can occur in offspring of female alcoholics. Some babies are born with abnormally small heads or mental deficiencies. Some babies may also be born with an addiction and experience withdrawal symptoms within the first week of life.

Malnutrition. Because alcoholics sometimes receive more than half of their total calories from alcohol itself, they are more likely to develop eating disorders. Many develop addictions to food, especially sweets, and become obese.

Liver Disease. Many alcoholics develop liver diseases, including alcoholic hepatitis and liver cirrhosis, which can be fatal.

Heart Disease. Alcohol directly poisons the heart muscles and can cause alcoholic cardiomyopathy.

Stomach Disease. Alcohol can cause gastritis and ulcers.

Lung Disease. Alcohol has been linked with greater incidences of tuberculosis, pneumonia, and emphysema.

Nerves. Alcohol increases the risk of polyneuritis (loss of sensation).

Blood and Marrow Disease. Alcohol increases the coagulation of blood, which can lead to anemia and blood and bone marrow defects.

Muscle Disease. Alcohol increases muscle weakness, cramping, and alcoholic myopathy (painful muscle contractions).

Cancer. Alcoholics tend to smoke more, which increases the risk of cancer of the mouth, esophagus, pancreas, and breast.

Impotence. Alcohol directly damages the nerves of the penis and brain, and causes atrophy of the testes in males. Because alcohol also damages the liver, the liver produces less testosterone and more estrogen.

individual and how much alcohol is consumed.

Chronic drinking can impair memory and cause degeneration of white brain matter, as well as brain damage and premature senility. Edlin and Golanty list obvious signs of alcohol intoxication as drowsiness, judgment errors, loss of inhibitions, poorly articulated speech, uncoordinated movement, and involuntary, rhythmic movements of the eyes.

At one time, it was believed that chronic drinking killed nerve cells in the brain which, once dead, could not regenerate or be replaced. A Danish study, however, found that alcohol does not kill the nerve cells, but disconnects them. According to an Associated Press report on November 12, 1993, the Danish scientists compared the brains of eleven severely alcoholic men who died to those of eleven dead men who were not alcoholics. Using a sophisticated technique, the scientists counted the number of nerve cells in tissue-thin slices of the neocortex, the outermost region of the brain. The number of nerve cells, according to Dr. Bente Pakkenberg, director of the Neurological Research Laboratory at the Bartholin Institute in

Vitamin, Mineral, and Botanical Treatments for Alcoholism

Zinc. Zinc supplementation, combined with vitamin C, greatly increases alcohol detoxification.

Vitamin A. Vitamin A deficiency, along with zinc deficiency, appears to be linked to alcoholism. Vitamin A supplementation inhibits alcohol consumption in experimental animals.

Amino Acids. Serum amino acid levels are abnormal in alcoholics, and restoration to normal levels generally helps these patients.

Vitamin C. Supplemental vitamin C helps reduce the effects of acute and chronic ethanol toxicity. Vitamin C increases white blood cell count, helps eliminate alcohol from the blood, and detoxifies the liver.

B Vitamins. Most alcoholics have a vitamin B deficiency. B vitamin supplements, especially thiamine (B2), may be helpful.

Selenium. Selenium, an important antioxidant, works synergistically with vitamin E to prevent alcohol-induced lipoperoxidation, or the oxidation of fats.

Fats. Alcohol induces essential fatty acid deficiency.

Glutamine. Supplementation of glutamine, an amino acid found in many proteins in the body, has been shown to reduce voluntary alcohol consumption in several studies.

Copenhagen, was "almost identical in the two groups." Nevertheless, the alcoholics did show significant damage to their white matter—the cells and fibers that support and nourish neurons, which carry signals throughout the brain. In the Danish study, the alcoholics' white matter was reduced by 11 percent in the outer brain region and 30 percent in a deeper area that contains the memory center. The findings suggest that cerebral damage caused by heavy drinking may be potentially reversible.

Conventional Treatments for Alcoholism

Conventional medicine has sometimes treated alcoholic patients with aversive drugs. One such drug, disulfiram (Antabuse), has proven helpful in deterring impulse drinking by blocking the metabolizing of alcohol.

People who have alcohol in their blood and take disulfiram normally experience headaches, flushing, and nausea within thirty minutes. While disulfiram effectively discourages people from drinking, in rare cases it can lead to a buildup of toxic substances and may have side effects such as impotence, liver damage, drowsiness, and fetal anomalies in pregnant women. Disulfiram cannot be used by persons with thyroid, liver, or kidney problems or diabetes, reports Steven Schroeder in his 1992 book, *Current Medical Diagnosis and Treatment.*

Alternative Treatments for Alcoholism

Holistic treatments focus on treating underlying psychological factors that may cause alcoholics to drink to excess. In the first stage of treatment, patients are forced to acknowledge that they have a chemical or psychological dependence on alcohol. Social support for both the patient and family is very important during this stage, and patients often choose to join groups such as Alcoholics Anonymous (AA). Programs such as AA always prohibit drinking, and although strict abstinence is not always followed, it has proven the safest and most effective treatment. This is largely because of the support, encouragement, and acceptance offered by those in the group.

Holistic practitioners also have treated alcoholism with various diets. In general, as explained by Michael Murray and Joseph Pizzorno in their *Encyclopedia of Natural Medicine,* these diets focus on stabilizing blood sugar levels by eliminating simple sugars and foods containing added sucrose, fructose, or glucose. Alcoholics crave calorie-rich, nutrient-poor foods, especially sugars that increase their desire for more alcohol. Therefore, these foods must be avoided, including all sweets, dried fruit, low-fiber fruits (grapes and citrus fruits), white flour, and instant potatoes. Meat normally is restricted, to keep protein and fat levels low, and brown rice, whole grains, vegetables, and legumes are used instead.

Holistic physicians may treat alcoholism with vitamin and mineral supplements. The type and amounts of supplements vary with each patient, and most treatment regimens are supervised by a licensed physician or nutritionist.

Alternative practitioners may prescribe botanical medicines that have been used successfully in limited clinical studies. XJL, an ancient Chinese herbal hangover remedy, may help reduce the desire for alcohol and limit excess drinking. In clinical trials conducted at the University of North Carolina, researchers found XJL, an herb that interacts with neurotransmitters in the brain, reduced the desire

for alcohol by up to 60 percent. Previous studies have shown that it effectively reduces hangover symptoms and inebriation levels. According to the September 21, 1993, issue of *Your Health,* investigators speculate that because of the way the herb interacts with the brain, XJL may be capable of reducing cravings for other illegal drugs as well.

Kudzu, an Asian vine, has been used widely in China and Japan since a.d. 200 to treat alcohol abuse. It is available in those countries in pill form, and consumed in tea. Dr. Bert Vallee at the Harvard Medical School has used an extract from the plant, its active ingredient (daidzin), to reduce voluntary alcohol consumption in laboratory animals by more than 50 percent. Daidzin produces no significant change in food intake or body weight, and Vallee says he hopes the drug will soon be ready for clinical testing in humans. "I believe we will come up with a pharmacological agent that will have beneficial effects without any deleterious effects," he says, as reported by the *Wall Street Journal* on November 2, 1993.

Holistic treatments for alcoholism usually incorporate an exercise program, to help alleviate the anxiety and depression caused by the disease. Murray and Pizzorno recommend that alcoholic patients exercise 20 to 30 minutes, five to seven times per week, at an intensity sufficient to raise their heart rate to 60 to 80 percent of maximum capacity for the given age group.

Caffeine

Caffeine is the most widely used drug in the United States. The average American consumes an estimated 150–225 milligrams of caffeine daily, 75 percent of which comes from coffee. A typical cup of coffee contains approximately 50 to 150 milligrams, while a cup of tea contains 50 milligrams and a 12-

Caffeine's Effects on the Body

Immune System Suppression. Overconsumption of caffeine (like alcohol) has been demonstrated to have unhealthy effects on the immune system.

Depression. Caffeine intake has been correlated with the degree of mental illness in psychiatric patients.

Heart Problems. Caffeine increases cholesterol levels and heart palpitations and aggravates hypertension.

Fibrocystic Breast Disease. There is strong evidence that overconsumption of caffeine (along with theophylline and theobromine) is linked to fibrocystic breast disease.

Blood Pressure. Even when consumed in moderate amounts, caffeine raises blood pressure. One study of 6,321 adults demonstrated a small but statistically significant elevation in blood pressure when comparing those who drank five or more cups a day to non-coffee drinkers.

ounce can of a cola drink contains approximately 35 milligrams. Some Americans consume in excess of 7,500 milligrams of caffeine per day, according to Murray and Pizzorno.

Although caffeine, a natural substance found in a variety of plants, is consumed by most Americans in coffee, it is also an ingredient in teas, cola drinks, kola nuts, chocolate, and many nonprescription stimulants, pain relievers, cough medicines, cold remedies, alertness tablets, and weight control pills.

In moderate amounts, caffeine increases alertness and physical and mental endurance. In high doses, however, it can produce nervousness, insomnia, tremors, and restlessness. What constitutes a high dose, as well as the effects of the dosage, varies substantially among individuals.

Treatment for Caffeinism

"Caffeinism" is a clinical syndrome in which people develop a mild psychological dependence on caffeine, and must consume increasing amounts to maintain their mental alertness.

Caffeinism is not difficult to treat. Holistic physicians may encourage patients to drink green tea, which is not roasted and therefore less toxic than coffee, is rich in flavonoid compounds, and may have antioxidant and antiallergy properties. The choice of which green tea to substitute for coffee should be made after consulting with a health practitioner, because some teas contain ephedra, camellia, or cola that can produce insomnia, anxiety, and hypertension. Coffee substitutes are usually prescribed in conjunction with a diet and exercise program.

In the late 1980s, it was believed that caffeine-containing foods, such as tea, coffee, cola drinks, and chocolate, might be responsible for the monthly breast pain and tenderness some women experience, because these substances contain methylxanthines (such as caffeine, theophylline, and theobromine), which are known to stimulate the overproduction of fibrous tissue and cyst fluid. However, various studies have yet to prove an association between methylxanthine and the development of these symptoms or breast cancer. Nevertheless, women with these symptoms who consume large amounts of coffee or chocolate should consult with a physician.

Amphetamines

Students who stay up all night to write term papers and truck drivers who are on the road for 24 hours at a time may well be familiar with amphetamines, chemical compounds that stimulate the sympathetic and central nervous systems and act as euphoriants. People using amphetamines experience increased alertness and elevation of mood and are able to do strenuous physical work. Most amphetamines, including dexedrine, benzedrine, and methedrine are taken orally, although some can be injected.

Amphetamines originally were developed by chemists to help people lose weight, overcome depression, and increase their intelligence. Very few of these benefits, however, have been clinically proven. Excessive intakes of amphetamines can produce headaches, irritability, dizziness, insomnia, panic, confusion, and delirium. In addition, users may experience a rebound crash after several hours, during which they sleep for long periods, and may become very tired or, in some cases, progress to depression.

Alternative Treatments for Amphetamine Dependency

Amphetamines are not physically addictive, but people can become psychologically dependent on the euphoric moods the drugs produce, as do people who use amphetamines to lose weight. In some cases, the dependency is difficult to treat because of the so-called "yo-yo cycle." People first use the drugs to stimulate their nervous system and to stay awake. Later, they may take a depressant to go to sleep. After they wake up, they need more of the stimulant to become alert again. Prolonged use can produce amphetamine psychosis, in which people experience auditory or visual hallucinations or delusions.

Cocaine's Effect on the Body

- Stimulates the central nervous system.
- Produces a short-lived high followed by depression and craving.
- Depletes the brain's supply of natural chemicals such as norepinephrine and dopamine.
- Acts as a local anesthetic to relieve pain and numb tissues.
- Constricts the blood vessels.
- Increases temperature, heart rate, and blood pressure.
- Depresses appetite.
- Relaxes and anesthetizes the throat, larynx, and lower respiratory tract.

The holistic treatment substitutes natural stimulants for amphetamines to break the first stage of the yo-yo cycle. If the abuser has a normal heart rate, aerobic exercise then is used to replace drug depressants so that the muscle system tires naturally. Gradually, through diet, exercise, botanical supplements, and psychological counseling, natural brain endorphins are activated and patients no longer require the amphetamines.

Cocaine

More than 25 million people in the U.S. have tried cocaine, 10 million regularly use the drug and half of them suffer serious problems. Each day, 5,000 Americans reportedly try cocaine for the first time. Twenty percent (more than 1 million) of those who continue to use it eventually become addicted, accord-

Dangers of Cocaine Addiction

- Snorting cocaine can cause perforated septums (tiny holes in the nasal membranes).

- Intravenous users often share needles and "works" and thus suffer the risk of hepatitis, AIDS, and other diseases.

- Smoking cocaine can seriously damage the lungs.

- Chronic use can produce affective disorder, schizophrenia, and personality disturbances.

- Other side effects include tremors, twitching, malnutrition, sexual dysfunction, insomnia, paranoia, auditory or visual hallucinations, psychosis, coma, strokes, seizures, liver damage, heart failure, and respiratory arrest.

- Sudden death can occur in otherwise healthy people.

ing to an article by Joseph Treaster in the *New York Times,* July 16, 1993.

Cocaine is derived from the leaves of the coca plant, which is found primarily in South America. After the plant is grown, the coca leaves are made into either a paste or a powder. Coca paste is popular in South America, and is smoked with tobacco or marijuana cigarettes. Most cocaine found in the U.S. is a white powder (cocaine hydrochloride) that is sniffed through the nose or mixed with water and injected.

"Freebase" is a purified, concentrated form of cocaine paste that is heated and smoked. It is chemically stronger than cocaine powder, which usually is mixed ("cut") with baking soda or other solvents. People addicted to cocaine powder often progress to freebase because it contains more pure cocaine. "Crack" is a rock form of freebase, prepared in vials or sticks, that is easier to sell and to smoke—either in a water pipe or after being added to tobacco or marijuana cigarettes.

Cocaine Withdrawal

Because cocaine is physically addictive, people attempting to withdraw from it often experience sweating, muscle tremors, accelerated heart rate, weight loss, malnutrition, sexual dysfunction, anxiety, panic, insomnia, paranoia, and hallucinations, according to Barbara Yoder in *The Recovery Resource Book.* As they report, even more serious side effects of withdrawal can include psychosis, coma, strokes, seizures, liver damage, heart failure, and respiratory arrest. Withdrawal symptoms usually occur within 24 to 48 hours of the last dose and may continue for seven to ten days.

Several conventional treatments have been partially successful in curing addiction or alleviating withdrawal symptoms. Buprenorphine, a painkiller, produces abstention in some addicts. Desipramine, an antidepressant, reduces cravings and helps abstention in many difficult-to-treat patients. Flupenothixol, also an antidepressant, promoted abstinence for an average of 24 hours in one clinical trial. Carbamazapine, an antiseizure drug, can reduce craving and prevents seizures brought on by chronic cocaine use, Yoder reports.

Alternative Treatments for Cocaine Addiction

Holistic treatment for cocaine addiction, similar to that for alcoholism, focuses on rebuilding the addict's immune system and preventing the depression that occurs during the withdrawal period. Normally the addict is given group and family therapy and least-invasive antidepressants.

A key component of alternative treatment is denying the patient access to more cocaine. Some physicians may decide to control all of the addict's funds and to require routine urine testing for cocaine. If patients find it impossible to stay away from cocaine, temporary hospitalization may be necessary. As any treatments must prevent relapse, most therapists try to prevent the cues that trigger cravings. The American Council on Science and Health, in an April 1990 report, states that long-term treatment must focus on helping the patient build a full and satisfying life without cocaine while coping with the stresses that could bring on a relapse. Recovery for cocaine addicts almost always requires intensive psychological support, and groups such as Narcotics Anonymous have been very effective, according to R. DiGregorio in the January 1, 1990, issue of *American Family Physician.*

Possible Health Dangers of Chronic Marijuana Use

- Marijuana increases heart rate and blood pressure.
- Marijuana produces slight depression of immune system functions.
- Marijuana may decrease alertness and intellectual abilities.
- Marijuana smoke contains carcinogens, and users risk developing lung cancer. There is no evidence that marijuana inhibits some kinds of cancer, although it can relieve pain and discomfort associated with cancer.
- Marijuana users sometimes develop bronchitis sinusitis, asthma, increased nasal secretions, stuffiness, frequent colds, sore throats, and chronic inflammations.

Marijuana and Hashish

Marijuana and hashish, products of the Cannabis sativa plant, have been used as medicines in many different cultures. Marijuana, which is the leaves of the plant, is smoked or added to foods and teas. Hashish is a concentrated form of marijuana made by burning cannabis leaves and collecting the leftover resins into a brown gummy powder.

Tetrahydrocannabinol (THC) is the psychoactive constituent of marijuana. When the plant is smoked, THC is inhaled into the lungs, absorbed into the blood, and transported throughout the body. A small amount of THC in the bloodstream produces a euphoric state. Many people experience a sense of relaxation, and occasionally an altered perception of space and time. Some speech

impairment may occur, along with short-term memory loss. Different subspecies of marijuana vary substantially in THC content. Female plants (sensimilla marijuana), for example, have no seeds and are reported to have ten times the concentration of THC as either male or hermaphrodite plants.

Physiological Effects of Marijuana and Hashish

THC can be highly addictive in some individuals. High doses have been known to produce anxiety, panic, hallucinations, and paranoias. Marijuana and hashish also may complicate prior mental health problems or negative mood swings. Nevertheless, long-term use has not been proven to cause permanent changes in brain function or chemistry, nor has either marijuana or hashish been found to lead inevitably to the use of other drugs, according to a 1991 report of the National Academy of Sciences on "Marijuana and Health."

Opiates

Opiates are a class of compounds extracted from the opium poppy, Papaver somniferum, which contains several different chemicals that are isolated or mixed together to produce heroin, morphine, codeine, or opium. All opiates can cause physical dependence and produce serious withdrawal systems.

Heroin, derived from morphine, is a semisynthetic narcotic first manufactured in 1889 by the Bayer pharmaceutical company. It was originally marketed as a pain reliever for chronic coughs and was later used to treat opium, alcohol, and morphine addictions. Heroin is now illegal in the U.S., although it is still produced illegally in the Southwest. It is inhaled, smoked, or injected, and is often cut with dangerous substitutes. The heroin typically sold on American streets, for example, often contains only 1 percent heroin—the rest consists of cornstarch, cleansing agents, or strychnine.

Heroin affects the body as soon as it enters the bloodstream and reportedly produces extreme states of euphoria. Prolonged use leads to addiction, and large doses can result in death. Heroin does not cause any fatal diseases and does not directly damage internal organs. Rather, it triggers a reaction in the brain's respiratory center that can cause a person to stop breathing. Many users die as a result of injecting it, because they either destroy their veins or contract serum hepatitis or HIV through contaminated needles. A pregnant woman addicted to heroin can transfer the drug to her fetus, which will become addicted even before it is born.

Withdrawal from heroin usually begins four to eight hours after the last dose and lasts about a week. The physical discomforts of withdrawal typically involve insomnia, diarrhea, cramps, nausea, vomiting, and painful involuntary muscle spasms.

Treatments for Heroin Addiction

There is no known cure for addiction to heroin. The current treatment relies on methadone, a synthetic narcotic that eliminates the desire for heroin but is also addictive. Once on a methadone maintenance program, however, heroin users can eventually live without heroin. Several new drugs which block the effects of heroin on the central nervous system also show promise, as do antidepressants such as Prozac.

Alternative medical therapies can help people undergoing methadone treatment strengthen their immune systems. Nutrition, vitamins, and botanicals can be used to alleviate the heroin withdrawal symptoms.

Psychedelic Drugs

Drugs that produce changes in a person's psychological perception of reality are defined as psychedelic. As these altered perceptions sometimes include visual hallucinations, these drugs are called hallucinogens. People under the influence of one of these drugs usually are aware that their hallucinations are caused by the drug and eventually will disappear. The most potent psychedelic is lysergic acid diethylamide, or LSD. Other psychedelic drugs include mescaline (peyote), STP, DMT, DET, PCP (phencyclidine hydrochloride), and psilocybin mushrooms.

Hallucinogens are extracted from more than 100 plants or synthetically produced in laboratories. Psychedelic plants include datura, harmine, kava, morning glory seeds, and nutmeg. Both natural and synthetic psyche-delics are usually ingested orally.

Hallucinogens normally take effect in 45 to 60 minutes, and can result in sweating, nausea, increased body temperature, and dilation of the pupils. Although many hallucinogens have not been fully researched, most of the available studies suggest that they are not addictive. They can, however, produce a psychological dependence. Hallucinogens do not appear to produce any withdrawal symptoms, and no conclusive evidence exists that they cause permanent physiological or genetic damage or birth defects.

Mescaline, the active component of the peyote plant, is grown primarily in Mexico. It is sold dried and sliced or sometimes purified into a powder called mescaline sulfate. Most so-called mescaline sold in tablets and capsules is LSD, PCP, or both. Mescaline has a bitter taste that can cause nausea or vomiting. Peyote is stronger than mescaline and contains other alkaloids, some of which are toxic. Psilocybin and psilocin are the active components of several species of mushrooms that grow in many areas of the world, and are very powerful drugs with effects comparable to those of LSD. They are not illegal and are sold without a prescription.

Angel dust, also known as PCP, originally was developed as an anesthetic. PCP either stimulates or depresses the central nervous system, depending on its dosage and in what form it is taken. It can trigger hallucinations in some people. Users normally take it to elevate their mood or to relax. Edlin and Golanty report that pure PCP is not physiologically addictive, although the PCP sold on the streets is often mixed with other drugs and can be lethal. PCP's physiological effects are summarized below.

Physiological Effects of PCP

- PCP can create such psychological effects as mental confusion, restlessness, disorientation, feelings of depersonalization, and violent or bizarre behavior.
- PCP can result in coma in high doses.
- PCP can interrupt breathing.
- PCP can impair muscular control and cause accidents such as falling from heights and drowning.

Central Nervous System (CNS) Depressant Drugs

CNS depressants constitute the largest class of prescription drugs sold in the U.S., and many are dangerous. Virtually all of them carry some potential for physical or psychological dependency, and some can be lethal in high doses. A large number have not been fully tested, and many of their side effects are still unknown, according to Edlin and Golanty.

They claim that the most widely used legal CNS drugs in the U.S. are tranquilizers. Valium, the best-selling drug in the world at one time, can cause ataxia (the loss of equilibrium and muscle coordination), vertigo, and drowsiness. It also reduces blood pressure and decreases sexual potency. Halcion, a legal sleeping pill, can cause serious side effects including confusion, hallucinations, and amnesia.

Psychologically, CNS depressants can produce a mild state of euphoria that helps some people relax and lose their inhibitions.

With prolonged use, many individuals become addicted to tranquilizers, and it can often take them years to cure their dependency. Withdrawal can be extremely painful psychologically, and users may experience deep depression and hallucinations.

Alternative Treatments for CNS Depressants

Holistic practitioners treat CNS depressant dependency with vitamin and mineral supplements, botanical medicines, and diet programs. The alternative treatment for each drug varies with its chemical nature. Treatment usually includes substituting a natural, nontoxic tranquilizer for the synthetic drug tranquilizer. Holistic physicians also use nutrition, exercise, and group therapy to alleviate the underlying psychophysiological factors involved. The initial difficult stages of withdrawal are eased most effectively when undertaken with medical advice and the assistance of a support group or counselor.

Nicotine

According to Edlin and Golanty, more than 400,000 Americans die each year as a result of smoking tobacco, while another 10 million suffer from diseases related to smoking. Cigarette smoking is responsible for 85 percent of lung cancers in the U.S, and heavy smokers suffer 20 times the rate of lung cancer than nonsmokers. Nevertheless, more than 50 million Americans continue to smoke cigarettes.

Even nonsmokers, especially children, can develop lung cancer by being exposed to tobacco smoke. According to the Environmental Protection Agency (EPA), children exposed to secondhand tobacco smoke are more likely to suffer lower respiratory tract infections, reduced lung function, and ear infections. The EPA and the Centers for Disease Control estimate that secondhand smoke annually causes three thousand deaths from lung cancer, 150,000 to 300,000 cases of bronchitis and pneumonia in youngsters, and asthma attacks in more than twice that number, the *New York Times* reported on November 7, 1993.

Nicotine is the principal component of tobacco products, although as many as 4,000 other chemical substances are released and carried in tobacco smoke, including carbon monoxide, methanol, nitrous dioxide, traces of mineral and radioactive elements, acids, and insecticides. There are several species of the tobacco plant, and the toxicity of particular brands of cigarettes or pipe tobacco varies depending on the soil and climate in which the species is grown and the chemicals with which it is treated.

Conventional Treatments for Nicotine Addiction

People who smoke tobacco can become either psychologically or physiologically addicted to nicotine. There are many therapies for treating nicotine addiction, and each year approximately 20 percent of the 50 million smokers in the U.S. attempt to give up smoking. More than 85 percent of all smokers who quit do so on their own, without the aid of smoking cessation programs or products, according to Yoder in *The Recovery Resource Book*. Most people who quit indicate in surveys that they did so because they were worried about cancer or other diseases they knew were linked to smoking.

The best way for people to permanently stop smoking depends on the nature of their addiction. People who are chemically addicted may need a chemically based therapy, such as nicotine gum or a nicotine-like drug that satisfies their dependence on nicotine. A significant number of American smokers successfully quit each year using gum therapies. Chewing gum replacements, when combined with psychological counseling, are successful in 38 percent of cases where addiction is cured.

Other chemical aids for smoking cessation, such as the nicotine patch, nicotine aerosol, or nasal nicotine solutions currently are being studied. However, the side effects of nicotine patches—which release a constant low-level stream of nicotine into the blood stream—are controversial. In 1992, for example, a Massachusetts hospital claimed it treated five heart attack victims who had been smoking while using the patches. Also, nicotine patches apparently do not supply a powerful enough jolt to overcome the need to smoke. After a person inhales a cigarette,

nicotine reaches the brain in only seven seconds, faster than injecting nicotine directly into a vein. In contrast, patches take nearly four hours to reach peak strength. For this reason, some manufacturers have begun to increase the nicotine in patches to equal the amount found in a pack of cigarettes. Nasal inhalers and sprays appear to be more effective. In one British study, 26 percent of smokers using a nasal spray to administer nicotine quit smoking, according to an article by Eben Shapiro in the November 8, 1993, *Wall Street Journal*. Whatever alternative is used, however, the key to success, according to Shapiro, appears to be a strong desire on the part of the user to stop smoking—a habit that is about 75 percent psychological.

Of those smokers who attempt to quit, only 6 percent are able to do so "cold turkey." However, a study conducted at the University of California, San Diego, from 1992 to 1993 showed that when smokers are encouraged to smoke less and quit intermittently, rather than making the difficult choice of stopping immediately, they have a good chance of eventually dropping the habit for good. Of those taking part in the study, 26.7 percent were able to stop smoking, approximately twice the rate of those trying to quit without the program. The study also found that restriction of smoking at home and at the workplace is a factor contributing to successful quitting. The study was based on interviews with 4,624 Californians who were asked about their smoking habits and history, and interviewed again eighteen months later, the Associated Press reported on November 14, 1993.

Alternative Treatments for Nicotine Addiction

Alternative treatments for nicotine addiction, as with other substance dependencies, incorporate vitamins and botanical supplements, nutrition, and exercise. If a person has a chemical addiction, a holistic physician may use nicotine gum along with vitamin supplements to help the lungs recover from the adverse effects of nicotine and to ease withdrawal symptoms. Dr. Leon Chaitow's detoxification program, as detailed in his book *The Body/Mind Detoxification Program,* recommends the following vitamin supplements: vitamin A, vitamin C, vitamin E, and one high potency B-complex vitamin. The herb obeline (oats) is also reported to be of great value in helping patients stop smoking.

Edlin and Golanty point to other alternative therapies that have proven successful for many people, including hypnosis, group therapy, and stress reduction techniques such as biofeedback and meditation.

In general, holistic therapies for nicotine addiction focus on changing smokers' lifestyles. The American Heart Association (AHA) now claims that smokers who quit dramatically reduce their risk of heart attacks and strokes. In particular, the AHA stresses that diet and vitamin supplements can help former smokers avoid the fatal diseases associated with smoking. In 1993, the AHA released a study in which female survivors of heart attacks or strokes cut their risks of further trouble by eating spinach, carrots, and other fruits and vegetables that contain vitamins C, E, B2, and beta-carotene. In the study, reported by Associated Press on November 9, 1993, researchers found that those whose diets included the highest quantities of these vitamins had a 33 percent lower risk of heart attack and a 71 percent lower risk of strokes.

Treating Drug Addiction with Acupuncture

Chaitow also claims that acupuncture and acupressure have been found effective in clin-

ical trials in which patients quit smoking. Experimental use of acupuncture to treat alcohol and drug addiction has already proven effective in drug treatment programs. The Elmwood Rehabilitation Center in Santa Clara, California, for example, has used acupuncture since 1991 to help patients cure their drug addictions. The city of San Francisco and approximately twelve counties in California offer acupuncture in their drug treatment services, as acupuncture apparently helps people through the difficult first stages of sobriety, according to Maira Alicia Gaura in an article in the *San Francisco Chronicle,* November 1, 1993. Eventually clients are moved into traditional counseling, education, and twelve-step programs.

Terry Rooney, who manages women's treatment services for Santa Clara County's Bureau of Alcohol and Drug Programs, suggests that acupuncture gives people "relief from classic withdrawal symptoms—anxiety, high blood pressure, high stress, tremors, hallucinations." It also helps them sleep and maintain their appetites. Opiate addicts often suffer severe stomach cramps and, according to Rooney, acupuncture relieves this symptom as well.

Dr. Michael Smith of Lincoln Hospital in the Bronx, New York, has used acupuncture for nearly two decades. He prefers acupuncture to help heroin, opium, and tranquilizer users because "Methadone and Valium are so addictive. The alternative drugs all create problems of their own. And there is no pharmaceutical treatment effective in quelling the cravings for cocaine." Acupuncture may have psychological benefits as well. The treatments are not threatening, help patients feel better immediately, and enable dialogue with the therapist to take place during the sessions in a relaxing way, Gaura reports.

Summary

Drugs taken under a physician's supervision may be helpful in treating some psychological and physical disorders. However, certain drugs can have hidden side effects and cause physiological or psychological dependency. Psychoactive drugs contain substances that can lead to addiction. Drug abuse is a serious problem in the U.S. A study conducted by researchers at Brandeis University, in Waltham, Massachusetts, for example, concluded that drug abuse was America's "number one health problem." According to the study, in the October 24, 1993, *New York Times,* more than 520,000 Americans die each year as a result of substance abuse, particularly cigarettes, alcohol, or drugs.

The physical and psychological addictions caused by most psychoactive drugs can be treated successfully with alternative medical therapies that combine nutrition, exercise, vitamin and botanical supplements, and changes in lifestyles. In fact, the importance of using holistic treatments for drug addictions was highlighted in the Brandeis study, which concluded that many drug-related deaths "could be reduced, if not eliminated, by changing people's habits."

Resources

References

"Alcoholism." *Your Health* (September 21, 1993).

American Council on Science and Health. "Cocaine: Facts and Dangers." (April 1990): 32–33.

Dicke, William. "Ancient Chinese Herbal Remedy Found to Curb Desire for Alcohol." *Wall Street Journal* (November 2, 1993).

Edlin, Gordon, and Eric Golanty. *Health and Wellness: A Holistic Approach.* Boston, MA: Jones and Bartlett Publishers, 1992.

DiGregorio, R. "Cocaine Update: Abuse and Therapy." *American Family Physician* (January 1, 1990): 250.

Gaura, Maira Alicia. "Drug Addicts Treated with Acupuncture." *San Francisco Chronicle* (November 1, 1993).

Murray, Michael, and Joseph Pizzorno. *Encyclopedia of Natural Medicine.* Rocklin, CA: Prima Publishing, 1991.

National Academy of Sciences. "Marijuana and Health." National Academy of Sciences, 1991.

Schroeder, Steven. *Current Medical Diagnosis & Treatment.* Norwalk, CT: Appleton & Lange, 1992.

Shapiro, Eben. "After Nicotine Patches: Sprays, Pill, Inhalers?" *Wall Street Journal* (November 8, 1993).

"Smoking Doubles Smoke Risk, Study Finds." Associated Press (November 9, 1993).

"Snuffing Out Secondhand Smoke." *New York Times* (November 7, 1993).

"Study: Alcohol Doesn't Kill Cells in Brain." Associated Press (November 12, 1993).

"Substance Abuse is Blamed for 500,000 Deaths." *New York Times* (October 24, 1993).

"Tapering Off Proves Better Way to Quit Smoking." Associated Press (November 14, 1993).

Treaster, Joseph. "Drug Use Making Comeback, Study Says." *New York Times* (July 16, 1993).

Yoder, Barbara. *The Recovery Resource Book.* New York: Simon & Schuster, Inc., 1990.

Organizations

Al-Anon
1372 Broadway, New York, NY 10018.

Alcoholics Anonymous
PO Box 459, Grand Central Station, New York, NY 10163.

American Cancer Society
1599 Clifton Rd. NE, Atlanta, GA 30329.

American Council on Alcoholism
8501 LaSalle Rd., Ste. 301, Towson, MD 21204.

American Council for Drug Education
204 Monroe St., Rockville, MD 20850.

American Lung Association
1740 Broadway, New York, NY 10019.

Hazelden Foundation
Box 11, Center City, MN 55012.

Johnson Institute of Rehabilitation
509 S. Euclid Ave., St. Louis, MO 63110.

National Clearinghouse for Alcohol and Drug Information
PO Box 2345, Rockville, MD 20852.

National Council on Alcoholism
12 W. 21st St., New York, NY 10010.

Nic-Anon
511 Sir Francis Drake Blvd., Greenbrae, CA 94904.

Office on Smoking and Health, Public Information Branch
Parklawn Bldg., 5600 Fishers Ln., Rockville, MD 20857.

Additional Reading

Al-Anon. *Al-Anon Is for Adult Children of Alcoholics.* New York: Al-Anon, 1987.

Alcoholics Anonymous. *Twelve Steps and Twelve Traditions.* New York, NY: Alcoholics Anonymous, 1953.

American Council on Alcoholism. *The Most Frequently Asked Questions About Drinking and Pregnancy.* Towson, MD: American Council on Alcholism, 1988.

Barringer, F. "Youthful Drinking Persists: With Teens and Alcohol, It's Just Say When." *New York Times* (June 23, 1991): Section 4.

Baum, Joanne. *One Step Over the Line: A No-Nonsense Guide to Recognizing and Treating Cocaine Dependency.* New York, NY: Harper & Row Publishers, Inc., 1985.

Fisher, Edwin B., Jr., et al. "Smoking and Smoking Cessation." *American Review of Respiratory Disease* (1990): 702–20.

Gold, Mark. *800-COCAINE.* New York, NY: Bantam Books, 1984.

———. *The Facts about Drugs and Alcohol.* New York, NY: Bantam Books, 1987.

Goodwin, Donald W. *Is Alcoholism Hereditary?* New York, NY: Ballantine Books, 1988.

Gordis, Enoch, et al. "Finding the Gene(s) for Alcoholism." *JAMA* (April 18, 1990): 2094–95.

Hannan, Deborah J., and Alan G. Adler. "Crack Abuse: Do You Know Enough About It?" *Postgraduate Medicine* (July 1990): 141–43, 146–47.

Jeanne, E. *The Twelve Steps for Tobacco Users.* Center City, MN: Hazelden, 1984.

Johnson Institute of Rehabilitation. *Alcoholism: A Treatable Disease.* St. Louis, MO: Johnson Institute of Rehabilitation.

Mumey, Jack. *The Joy of Being Sober.* Chicago, IL: Contemporary Books, 1984.

National Clearinghouse for Alcohol and Drug Information. *Alcohol and the Body.* Rockville, MD: National Clearinghouse for Alcohol and Drug Information, 1988.

RESOURCES

———. *Facts about Alcohol.* Rockville, MD: National Clearinghouse for Alcohol and Drug Information, 1988.

National Institute on Drug Abuse. *Cocaine/Crack: The Big Lie.* National Institute on Drug Abuse, 1989.

———. *When Cocaine Affects Someone You Love.* National Institute on Drug Abuse, 1989.

Pike, Ronald F. "Cocaine Withdrawal: An Effective Three-Drug Regimen." *Postgraduate Medicine* (March 1989): 115–16, 121.

Rogers, Jacqueline. *You Can Stop Smoking.* New York, NY: Pocket Books, 1987.

Weiss, Roger D. *Cocaine.* Washington, DC: American Psychiatric Press, 1987.

Wolf, Phillip A., et al. "Cigarette Smoking as a Risk Factor for Stroke." *JAMA* (February 19, 1988): 1025–29.

RESOURCES

Chapter 11

MENTAL HEALTH DISORDERS

Everyone periodically experiences emotional stress, and most people develop ways to cope successfully with these episodes. Some people, however, for psychological or physiological reasons, cannot control their thoughts, moods, fears, or emotional reactions to stressful life experiences. These people suffer from a variety of mental health disorders, including depression, panic disorders, or psychotic states such as schizophrenia. Each disorder is distinguished by specific symptoms, yet all usually involve some abnormalities in brain biochemistry. This chapter discusses causes of, and alternative treatments for, the most common of these disorders, including depression, phobias, panic disorders, schizophrenia, and insomnia.

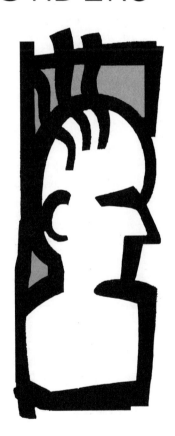

Depression

According to the U.S. Department of Health and Human Services, approximately 1 in 20 Americans (more than 11 million people) suffers from depression in a given year, and for nearly two-thirds, the condition goes undiagnosed and untreated. The annual cost of depression in America is an estimated $43.7 billion, including the costs of suicide, days lost from work, and productivity impairment on the job caused by such symptoms as poor concentration and memory, indecisiveness, apathy, and a lack of self-confidence. The director of the National Institute of Mental Health (NIMH), Dr. Frederick Goodwin, stated in the December 3, 1993, edition of the *New York Times* that among major diseases, clinical depression ranks second only to advanced coronary heart disease in the total number of days patients spend

DEPRESSION

Symptoms of Depression

The American Psychiatric Association (APA) lists the following symptoms to help people determine if they are depressed. According to the APA, if people have five of these symptoms, they definitely are depressed; if they have four, they are likely to be suffering from depression. The APA advises that people who experience these symptoms for at least one month should seek professional medical help.

- Poor appetite with weight loss, or increased appetite with weight gain.
- Insomnia.
- Physical hyperactivity or inactivity.
- Loss of interest or pleasure in usual activities, or a decrease in sexual drive.
- Loss of energy and feelings of fatigue.
- Feelings of worthlessness, self-reproach, or inappropriate guilt.
- Diminished ability to think or concentrate.
- Recurrent thoughts of death or suicide.

in the hospital or disabled at home. Goodwin told *Times* columnist Daniel Goleman: "Major depression is far more disabling than many medical disorders, including chronic lung disease, arthritis and diabetes."

Many life events can cause depression and, in fact, transitory feelings of sadness or discouragement are perfectly normal, especially during difficult times. Ordinarily, most people are able to overcome a temporary

depression within several weeks. People who cannot boost their spirits, however, experience a continuous cycle of depression in which they think increasingly negative thoughts. They often withdraw from their friends and family and lose interest in activities that once brought them pleasure. This withdrawal reinforces their feelings of worthlessness, helplessness, gloom, and futility. Many depressed people also are afflicted with vague physical symptoms or complaints such as stomach aches or pain in the joints. Untreated, the disorder may last six months or more.

Three types of depression were identified by the NIMH in its 1989 publication, *Plain Talk About Depression*. People with major depression are defined as those who have difficulty working, sleeping, eating, or enjoying once pleasurable activities. This form of depression is episodic, and usually occurs only a few times in a lifetime. Dysthymia, a less severe type of depression, involves long-term chronic symptoms that do not disable people from working, but that nevertheless prevent them from feeling good about themselves or their life. The third type of depression is called bipolar disorder (formerly known as manic depression). Bipolar disorders involve cycles of depression (lows) followed by elation (mania). The mood switches can be quite dramatic and rapid—and a person's judgment and thinking abilities may become irresponsible. This is the most serious form of depression and often is a chronic or recurring condition.

The three major forms of conventional treatment for depression are antidepressant medicine (which corrects brain chemistry imbalances), psychotherapy (which is most helpful for those whose personality and life experiences are the main causes of their illness), and a combination of antidepressant medicine and psychotherapy. There are now more than 20 antidepressants available, the most popular of which—Prozac—is prescribed to more than 5 million Americans.

Causes of Depression

According to the U.S. Department of Health and Human Services, in an April 1993 publication entitled *Depression Is a Treatable Illness: A Patient's Guide,* major depressive disorders are not caused by single factors. They are instead brought about by a combination of biochemical, genetic, and psychological factors. Certain life conditions, such as extreme stress or grief, may trigger a natural psychological or biological tendency toward depression. In some people, depression occurs even when life is going well.

The U.S. Public Health Service also suggests that drinking too much alcohol or using drugs can cause depression. When the drug and alcohol use is stopped, the depression usually goes away. Additionally, about 10 to 15 percent of all depression is caused by general medical illness (such as thyroid disease, cancer, or neurologic disease) or by medicines that patients take for those diseases.

It is thought that a disruption in the normal interplay between certain chemicals in brain cells and the neurotransmitters (natural substances that facilitate the passage of impulses from one nerve cell to another) plays an important part in the onset of depression. Of the 100 neurotransmitters scientists have thus far identified, two of them—norepinephrine and serotonin—appear to be most closely tied to depression. Depression also appears to be partly genetic, and scientists hope that once they identify the genes that are associated with it, they can design more effective therapies.

Psychological traumas such as the loss of a parent during childhood, chronic stress, rejections, and failures may contribute to depression. People with certain types of personalities—those with low self-esteem or who tend to be dependent on others, for example—are more vulnerable to depression.

Medical problems can trigger depression in some people. Persons who suffer strokes, thyroid disorders, hepatitis, viral pneumonia, or cancer, for example, are more likely to become depressed. Specific vitamin and mineral deficiencies also may bring on depression in some people. Medications, including barbiturates, tranquilizers, heart drugs, hormones, blood pressure medications, painkillers, arthritis drugs, and even some antibiotics, have been linked with depression, as has chronic alcohol use, according to an article in the November 1990 issue of *The Johns Hopkins Medical Letter: Health After 50* entitled "Depression: Lifting the Cloud."

Depression in the Elderly

Cerebral circulation gradually declines as people get older, which can cause symptoms of depression and mental confusion in the elderly. This is complicated by the fact that elderly people tend to exercise less and may not be able to maintain a healthy diet of natural, unprocessed foods. As a result, older people become more susceptible to the adverse psychological side effects of medications they may be taking for high blood pressure, cancer, or arthritis. Their low moods of depression sometimes are misdiagnosed as Alzheimer's disease or senility and, as a result, appropriate therapy is not sought or provided.

Treatments for Depression

Depression is one of the most treatable mental disorders. Between 80 and 90 percent of all depressed people respond to treatment, according to the NIMH. The holistic approach to treating depression is to first determine what nutritional, environmental, social, and psychological factors may be related to the depressive cycle. A complete medical examination usually is given to identify the overall health of clients, whether they are suffering from illnesses such as hypothyroidism that can bring on depression, and whether they are taking any medications that may contribute to their condition. The evaluation should also include a psychiatric history to outline a patient's emotional background, and a medical status examination to uncover changes in mood, thoughts, patterns of speech, and memory that are symptomatic of depression.

Botanical Therapies. St. John's Wort (hypericum perforatum) appears to relieve minor depression. Researchers have discovered that components in St. John's Wort alter brain chemistry in a way that improves mood. In one clinical study of 15 women with depression cited by Michael Murray and Joseph Pizzorno in the *Encyclopedia of Natural Medicine,* a standardized extract of St. John's Wort significantly reduced symptoms of anxiety, depression, and feelings of worthlessness. The extract also greatly improves the quality of sleep because it relieves both insomnia and hypersomnia (excessive sleep). Additionally, as noted in Chapter 5, ginkgo biloba extract has been effective in treating insufficient blood and

oxygen supply in the brain associated with common symptoms of depression.

Increasing serotonin levels also can help reduce the symptoms of manic depression. Dr. Hugh Riordan, director of the Center for the Improvement of Human Functioning International, suggests in *Alternative Medicine: The Definitive Guide* that people who experience recurring cycles of depression may benefit from drinking walnut tea, which is high in serotonin, an amino acid believed to elevate moods.

Deep Breathing Exercises. Riordan also uses deep breathing exercises to prevent the depressive stage of bipolar disorder. He claims that many studies show that a nondepressed person breathes in six times more air than a depressed person does. Deep breathing exercises increase the amount of air breathed in, raise oxygen levels in the brain, and appear to elevate moods.

Exercise. Exercise is extremely important in preventing and treating depression. A 1988 study by C.E. Ross and D. Hayes, summarized by Murray and Pizzorno in the *Encyclopedia of Natural Medicine,* found that regular exercise reduces stressful emotions associated with depression, reduces muscle tension and anxiety levels, and increases self-confidence and emotional stability. This effect is due to enhanced cerebral circulation resulting from general cardiovascular improvement. As a result, many psychiatrists now encourage their able-bodied patients to take up moderate aerobic exercises such as jogging, walking, or cycling. Regular exercise not only alleviates depression, but also improves concentration, memory, creativity, and mental agility. Physicians normally advise depressed patients to exercise three times a week at a level that elevates their heart rates by 50 percent.

Homeopathic Therapies. According to Dana Ullman in *Discovering Homeopathy,* homeopaths treat both depression and anxiety disorders using a holistic approach. Homeopaths will prescribe individually chosen medicines. When appropriate, they provide basic information on nutrition, exercise, stress management, and lifestyle changes. They also may provide psychological counseling to help the patient deal with the "emotional and mental state" they may be experiencing. Homeopaths, according to Ullman, view human nature as basically creative, and they attempt through different therapies to help the "body and mind adapt to and deal creatively with internal and external stresses."

Lithium. Lithium carbonate, a prescription drug containing lithium, also effectively balances mood swings in patients suffering from bipolar disorder. According to an article in the November 1990 issue of *The Johns Hopkins Medical Letter: Health After 50* entitled "Depression: Lifting the Cloud," lithium is a powerful mood stabilizer and can be used safely without severe side effects. It is not a sedative and prevents extreme high and low mood swings. The article claims that 80 percent of all people suffering from bipolar disorder can be treated successfully with balance-restoring medications. People who regularly take lithium usually suffer fewer

attacks—and the attacks are less severe. If taken in excess, however, lithium can cause intoxication and uncomfortable side effects such as nausea, hand tremors, thirst, fatigue, and muscle weakness. These side effects, if persistent, usually can be alleviated by taking a smaller dose. According to Dr. Roger Kennedy, internist and bioethicist at Kaiser Permanente Medical Center in Santa Clara, persons on lithium may be unable to conserve water, which may result in dehydration and lithium toxicity.

Massage Therapy. Massage therapy has been used to treat depression brought on by trauma. The Touch Research Institute (TRI) at the University of Miami Medical School studied the effect of massage on patients whose depression arose from trauma. The researchers, according to an article by Meredith Ruch in the November/December 1993 issue of *Natural Health,* found that depressed patients had consistently lower levels of stress-related hormones—specifically cortisol and norepinephrine—and were more alert, less restless, and better able to sleep after a 30-minute massage.

Nutritional Therapies. Nutritional therapies may help some individuals because unbalanced diets, food sensitivities, nutrient deficiencies, and food allergies all have been linked to depression. Many patients who complain of depression, according to Dr. Harvey Ross, an orthomolecular psychiatrist in Los Angeles quoted in *Alternative Medicine: The Definitive Guide,* also have hypoglycemia, or low amounts of sugar in their blood. He suggests that depressed people who think they might be hypoglycemic start an individualized diet plan that eliminates simple sugars. He recommends a high-protein, low-carbohydrate diet. In addition to three meals daily, he advises patients to eat smaller snacks every two hours between meals until bedtime. After four months on this diet, Ross recommends that people suffering from depression begin a maintenance diet that avoids processed foods and sugars and adds no more than three servings of fruit a day.

Dr. Leon Chaitow, author of *The Stress Protection Plan,* suggests that one common cause of depression is the excessive use of aspartame, the artificial sweetener widely used in diet colas and foods. He claims that aspartame can cause an allergic or food sensitivity that leads to depression.

James F. Balch and Phyllis Balch stress in *Prescription for Nutritional Healing* that patients suffering from depression, especially bipolar disorder (manic depression) should follow a dietary plan that consists of vegetables, fruits, nuts, seeds, beans, and legumes. Foods that contain sugar or its byproducts should be avoided, along with alcohol, soda, caffeine, and dairy products. All foods that have nitrates, such as additives or food colorings, as well as processed foods, also should be eliminated.

Psychotherapy. A key component of the alternative approach to mental disorders is correctly diagnosing the underlying cause of depression. Psychotherapy can be very helpful, especially if the patient does not have a major personality disorder, related medical problems, or a history of psychosis. Psychotherapists help clients define the psychological or physiological cause of their depression, assist them in setting goals for the outcome of therapy, and monitor how well the goals are being achieved. The final step involves empowering the client to make lifestyle changes that will prevent the depression from recurring. Not all patients can be helped with psychotherapy counseling alone, and a combined approach using psychotherapy and drug therapy may be useful in those cases, according to G. Tollepson in the November 1990 issue of *American Family Physician.*

American health professionals are growing more concerned about the increase of depression in children. It was once thought that childhood and adult depression were unrelated—that a child who was regularly depressed would not necessarily become depressed as an adult. However, a recent study conducted by Dr. Maria Kovacs, a psychologist at Western Psychiatric Institute and Clinic in Pittsburgh, which was reported in the January 11, 1994, issue of the *New York Times,* found that 75 percent of children between the ages of eight and thirteen who became depressed had recurrences of depression in their adult years. According to Kovacs, one of the symptoms of depression in children is their inability or unwillingness to talk about their sadness. They are typically irritable, impatient, cranky, and angry, especially towards their parents.

The best therapy for children suffering from depression usually involves helping them learn more positive ways of reacting to their difficulties. Dr. Gregory Clark, a psychologist at Oregon Health Sciences University, found that 25 percent of students in one high school had a low-level depression, as the *New York Times* goes on to report. Seventy-five students subsequently attended eight weeks of after-school classes in which they learned to change the thinking patterns that lead to depression, improve their skills in making friends and reducing conflict with their parents, and find enjoyable social activities. By the end of the sessions, 55 percent had recovered from their mild depression (about twice as many as in a comparison group that did not attend the classes)—and of that 55 percent, only 14 percent later became seriously depressed.

The *New York Times* article concluded that group therapy also appears to be successful in preventing children from becoming depressed. One experiment led by Dr. Martin Seligman of the University of Pennsylvania proved that it is possible to prevent the emergence of depression in children who are not yet depressed but thought to be at risk because they feel at odds with their parents and show other early signs. In the program, 69 children from ten to thirteen years of age met in small groups once a week for 12 weeks in special afternoon classes. They learned to handle interpersonal disputes; to understand and control moods such as anxiety, sadness, and anger; and to alter pessimistic beliefs that can lead to depression. A year later, 44 percent of the children who did not take the classes developed depression, compared with only 22 percent of the children who had attended the classes.

Vitamin and Mineral Therapies. A substantial amount of research, as discussed in Chapter 3, has shown that deficiencies in vitamins B1, B3, B9, and C may be specifically linked to depression. Several mineral deficiencies, including magnesium and zinc, as described in Chapter 4, also may contribute to depression. As a result, some holistic physicians and nutritionists now believe that sufferers of depression may benefit from vitamin, mineral, and amino acid supplements. However, vitamin and mineral supplements should always be supervised by a physician or alternative health practitioner.

Insomnia

Sleep patterns vary widely among individuals, and although insomnia is not a psychotic disorder like schizophrenia, it has become a chronic mental health problem for an increasing number of Americans. Dr. Sanford Auerback, director of the Sleep Disorders Center at Boston University, estimates in the July/August 1993 issue of *Natural Health* that as many as 15 to 17 percent of Americans suffer from chronic, untreated sleep disorders such as insomnia. A

pamphlet compiled by the American Sleep Disorders Association entitled *How Much Sleep Do You Need?* claims that accidents and loss of productivity due to sleep deprivation cost the U.S. $50 billion per year. As a result of these disturbing trends, President Clinton has signed legislation creating a new National Center for Sleep Disorders at the National Institutes of Health.

Most researchers now think that few people can subsist regularly on less than seven hours a night—the minimum amount of sleep needed to promote continuous daytime alertness. By this definition, many Americans are sleep deprived. Coffee, tea, chocolate, soft drinks, and other foods or drugs containing caffeine are believed to be important factors that prevent people from obtaining an adequate amount of sleep. Nicotine also is a stimulant that prevents normal sleeping behavior.

Treatments for Insomnia

Botanical Therapies. Several plants have sedative effects, including passion flower (passiflora incarnata), hops (humulus lupulus), skullcap (scutellarea latriflora), chamomile (matricaria chamomilla), and valerian (valeriana officinalis). In a large double-blind study involving 128 subjects, reported in a 1992 issue of *Psychopharmacology* (Volume 108, No. 3), valerian root improved the patients' subjective ratings for sleep quality and sleep latency (the time required to get to sleep), and did not leave them feeling lethargic the following morning.

Exercise. When the body is exercised, it becomes naturally fatigued—and most people who exercise regularly find it much easier to fall asleep naturally. H. Kaplan, in his book *Modern Synopsis of Comprehensive Textbook of Psychiatry*, cites several studies indicating that regular aerobic exercise helps promote healthy sleeping patterns. However, exercise

Guidelines for Getting a Good Night's Sleep

The National Institute on Aging suggests the following sleep strategies for people who experience difficulty falling asleep at night:

- Exercise in the morning or afternoon, not immediately before bedtime.
- Avoid coffee, colas, or teas within three hours prior to bedtime.
- Alcohol and cigarettes distort sleep, so avoid them.
- Relax for an hour or so before going to bed. Read, listen to music, or take a warm bath.

- Consciously relax each muscle area progressively when going into bed. Start with the toes and move toward the head.
- Try to adjust the internal sleep clock by getting some exposure to natural light in the afternoon.
- Keep the bedroom quiet and dark and set the temperature to a comfortable level.
- If a nap is needed, it should be taken in the afternoon rather than in the morning or early evening.

should not be performed just before bedtime. It should be of moderate intensity and last a minimum of 20 minutes to achieve the aerobic effect of a heart rate between 60 to 75 percent of maximum.

Homeopathic Therapies. Dr. Stephen Cummings and Dana Ullman in *Everybody's Guide to Homeopathic Remedies* suggest that homeopathic formulas can be very helpful for occasional insomnia, including nux vomica, coffea pulsatilla, passiflora, arnica, and chamomilla. They advise patients with recurrent or chronic insomnia to seek professional homeopathic care.

Hormone Therapy. Melatonin is a hormone produced by the pineal gland in the brain that regulates the body clock and induces sleep. As reported in the April 1994 issue of *Your Health,* a synthetic version of melatonin has been used successfully to treat insomnia. Neuroscientist Richard Wurtman of the Massachusetts Institute of Technology gave subjects either melatonin or an inert placebo substance, placed them in a dark

room at midday, and told them to close their eyes for 30 minutes. In the stressful environment of having to sleep on demand, it took the volunteers with the placebo 25 minutes to fall asleep. Those who took melatonin were able to fall asleep within 5 to 6 minutes. Judith Vaitukaitis of the National Center for Research Resources is quoted in the article as suggesting that melatonin may be a natural, nonaddictive agent that could improve sleep for millions of Americans.

Sleep Therapy. Sleep therapy may be able to help insomniacs sleep better. An experimental study at the Medical College of Virginia, reported in the September/October 1991 issue of *Natural Health,* placed 24 adults (average age: 67) who had suffered from insomnia for an average of 13 years on an 8-week program of sleep therapy. Before, during, and after the study, participants kept a sleep diary in which they recorded their sleep patterns and their emotional reactions to sleep. During the 8-week program, researchers instructed participants to use their beds only for sleep and sex, and to forego reading, watching television, or eating in bed. After the 8 weeks, more than half of the participants reported that they were sleeping better with fewer awakenings. Although almost 50 percent had used sleeping pills before the study, none resumed these medications in the year following therapy.

Panic Disorders and Phobias

Everyone occasionally is frightened by something, and most people learn to overcome common fears or learn to live with them. Some people, however, suffer from intense fears (phobias) or panic disorders that they cannot control and that can seriously disrupt their lives. According to the NIMH pamphlet, *Useful Information on Phobias and Panic,* panic disorders afflict approximately 3 million Americans. Victims usually report experiencing intense, overwhelming terror for no apparent reason. The fear is accompanied by sweating, heart palpitations, hot or cold flashes, trembling, choking, shortness of breath, chest discomforts, and dizziness. People suffering such an attack for the first time often rush to a hospital, convinced that they are having a heart attack.

People who suffer from simple phobias have fears of specific objects or situations. Common examples include fear of heights (acrophobia), fear of open spaces (agoraphobia), fear of enclosed spaces (claustrophobia), fear of dirt and germs (mysophobia), fear of snakes (ophediophobia), and fear of animals (zoophobia). Simple phobias, especially fears about animals, are common in children, but they are known to occur at all ages. The recognition by most phobics that their fears are unreasonable does not make them feel any less anxious, although their phobias normally do not interfere with daily life.

People with social phobias are intensely afraid of being watched and judged by others, which manifests as shyness or avoidance of social situations such as public speaking, eating in public, or going to parties. Social phobias usually begin between the ages of 15 and 20 and, if left untreated, continue through much of a person's life. Sufferers may have difficulty breathing in such situations, or fail to remember what to say or how to act appropriately.

Causes of Panic Disorders and Phobias

Scientists do not agree on what causes panic disorders. They appear to run in families, which suggests the disorder is partly genetic in origin. Psychotherapists believe that disordered thinking in some people produces an anxiety level that can trigger panic attacks. Biochemical theories point to possible physical defects in a person's autonomic nervous system. General hypersensitivity in the nervous system, for example, can increase arousal. Chemical imbalances created by caffeine, alcohol, or other agents can also trigger these symptoms.

Treatments for Panic Disorders and Phobias

Biofeedback and Relaxation. Many people who suffer from anxiety, panic attacks, and phobias show patterns of hyperventilation and shallow breathing. Chaitow notes that these people often report a sense of oppressive pressure on the chest and an inability to take a full breath. According to Chaitow, biofeedback, relaxation exercises (such as yoga, meditation, or tai chi), and visualizations can help stimulate the relaxation response. Once sufferers are relaxed, they can retrain their breathing habits, decrease their hyperventilation, and stimulate a more positive mental state. These techniques, Chaitow relates, are widely used in Europe to treat chronic phobias and anxiety.

Homeopathic Therapies. Ullman describes two psychotherapeutic treatments that he considers homeopathic in their approach to treating phobias: "paradoxical intention" and "therapeutic double-blind." Both approaches aim at dislodging the symptoms and setting in motion the natural healing process of the brain. The homeopathic therapist encourages the patient to pretend to experience the problematic emotional state. If the patient has a phobia of snakes, for example, the therapist asks him to pretend to see a snake and to pretend to feel afraid. Ullman states that this method is considered effective if the client is unable to produce the fear at will and afterwards, as a result, is less susceptible to having the phobia at other times.

Psychotherapy. Psychotherapy helps people think and act appropriately by making the feared object or situation less threatening through group support and desensitization. Group therapy, with or without individual therapy, is valuable for those with low self-esteem because they may find it easier to accept criticism or guidance from group members than from a therapist. Family members and friends can play an important role in the treatment process if they provide support, assistance, and encouragement.

Schizophrenia

The NIMH, in its pamphlet entitled *Schizophrenia: Questions and Answers,* estimates that at least 2 million Americans suffer from the disabling symptoms of schizophrenia. The economic costs of the disease, in terms of patient care and lost productivity, are estimated to run as high as $20 billion a year.

Schizophrenia, according to the NIMH, can be one psychotic disorder or many different disorders. To be psychotic means to be out of touch with reality, or unable to separate real from unreal experiences. There are several degrees of schizophrenia ranging from mild schizophrenic disorder (paranoia) to severe chronic, deteriorating schizophrenia. People with mild schizophrenia have infrequent psychotic episodes and can lead relatively normal lives during the interim periods. Chronic schizophrenics, on the other hand, tend to suffer from prolonged depression, personality problems, fatigue, mental derangement, or hallucinations. They usually cannot lead normal lives and require long-term treatment, which often necessitates institutionalization and controlled medication to alleviate the symptoms. Some schizophrenics suffer from hallucinations or sense things that in reality do not exist, such as hearing voices.

Another group of schizophrenics experiences delusions, or false personal beliefs that are not subject to reason or contradictory evidence. These people feel they are being persecuted, watched, or followed by other people, or they have delusions of grandeur. Another class of schizophrenics suffers from disordered thinking. They may not be able to think clearly, or may experience thoughts that they cannot control. Schizophrenics also sometimes exhibit what is called "inappropriate affect"—that is, they show emotions that are inconsistent with their own speech or thoughts. For example, schizophrenics may say they are being persecuted by demons and then laugh. They also may exhibit prolonged extremes of elation or depression. In these cases, the NIMH urges physicians to determine whether the patient is schizophrenic or suffering from bipolar disorder.

According to the NIMH's pamphlet, *Useful Information on Paranoia,* paranoid schizophrenia is characterized by suspiciousness (or mistrust) that is either highly exaggerated or not warranted at all. Extreme paranoid schizophrenics often experience bizarre delusions or hallucinations. They may claim to hear voices that others cannot hear, or believe that their thoughts are being controlled or broadcast aloud. In contrast, people with milder paranoid disorders may experience delusions of persecution or delusional jealousy, but not hallucinations. These people usually can live a relatively normal existence because, apart from occasional delusions, their thinking remains clear and orderly.

Causes of Schizophrenia

Scientists do not know precisely what causes schizophrenia. It was once thought that traumatic events such as family divorce, the loss of a parent, or other tragedies caused the disorder. Recently, genetic scientists have speculated that schizophrenia is hereditary. A study by the NIMH seems to indicate it is not. As related in the March 22, 1990, issue of the *New England Journal of Medicine,* scientists used sophisticated scanning devices to examine the brain structure of 15 pairs of identical twins (one schizophrenic, the other normal) and discovered subtle anatomical differences. In the mentally ill twin, the fluid-filled brain cavities called ventricles were consistently found to be enlarged, indicating that the tissue had either shrunk or developed abnormally. In addition, regions of the brain responsible for thinking, memory, concentration, decision making, and higher mental abilities were abnormally smaller in the schizophrenic twin. Since the genetic material of identical twins is identical molecule for molecule, researchers concluded that the development of the illness must be nongenetic. It is not known whether schizophrenia is caused by a virus, chemical exposure to a toxin, or a metabolic defect, although some experts postulate that it could be partially induced by complications during birth or a head injury.

Whatever the origin of the disorder, scientists agree that altered brain structure and chemistry play a role in schizophrenia. For this reason, holistic physicians usually give schizophrenic patients a complete physical examination, including laboratory tests, to determine the underlying cause (or causes) of their specific disorder.

Treatments for Schizophrenia

Botanical Therapies. Dr. Q. Ma reports in the April 1991 issue of the *Chinese Journal of Integrated Traditional & Western Medicine* that xin shen ling (XSL), a Chinese immunological herbal formula, may prevent relapses of schizophrenia. Thirty Chinese patients suffering from chronic schizophrenia were given XSL rather than neuroleptic medications because these had not proved effective. Sixty-seven percent of the patients clinically improved after six weeks of herbal treatment with XSL.

Medications. One promising treatment for schizophrenia is the antipsychotic drug Clozapine, which has been approved by the FDA for nationwide use. Designed only for schizophrenics who fail to respond to the standard antipsychotic drugs, or who suffer from negative side effects such as anxiety or insomnia, Clozapine appears to counteract excess dopamine in the brain, which is associated with the disorder's symptoms. Clozapine, however, can cause a potentially fatal condition called agranulocytosis, in which the body's ability to produce infection-fighting white blood cells is impaired, as reported by science editor David Perlman in the March 2, 1990, edition of the *San Francisco Chronicle.* Because of that risk, all doctors prescribing the drug must require patients to undergo a white blood cell count every week while taking the medication, so that the medication can be stopped if white cells drop to a dangerously low level.

Vitamin and Mineral Therapies. Dr. Abraham Hoffer, president of the Canadian Schizophrenia Foundation, has successfully treated schizophrenics with megavitamins. Writing in a 1993 issue of the *Journal of Orthomolecular Medicine,* he demonstrates that vitamin B3 (nicotinic acid or nicotinamide) can double the recovery rate of acute schizophrenics. After 10 years of vitamin treatments, 11 of Hoffer's 26 schizophrenic patients are working, two are married and looking after their families, two are single mothers caring for their children, and three are managing their own businesses.

The orthomolecular treatment of schizophrenia developed by Hoffer and others appears remarkably more successful than traditional psychiatric treatment. A followup study of schizophrenics treated by psychiatrists, for example, reported by E. Johnstone in a 1991 issue of *The British Journal of Psychiatry,* showed that only 5 percent of schizophrenics treated by psychiatry showed significant recovery. Hoffer believes that nutritional and orthomolecular therapies combining nutritious foods, vitamins, minerals, and amino acids will soon become the standard treatment for schizophrenia.

Dr. William Walsh of the Carl Pfeiffer Treatment Center in Naperville, Illinois, reports in *Alternative Medicine: The Definitive Guide* that schizophrenia may be related to histamine levels in the blood. He has found that schizophrenics with low histamine levels are much easier to treat with nutritional therapies than those with elevated histamine levels. His medical staff gives folate and nutrients that eliminate excess copper and lower histamine levels. Nervousness, depression, and hallucinations often disappear after several months of treatment. Paranoid symptoms, however, may take as long as a year to subside.

For schizophrenic patients with elevated histamine levels, Walsh's treatments focus on megadoses of calcium that help release excess histamines from body cells. Megadoses of the amino acid methylamine also help eliminate unnecessary histamines. Schizophrenics with high levels of histamines must avoid niacin, folic acid, and green leafy vegetables. In each case, Walsh recommends individual nutritional counseling. Some adult psychotic patients have an excess of copper that may produce a schizophrenic syndrome. Copper excess has been linked to learning and behavioral disorders in children, and Walsh advises that copper levels be decreased in schizophrenic patients.

Summary

Like all other body organs, the human brain is composed of molecules and cells whose functioning is influenced by many factors. Brain tissues can be affected by injury, infectious disease, inherited genetic errors, chemical toxins, and stressful events. When, as a result of one or a combination of these factors, the brain becomes biochemically unbalanced, depression, phobias, and psychotic disorders such as schizophrenia can result.

Mental disorders can pose tragic problems for sufferers and their families. Fortunately, major advances have been made in noninvasive treatment of these disorders. Scientists have begun to map the brain and to identify the specific neurotransmitters that are responsible for emotions—and for mental disorders such as depression, schizophrenia, anxiety, and panic disorders. This chapter has suggested that alternative therapies such as nutrition, vitamins, minerals, amino acids, hormones, botanical medicines, exercise, and massage, when used in a combination with psychotherapy, behavioral therapy, or psychoanalysis, can help treat psychological disorders. The goal of holistic treatment is to return the patient to natural, total mind/body health as quickly as possible in the least invasive way.

Resources

References

American Psychiatric Association. *Diagnostic and Statistical Manual of Mental Disorders* (DSM-IIIR). Washington, DC: American Psychiatric Association, 1993.

Balch, James F., and Phyllis Balch. *Prescription for Nutritional Healing.* Garden City Park, NY: Avery Publishing Group, 1993.

The Burton Goldberg Group. *Alternative Medicine: The Definitive Guide.* Puyallup, WA: Future Medicine Publishing, Inc., 1993.

Chaitow, Leon, M.D. *The Stress Protection Plan.* HarperSanFrancisco: HarperCollins, 1992.

Cummings, Stephen, M.D., and Dana Ullman. *Everybody's Guide to Homeopathic Medicines.* Los Angeles, CA: Jeremy P. Tarcher, Inc., 1991.

"Depression: Lifting the Cloud." *The Johns Hopkins Medical Letter: Health After 50* (November 1990): 4–5.

Freudenheim, Milt. "The Drug Makers Are Listening to Prozac." *New York Times* (January 9, 1994): 7.

Goleman, Daniel. "Childhood Depression May Herald Adults' Ills." *New York Times* (January 11, 1994): D7.

————."Depression Costs Put at $43 Billion." *New York Times* (December 3, 1993): A9.

————. "Scientists Trace Voices in Schizophrenia." *New York Times* (September 22, 1993): 7.

Hoffer, Abraham, M.D. "Chronic Schizophrenic Patients Treated Ten Years or More." *Journal of Orthomolecular Medicine* (1993, Volume 8): 121–23.

"How to Get a Better Night's Sleep." *Natural Health* (September/October 1991): 21.

"How Much Sleep Do You Need?" *Natural Health* (July/August 1993): 21.

Johnstone, E. "Disabilities and Circumstances of Schizophrenic Patients: A Follow-up Study." *The British Journal of Psychiatry* (1991, Volume 159, Supplement 13): 3–46.

Kaplan, H. *Modern Synopsis of Comprehensive Textbook of Psychiatry.* Baltimore, MD: Williams & Wilkens, 1985.

Lader, M. "Rebound Insomnia and Newer Hypnotics." *Psychopharmacology* (1992, Volume 108): 248–55.

Ma, Q. "Immunological Study of Inefficiency Schizophrenics with Deficiency Syndrome Treated with Xin Shen Ling." *Chinese Journal of Integrated Traditional & Western Medicine* (April 1992).

Margolis, Simeon, and Hamilton Moses III. *The Johns Hopkins Medical Handbook.* New York, NY: Medletter Associates, Inc., 1992.

Mesulam, Marsel. "Schizophrenia and the Brain." *New England Journal of Medicine* (March 22, 1990): 842–45.

Murray, Michael, and Joseph Pizzorno. *Encyclopedia of Natural Medicine.* Rocklin, CA: Prima Publishing, 1991.

National Alliance for the Mentally Ill. *Clozapine.* Arlington, VA: National Alliance for the Mentally Ill, 1990: 2–3.

Perlman, David. "New Study, New Drug for Schizophrenia." *San Francisco Chronicle* (March 22, 1990): A17.

Posner, M. "Depression among Women Is Widespread, Survey Says." *Reuters* (July 15, 1993).

Ross, E.E., and D. Hayes. "Exercise and Psychological Well-Being in the Community." *American Journal of Epidemiology* (1988, Volume 127): 762–71.

Ruch, Meredith. "Feeling Down? Study Shows Massage Can Lift Your Spirits." *Natural Health* (November/December 1993): 48–49.

Tollepson, G. "Recognition and Treatment of Major Depression." *American Family Physician* (November 1990): 65S.

U.S. Department of Health and Human Services. *Depression Is a Treatable Illness: A Patient's Guide.* Washington, DC: U.S. Department of Health and Human Services, 1993.

Ullman, Dana. *Discovering Homeopathy.* Berkeley, CA: North Atlantic Books, 1989.

Waldholtz, M. "Study of Fear Shows Emotion Can Alter Wiring of the Brain." *Wall Street Journal* (October 29, 1993): B8.

Wartik, Nancy. "Depression." *American Health* (December 1993): 40–45.

"What Twins Tell Us about Schizophrenia." *U.S. News & World Report* (April 2, 1990): 13–14.

Organizations

American Psychiatric Association
1400 K St. NW, Washington, DC 20005.

Disabled American Veterans
807 Maine Ave. SW, Washington DC 20024.

National Alliance for the Mentally Ill
1901 N. Fort Myer Dr., Ste. 500, Arlington, VA 22209.

National Depressive and Manic Depressive Association
Merchandise Mart, Box 3395, Chicago, IL 60654.

National Foundation of Depressive Illness
245 7th Ave., 5th Fl., New York, NY 10001.

National Institute of Mental Health
Parklawn Bldg. 15C-05, 5600 Fishers Ln., Rockville, MD 20857.

National Mental Health Association
1201 Prince St., Alexandria, VA 22314-2971.

Phobia Society of America
PO Box 2066, Rockville, MD 20852-2066.

Additional Reading

American Psychiatric Association. *Let's Talk Facts About Panic Disorder.* Washington, DC: American Psychiatric Association, 1989.

———. *Manic-Depressive Disorder.* Washington, DC: American Psychiatric Association, 1990.

Griest, J. *Anxiety and Its Treatment: Help is Available.* Washington, DC: American Psychiatric Press, 1986.

National Alliance for the Mentally Ill. *Mood Disorders: Depression and Manic Depression.* Arlington, VA: National Alliance for the Mentally Ill, n.d.

National Institute of Mental Health. *Bipolar Disorder: Manic-Depressive Illness.* ADM 89-1009. Rockville, MD: National Institute of Mental Health, 1989.

———. *Depressive Disorders: Treatments Bring New Hope.* ADM 89-1491. Rockville, MD: National Institute of Mental Health, 1989.

———. *Helpful Facts about Depressive Disorders.* ADM 87-1536. Rockville, MD: National Institute of Mental Health, 1987.

RESOURCES

———. *Schizophrenia: Question and Answers*. ADM 86-1457. Rockville, MD: National Institute of Mental Health, 1986: 1–4.

———. *Useful Information on Paranoia*. Rockville, MD: National Institute of Mental Health, 1989: 1–10.

———. *Useful Information on Phobias and Panic*. ADM 89-1472. Rockville, MD: National Institute of Mental Health, 1989: 5–11.

Sheehan, D. *Anxiety Disease and How to Overcome It*. New York, NY: Scribner Educational Publishers, 1984.

Torrey, Fuller. *Surviving Schizophrenia: a Family Manual*. Revised Edition. New York, NY: Harper & Row Publishers, Inc., 1987.

Wilson, R. *Don't Panic: Taking Control of Anxiety Attacks*. New York, NY: Harper & Row Publishers, Inc., 1987.

RESOURCES

Chapter 12

COMMON MALE
HEALTH PROBLEMS

The most common health problems in men involve disorders of the genitourinary system, which includes the bladder, urethra, prostate gland, penis, and testicles. These disorders may involve infections, weakening of organs, or sexual diseases. For that reason, special attention must be paid to the health of the system in order to maintain normal sexual functioning, proper elimination, and sustained immune resistance. This chapter discusses alternative treatments for common male problems, including low sexual energy and impotence, enlarged prostate (benign prostatic hypertrophy), and prostatitis.

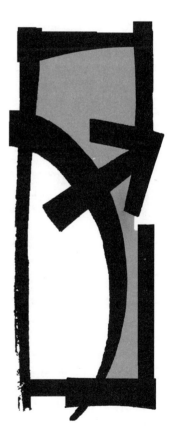

Impotence

As reported by Lawrence Altman in the December 22, 1993, edition of the *New York Times,* the largest study of impotence since the Kinsey report more than 40 years ago suggests that 19 million men from 40 to 70 years of age in the U.S., out of a total of more than 37 million (or 52 percent), may either be impotent or have experienced the problem. That is almost double the current estimate of 10 million, according to the study's senior author, Dr. John McKinlay, who directs the New England Research Institute in Watertown, Massachusetts.

The frequency of impotence reported in the study steadily increased with age. At the age of 40, 5 percent of respondents reported complete impotence. By age 70, the prevalence of complete impotence tripled to 15 percent.

Impotence (technically called male erectile dysfunction), or the inability to sustain an erection, once was linked solely to

IMPOTENCE

Therapies for Impotence

Botanicals: Ask your physician or herbalist about taking coryanthe yohimbe, ginkgo biloba, Siberian ginseng, unicorn root, dong quai, goldenseal, licorice, and saw palmetto supplements.

Nutrition: Reduce fats and increase whole grains and beans, fresh vegetables and fruit, fish, seeds, and nuts.

Vitamins and Minerals: Take vitamins A and B5, magnesium, copper, or zinc supplements.

Other Remedies: Consult your physician about cell therapy, exercise, psychotherapy, injections, or vacuum suction devices.

Other factors contributing to impotence include neurological disorders caused by injury or brain disease, high blood cholesterol, or low levels of the male hormone, testosterone. In addition, it can result from using heroin or other recreational drugs. About 25 percent of impotence cases are a result of medications taken for other conditions. More often, however, impotence problems are caused by a fear of sexual performance (including anxiety about the ability to get an erection), or the wish not to be sexually intimate with a particular partner.

Treatments for Impotence

Each case of impotence varies with the individual's environment, age, sexual history, diet, and level of exercise. A holistic physician may prescribe a low-fatty-acid diet, aerobic exercise, and vitamin, mineral, and botanical supplements to try to correct the condition.

Botanical Therapies. Botanical medicines, in some cases, may offer many of the same therapeutic benefits for impotence as do prescription drugs—and without severe side effects. In *Alternative Medicine: The Definitive Guide,* naturopath Dr. Tom Kruzel of Gresham, Oregon, reports that the botanicals coryanthe yohimbe and ginkgo biloba often are used to treat impotence because of their ability to stimulate vascular flow to the penis. Coryanthe yohimbe also increases libido and decreases the latency period between ejaculations. Kruzel cites a study in the December 1991 *Townsend Letter for Doctors* which found that ginkgo biloba extract increased penile blood flow in a group of patients who had not responded to traditional drug therapies. Half the group regained potency within six months.

N. Farnsworth, writing in *Economic and Medicinal Plant Research,* reports that

emotional causes or to a natural decline in sexual energy due to aging. However, according to McKinlay, it is now thought that the condition has many other causes as well, including medical conditions such as heart disease, diabetes, and high blood pressure; smoking; alcohol consumption; lack of exercise; depression; and repression of anger.

For example, McKinlay notes that men who take drugs for high blood pressure experience varying degrees of impotence. However, two classes of antihypertensive drugs are less likely to cause this condition. One group is known as ACE inhibitors, including captopril (Capoten), enalapril (Vasotec), and lisinopril (Prinivil, Zestril). The other group, called calcium channel blockers, includes diltiazem (Cardizem), nacardipine (Cardene), nifedipine (Procardia), and verapamil (Calan, Isoptin).

Siberian ginseng or panax ginseng has been used in Chinese medicine as an aphrodisiac. Its American counterpart, eleuthrococus senticosus, does not appear to possess the same stimulating properties, but, according to Farnsworth, is safer to use over an extended period of time.

H. Felter, in the *Eclectic Materia Medica,* reports on several studies which suggest that unicorn root (aletris farinosa) is an effective botanical medication for impotence in men. It also has been used to promote fertility in both females and males. Saw palmetto (serenoa repens) may be used to treat impotence and prostate problems, according to Felter, especially when it is combined with other botanical medicines. Dong quai, ginseng, goldenseal, and licorice have been used in Europe as aphrodisiacs, although the Food and Drug Administration (FDA) has not approved them for use in the U.S.

Cell Therapy. Dr. Peter Stephan of the Stephan Clinic in London reports in *Alternative Medicine: The Definitive Guide* that cell therapy has successfully treated impotence in clinical trials in England. Stephan removes cells of erectile tissue from patients' testicles, prostate, or pituitary gland and injects them into the penis. A study using his procedure was conducted with 3,500 men (ranging in age from 22 to 76 years) suffering from sexual disorders, and resulted in a 76 percent success rate.

Exercise. Exercise, especially aerobic exercise, is an important part of maintaining a healthy sexual response. By increasing blood flow to the heart, exercise boosts sexual energy. Jane Brody, in the August 4, 1993, edition of the *New York Times,* cites several large studies of men and women that have demonstrated the positive effects of regular exercise on sexual energy. As a relaxant, body toner, energy booster, antidepressant, and confi-

dence builder, exercise is one of the most accessible, safe, and effective treatments for impotence. Many holistic physicians use exercise to build sexual confidence in their patients.

Homeopathic Therapies. F. Ellingwood, writing in *American Materia Medica, Therapeutics and Pharmacognosy,* describes several homeopathic treatments for male impotence. He suggests that strychnos nux vomica is especially effective in cases where patients have an excess of alcohol, cigarettes, or dietary indiscretions. Male patients with symptoms of impotence should consult a licensed homeopath, as this formula contains small amounts of strychnine alkaloids that can be toxic.

Nutritional Therapies. According to James F. Balch and Phyllis Balch in *Prescription for Nutritional Healing,* diet is one of the most critical factors in male sexuality because androgen levels are directly influenced by the type and amounts of foods men eat. A diet that reduces calories and increases sexual vigor normally includes whole grains and beans, fresh vegetables and fruit, fish, seeds, and nuts. These foods are rich in vitamin E (essential for sexual hormone production and normal erections), as well as minerals such as zinc (which maintains hormonal balance) and the trace elements critical to a normal sex drive.

One important dietary measure for preventing and treating impotence is reducing the percentage of calories men consume as fats. High LDL ("bad") cholesterol levels contribute to both heart disease and high blood pressure, conditions that are directly associated with impotence problems. Conversely, McKinlay found in his study that low levels of high-density lipoprotein (HDL), the "good" form of cholesterol, also were significantly correlated with impotency.

Psychotherapy. Alternative treatments focus on determining what psychological or physiological factors are responsible for erection problems. Psychotherapy or behavioral therapy is used, especially when no physical cause for impotence can be detected. Psychological factors, including low self-esteem, anxiety, and communication problems with one's sexual partner, often contribute to the condition. For best results, the man's sexual partner should be involved in the therapy. In McKinlay's study, men who scored highest on measures of anger had the greatest risk of moderate or complete impotence. Men who were highly depressed were four times as likely to be moderately or completely impotent as were men who were not depressed.

Traditional Chinese Medicine (TCM).

Impotence and premature ejaculation are considered by Chinese physicians to be caused primarily by stress and nutritional imbalances. According to Kruzel, quoted in *Alternative Medicine: The Definitive Guide,* "impotence due to low hormone output is considered a deficiency of kidney yang, while premature ejaculation is viewed as an inability to withhold the semen and is considered a deficiency of the kidney storage vessel."

TCM uses acupuncture and botanical medicines to enhance blood flow. As noted, panax ginseng has long been regarded as an aphrodisiac in Chinese medicine. However, panax ginseng is not recommended for long-term use, and eleutherococcus senticosus often is substituted for it. S. Dharmananda suggests in his book *Your Nature, Your Health—Chinese Herbs in Constitutional Therapy* that lyceum berries are used to treat sexual dysfunctions, including impotence. Other botanicals, such as cascata and lotus seed, also enhance sexual function and eliminate premature ejaculation.

Vitamin and Mineral Therapies. Balch and Balch state that vitamin supplements play an important role in increasing and maintaining sexual energy. Vitamin A, for example, is necessary for maintaining healthy testicular tissue and sex hormone production and helps prevent cancer of the sexual organs. Good sources include liver, eggs, fortified milk, carrots, tomatoes, apricots, cantaloupe, fish, and dark-green leafy and yellow vegetables.

Vitamin B5 (pantothenic acid) found in whole grains, beans, eggs, nuts, organ meats (liver), peanuts, and broccoli regulates the adrenal cortex and increases sexual secretions. Vitamin C also is required for sexual stamina.

Magnesium found in whole grains, raw leafy vegetables, and nuts (especially cashews and almonds) plays a major role in sex organ sensitivity, healthy ejaculation, and orgasm. Copper and zinc deficiencies may lead to impotence or sexual dysfunction and/or infections. Large concentrations of zinc are located in the male prostate gland (and the female ovaries). Good natural sources include oysters, nuts, beans, eggs, raisins, corn oil, margarine, crab meat, liver, and whole wheat bread.

Other Treatments. Simeon Margolis and Hamilton Moses III report in *The Johns Hopkins Medical Handbook* that if nutrition, exercise, and psychological counseling do not produce results, physicians may prescribe other procedures, including vacuum suction devices or injections, as a last resort. In the first option, a vacuum or mechanical suction device is placed around the penis. As air is drawn out of the chamber of the instrument, it creates a vacuum that draws blood into the penis, causing an erection. This procedure is relatively safe, low cost, and noninvasive, and has no documented side effects. Papaverine injection therapy may be prescribed in cases of chronic impotence. This experimental drug increases blood flow to the penis and keeps it firm for several hours. However, as papaverine may have adverse side effects, its use should be supervised by a physician.

Premature Ejaculation

According to David Zimmerman, in *Zimmerman's Complete Guide to Nonprescription Drugs,* about 10 percent of U.S. males suffer from premature ejaculation, which means that orgasm occurs when the penis first enters a woman's vagina, or even before. The majority of men, in contrast, climax about two minutes after entering the vagina. Males who consistently reach climax too soon should consider counseling to determine if any psychological factors may be contributing to this condition.

Treatments for Premature Ejaculation

Ejaculation is a reflex activity that a man can learn to control in a manner similar to controlling bladder function. The key is to become aware of the bodily sensations that signal the onset of ejaculation and to modulate arousal. Holistic physicians usually begin treatment by trying to identify the physical or psychological factors that have been linked to premature ejaculation. Patients who practice coitus interruptus for birth control may be conditioned to ejaculate outside the vagina. In other men, early ejaculation can be caused by anxiety and fear about their sexual adequacy.

According to Zimmerman, the FDA has approved benzocaine and lidocaine as safe, over-the-counter treatments for premature ejaculation. Benzocaine temporarily diminishes penile sensation and thereby helps men delay orgasm. Lidocaine usually is sold in an aerosol spray dispensed from a dose-metered container that delivers measured amounts.

Repeated use, however, may irritate the skin. Condoms also may help delay orgasm by reducing sensitivity. In his book *Your Nature, Your Health—Chinese Herbs in Constitutional Therapy,* Dharmananda reports that lyceum berries, cascata, and lotus seed are natural botanicals that have been found to eliminate premature ejaculation.

Physical Therapies. In certain cases, a physician may prescribe the "squeeze technique." In this procedure, the partner manually stimulates the penis just before the point of ejaculation. To stop the ejaculation, the partner presses a thumb against the underside of the penis with sufficient pressure to deter ejaculation.

Prostate Enlargement

The prostate, the male sex gland beneath the urinary bladder, is the most common site of disorders in the male genitourinary system. The doughnut-shaped gland encircles the urinary outlet, or urethra. Contraction of the muscles in the prostate squeezes fluids into the urethral tract during ejaculation.

According to Balch and Balch in *Prescription for Nutritional Healing,* one-third of American men over the age of 50 develop a prostate enlargement, or benign prostatic hypertrophy—BPH. An enlarged prostate is not cancerous, but can cause disability and even serious illness if left untreated. If the prostate becomes too large, it presses against the urethral canal and interferes with normal urination. As a result, urine may back up in the kidneys, which subsequently can become damaged both by excessive pressure and by contaminated urine.

Symptoms of BPH typically include progressive urinary frequency, nighttime awakening to empty the bladder, pain, burning, difficulty in starting and stopping urination, and

Therapies for Prostate Enlargement

Botanicals: Ask your physician or herbalist about taking saw palmetto, pygeum bark, horsetail, or corn silk supplements.

Nutrition: Avoid spicy foods, foods high in fat and carbohydrates, caffeine, alcohol, and tobacco. Consume whole grains, nuts, seeds (especially pumpkin seeds), and vegetables.

Vitamins and Minerals: Take vitamins C and B, magnesium, zinc, garlic, or primrose oil supplements.

Other Remedies: Consult an Ayurvedic physician who may recommend yoga postures (especially the ashiwin mudra), or botanicals such as triphala, amla, neem, and shilajit.

an inability to empty the bladder fully. The condition, if left untreated, is likely to result in kidney infection because of the kidneys being filled with contaminated urine. Bladder infections such as cystitis commonly occur as well.

Treatments for Prostate Enlargement

Antibiotics and analgesics sometimes are prescribed for BPH. In addition, a new drug, finasterid (Proscar), shrinks the prostate by interfering with production of the hormone that stimulates growth. In one controlled clinical trial involving 1,645 men, as cited in *Consumer Reports Health Answer Book,* about one-third experienced greatly improved urinary flow after a year on the drug, while another third had at least some relief. Side

effects, including impotence, decreased libido, and decreased volume of ejaculation, were minimal (occurring in only about 4 percent of participants).

Balch and Balch note that another drug, leuprolide, may shrink enlarged prostates. However, they warn that side effects can include impotence, decreased libido, and even hot flashes, and counsel men not to take the drug if they are concerned about potency.

Acupuncture. Acupuncture treatment for BPH has been developed by naturopath Rick Marinelli of Beaverton, Oregon, as described in *Alternative Medicine: The Definitive Guide.* Marinelli uses acupuncture, herbal medicines, and Traditional Chinese Medicine (TCM) to reduce prostate swelling. According to Marinelli, some patients see improvement within the first three to six weeks of combined therapy.

Ayurvedic Medicine. Dr. Virender Sodhi, director of the American School of Ayurvedic Sciences in Bellevue, Washington, claims that Ayurvedic medicine has proved effective in treating BPH. In *Alternative Medicine: The Definitive Guide,* he advises patients to practice exercises such as the ashiwin mudra, which is the squeezing and relaxing of the anal sphincter, to help relieve congestion and aid circulation in the prostate gland. His patients also take several Ayurvedic botanical medicines, including triphala, amla, neem, and shilajit.

Botanical Therapies. Berries from the saw palmetto plant have been shown to relieve BPH symptoms and stimulate immune function in clinical studies, as reported by Morton Walker in the February/March 1991 *Townsend Letter for Doctors.* Berries from the plant contain approximately 15 percent saturated and unsaturated fatty acids, which significantly reduce prostatic swelling in BPH patients.

The bark of the pygeum africanus tree, taken in powder form, has been used in Europe for centuries to treat urinary disorders. Clinical trials in humans, according to Kruzel in the August 1991 issue of *Health Review Newsletter,* have clearly shown this herb can reduce prostate swelling associated with BPH with no toxic side effects, even when administered in large doses and for prolonged periods of time.

In *Alternative Medicine: The Definitive Guide,* Kruzel reports one case in which a 68-year-old man with BPH and a bladder stone reduced prostatic swelling within 10 days using a formula that included saw palmetto extract, prostate glandulars, pygeum africanus, horsetail, and corn silk. According to Kruzel, this formula also can decrease blood in the urine and increase urinary flow.

Balch and Balch report that flower pollen has been used to treat prostatitis and BPH in Europe since the early 1960s. It is not known how bee pollen reduces prostate swelling, although it has been shown to be quite effective in treating BPH in several double-blind clinical studies.

Balch and Balch also claim that drinking tea made from equal quantities of gravel root, sea holly, and hydrangea root three times a day will reduce the discomfort of urination in BPH sufferers. Marshmallow leaves may be added to this mixture if burning and pain persist. Other beneficial teas can be made from the diuretic herb buchu (which should not be boiled, however), and from corn silk.

Nutritional Therapies. An increasing number of nutritionists and physicians now believe that most prostate problems, including BPH, are caused by dietary imbalances that can be reversed with low-fat diets. Kruzel advises men with BPH to avoid spicy foods, foods high in fat and carbohydrates, caffeine, alcohol, and tobacco. These can be irritants and negate the effects of essential vitamins and minerals such as vitamins C and E and zinc, which are necessary for the production of semen.

Kurt Butler and Lynn Rayner suggest in *The Best Medicine: The Complete Health and Preventive Medicine Handbook* that inadequate intake of essential fatty acids such as linoleic acid promotes prostate enlargement, and recommend consumption of whole grains, nuts, seeds, and vegetables. Balch and Balch claim that the high level of zinc obtained by eating one ounce of raw pumpkin seeds or taking pumpkin seed oil capsules on a daily basis is helpful for almost all prostate disorders.

Vitamin and Mineral Therapies. According to *Alternative Medicine: The Definitive Guide,* vitamin and mineral supplementation is beneficial. Vitamin C is a major component of the seminal vesicles and prostate gland, and high amounts are found in prostatic secretions. Vitamin E also is present and, due to its fat solubility, acts as an antioxidant and stabilizes membranes and lipids. Vitamin B and magnesium may relieve BPH, as these have been shown to be deficient in most BPH patients. Garlic can help supply the body with vitamins and minerals and prevent infection of the prostate.

Zinc supplements appear to reduce dihydrotestosterone levels in the prostate, and help to shrink the gland. According to Michael Murray and Joseph Pizzorno in the *Encyclopedia of Natural Medicine,* zinc picolinate and zinc citrate are the best forms to use. However, Butler and Rayner warn that men should not take large doses of zinc indefinitely.

According to *Alternative Medicine: The Definitive Guide,* essential fatty acids such as fish oils, olive oil, evening primrose oil, and eicosapentaenoic acid (EPA) are needed in large amounts for normal functioning of the prostate gland. Used as supplements, these acids can help normalize prostatic functioning.

Prostatitis

Many males between the ages of 20 and 50 suffer acute or chronic inflammation of the prostate gland—or prostatitis. The condition is usually caused by a bacterial infection elsewhere in the body that has invaded the prostate. Noninfective forms of prostatitis may be associated with autoimmune disorders. Prostatitis can partially or totally block the flow of urine out of the bladder, resulting in urine retention. This causes the bladder to become distended, weak, tender, and susceptible to infection due to the increased amount of bacteria in the retained urine.

Some symptoms of acute prostatitis detailed by Butler and Rayner include fever, chills, frequent urination accompanied by a burning sensation, pain between the scrotum and rectum, fatigue, and blood or pus in the urine. Symptoms of chronic prostatitis are frequent and burning urination with blood in the urine, lower back pain, and impotence. As prostatitis becomes more advanced, urination is increasingly difficult.

It is important for men who suffer from any of these symptoms to see a physician, because the condition may progress to more severe complications, including kidney infection, orchitis (painful swelling of the testicles), and epididymitis (inflammation of the epididymis, a tube along the back of the testicles). Bladder outlet obstruction and prostate stones also may occur if chronic prostatitis remains untreated.

Treatments for Prostatitis

Ayurvedic Medicine. Sodhi describes a typical Ayurvedic treatment for prostatitis in *Alternative Medicine: The Definitive Guide* that combines three procedures. First, he advises patients to reduce sexual activity if their infection is caused by sexual overstimulation. Second, he counsels them to drink large amounts of water so they urinate more frequently. He also suggests they practice the ashiwin mudra exercise and soak their testicles in cold water. Finally, Sodhi recommends taking antibiotic botanicals such as neem, amla, and shilajit. In certain cases, he prescribes a berberine extract and zinc supplements.

Botanical Medicines. Felter reports in the *Eclectic Materia Medica* that an evergreen plant, pipsissewa (chimaphilia umbellata), is effective in treating urinary tract disorders, including prostatitis. The plant contains arbutin, the active ingredient in uva ursi, which combats infections of the urinary tract and increases blood flow to the prostate gland. He also suggests that horsetail has effectively treated acute prostatic infection. Purple coneflower has been used against prostatitis and often is combined with delphinia staphysagria, thuja occidentalis, and anemone pulsatilla. According to Felter, these botanical agents decrease pain, irritation, prostate swelling, and impotence associated with prostatitis.

Balch and Balch agree that horsetail, an astringent, can be used if small amounts of blood are passed and can help alleviate frequent urination at night. Other herbs to treat these symptoms are goldenseal, parsley, juniper berries, slippery elm bark, and ginseng, which Balch and Balch describe as a tonic for male reproductive organs.

Homeopathic Therapies. Kruzel reports that homeopathy has been used to treat all forms of prostatitis, especially chronic prostatitis unresponsive to antibiotics. For example, a 38-year-old man with severe aching pains in his hips, thighs, testicles, and prostate gland had been given antibiotics and later nonsteroidal anti-inflammatory medication over the course of several years without experiencing any pain relief. After one month of homeopathic treatment with berberis 30C the patient was 60 percent better—and after three months, he was pain free.

Hydrotherapy. Balch and Balch claim that, in some cases, hydrotherapy effectively increases circulation in the prostate region. One treatment is to sit in a tub that contains the hottest water tolerable for 15 to 30 minutes once or twice a day. Men may also stand in a shower and spray their lower abdomen and pelvic area with warm water for 3 minutes, and then cold water for 1 minute. A third treatment is to sit in hot water while putting the feet in cold water for 3 minutes, and then to sit in cold water while immersing the feet in hot water for 1 minute. Balch and Balch also recommend drinking two to three quarts of spring or distilled water daily to stimulate urine flow, which helps prevent retention, cystitis, and kidney infection.

Traditional Chinese Medicine (TCM). Kruzel, again in *Alternative Medicine: The Definitive Guide,* states that prostatitis is regarded in TCM as a condition of damp heat in the prostate and urinary tract, and acupuncture is not considered effective in treating it. However, Chinese botanical medicines that contain polyporus, akebia, or the cephalanoplos or dianthus formulas have successfully neutralized prostatic infections.

Summary

Prevention of common male health problems associated with the genitourinary tract is the wisest approach for men of all ages. Periodic examinations coupled with blood tests to detect levels of prostatic specific antigens provide the best method of early detection for prostate enlargement, prostatitis, and other genitourinary problems. In fact, the American Cancer Society recommends that males over the age of 40 receive annual examinations. High-fat diets, especially diets high in animal fats, often are linked to these disorders. A low-fat diet with a balance of protein is recommended for men older than 30. Lifestyle changes, especially those associated with sexual habits, are also important in preventing genitourinary problems. If these problems do occur, changes in dietary habits, along with homeopathic therapies, hydrotherapy, Traditional Chinese Medicine, Ayurvedic therapies, and vitamin, mineral, and botanical supplements, may be effective methods of treatment.

RESOURCES

Resources

References

Altman, Lawrence. "A Study of Impotence Suggests Half of Men Over 40 May Have Problem." *New York Times* (December 22, 1993): B9.

Balch, James F., and Phyllis Balch. *Prescription for Nutritional Healing.* Garden City Park, NY: Avery Publishing Group, 1993.

Brody, Jane. "Science Finds No Magic in Age-old Aphrodisiacs." *New York Times* (August 4, 1993): B7.

Brown, D. "Literature Review—Ginkgo Biloba; Phytotherapy Review & Commentary." *Townsend Letter for Doctors* (December 1993).

The Burton Goldberg Group. *Alternative Medicine: The Definitive Guide.* Puyallup, WA: Future Medicine Publishing, Inc., 1993.

Butler, Kurt, and Lynn Rayner. *The Best Medicine: The Complete Health and Preventive Medicine Handbook.* New York, NY: Harper & Row Publishers Inc., 1985.

Dharmananda, S. *Your Nature, Your Health— Chinese Herbs in Constitutional Therapy.* Portland, OR: Institute for Traditional Medicine and Preservation of Health Care, 1986.

Ellingwood, F. *American Materia Medica, Therapeutics and Pharmacognosy.* Portland, OR: Eclectic Medical Publications, 1983.

Farnsworth, N. "Eleuthrococcus Senticosus: Current Status as an Adaptogen." *Economic and Medicinal Plant Research* (1985): 156–215.

Felter, H. *The Eclectic Materia Medica.* Portland, OR: Eclectic Medical Publications, 1983.

Kruzel, T. "What Is the Prostate and Why Is It Doing This to Me?" *Health Review Newsletter* (August 1991): 8–10.

Leff, Jonathan, and the editors of *Consumer Reports. Consumer Reports Health Answer Book.* Yonkers, NY: Consumers Union of United States, Inc., 1993.

Margolis, Simeon, and Hamilton Moses III. *The Johns Hopkins Medical Handbook.* New York, NY: Medletter Associates, Inc., 1992.

Murray, Michael, and Joseph Pizzorno. *Encyclopedia of Natural Medicine.* Rocklin, CA: Prima Publishing, 1991.

Walker, Morton. "Seronoa Repens Extract (Saw Palmetto) Relief for Benign Prostatic Hypertrophy." *Townsend Letter for Doctors* (February/March 1991): 67.

Zimmerman, David. *Zimmerman's Complete Guide to Nonprescription Drugs.* Detroit, MI: Gale Research Inc. and Visible Ink Press, 1993.

Organizations

Alan Guttmacher Institute
11 5th Ave., New York, NY 10003.

Association for Voluntary Sterilization Inc.
112 E. 42nd St., New York, NY 10168.

National Institute of Allergy and Infectious Diseases
9000 Rockville Pke., Bethesda, MD 20205.

Additional Reading

Cummings, Stephen, M.D., and Dana Ullman. *Everybody's Guide to Homeopathic Medicine.* New York, NY: St. Martin's Press, 1991.

"Impotence Can Often Be Avoided, Study Finds." *San Jose Mercury News* (May 25, 1994): 7C.

Reid, Daniel. *Chinese Herbal Medicine.* Boston, MA: Shambhala Publications Inc., 1993.

Watson, Cynthia Mervis. "Exercise Aphrodisiacs." *Fitness* (November/ December 1993): 38–39.

RESOURCES

Chapter 13

COMMON FEMALE HEALTH PROBLEMS

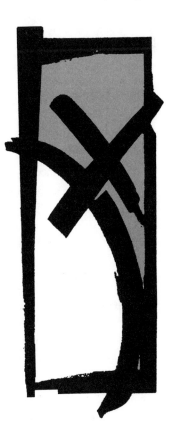

In 1900, the average life expectancy for a woman in the United States was 50 years. Today, that average has increased to almost 80 years, which means that American women can expect to live a third of their lives after menopause. With 40 million women now in or past menopause, and another 20 million due to reach that stage of life in the next decade, the subject has become one of national concern. In addition to menopause, this chapter discusses alternative therapies for preventing and treating common female health problems, including dysmenorrhea, fibrocystic breast disease, premenstrual syndrome, and vaginitis.

While conventional practitioners often have used invasive medical procedures (the two most dramatic being breast removal and hysterectomies) to treat symptoms and diseases affecting women's health, alternative medicine offers a variety of therapeutic and preventive approaches (including diet, vitamin and mineral supplementation, exercise, and stress management) to help women regain their health and maintain their overall well-being.

Fibrocystic Breast Disease

Fibrocystic breast disease (FBD), also known as cystic mastitis, is a noncancerous condition marked by the presence of nodules or cysts (sacs filled with fluid), which may or may not be accompanied by pain and tenderness. It can occur in one or both breasts, with the cysts spread throughout the breasts or located in one general area. The lumps can be firm or soft, and may change in size. FBD typically is cyclical, and usually disappears during pregnancy and nursing.

Dr. Susan Love, associate professor of clinical surgery at UCLA and director of the Breast Center in Los Angeles, estimates in *Alternative Medicine: The Definitive Guide* that FBD occurs in 80 percent of premenopausal women. While FBD can develop at any age, it is most likely to appear between the age of 30 and menopause.

The cause or causes of FBD are unknown, but according to James F. Balch and Phyllis Balch in *Prescription for Nutritional Healing,* the Medical College of Pennsylvania claims that an iodine deficiency is a common reason. Other factors include an imbalance of the female sex hormones and abnormal breast milk production (caused by high amounts of the hormone estrogen).

The benign cysts that develop in women with FBD may be tender and move freely, unlike cancerous lumps, which usually do not move freely, generally are not tender, and do not go away. FBD is considered a low risk factor for breast cancer.

To diagnose FBD, a physician uses a needle to remove fluid from the cysts in a simple office procedure. A mammogram usually is taken to rule out cancer. If FBD is diagnosed, treatment focuses on relieving pain and tenderness, and reducing or eliminating the cysts. Conventional options for severe symptoms include hormonal therapies (including birth control pills, danocrine, bromocriptine, and tamoxifen, an antiestrogen drug), which can have undesirable side effects such as weight gain, growth of facial and bodily hair, headaches, fatigue, blood clots, depression, and nerve problems.

The drug danazol, a hormone, has been successful in shrinking FBD lumps, according to Balch and Balch. Approximately 60 percent of women who use it report less pain and breast tenderness within several weeks.

However, danazol is not effective for all women and may have some side effects.

Treatments for Fibrocystic Breast Disease

Botanical Medicines. Balch and Balch indicate that echinacea, goldenseal, mullein, pau d'arco, poke root, and red clover may be helpful in treating FBD, and report good results with primrose oil in reducing the size of the cysts. They also recommend daily supplementation of germanium and kelp. David Hoffman, past president of the American Herbalist Guild, suggests in *Alternative Medicine: The Definitive Guide* that herbal squaw vine, mullein, pau d'arco, and red clover can reduce swelling. Dandelion also is used for breast sores, tumors, and cysts, while parsley reduces swollen breasts.

Tori Hudson, academic dean at the National College of Naturopathic Medicine in Portland, Oregon, reports in the May 1994 *Townsend Letter for Doctors* that she has successfully used botanical diuretics to treat FBD, including taraxacum leap, foeniculum, angelica, macrotys, and arctium. Hudson claims she has never had an FBD patient who did not respond to natural botanical therapies. She also recommends evening primrose oil, iodine, flax seed oil, and methionine.

Hormone Therapy. Dr. John Lee, a physician and educator in Sebastopol, California, states in *Alternative Medicine: The Definitive Guide* that applying natural progesterone cream directly to the skin usually causes breast cysts to disappear. He advises women to use progesterone cream starting on the fifteenth day of their monthly cycle and continuing until the twenty-fifth day.

Nutritional Therapies. Balch and Balch recommend that women consume a low-fat, high-fiber diet of raw foods, beans, seeds, nuts, and whole grains to treat FBD. They advise eating bananas, grapes, grapefruit, apples, yogurt, and fresh vegetables at least three times a day. They also suggest avoiding animal fats, cooking oils, fried foods, salt, sugar, white flour, tobacco, and caffeine.

Research proving that the avoidance of caffeine helps treat benign FBD symptoms is inconclusive. However, one study by Dr. John Peter Minton of the Department of Surgery at Ohio State University College of Medicine, cited by Balch and Balch, found that women suffering from FBD who eliminated caffeine-containing substances from their diets had a high rate of disappearance or elimination of breast cysts.

Vitamin and Mineral Therapies. Hudson suggests in the May 1994 *Townsend Letter for Doctors* that vitamin E regulates the synthesis of specific proteins and enzymes required to prevent and treat FBD. Hudson advises women with FBD to start a combined supplementation program of vitamin E, beta-carotene, vitamin B-complex, choline, and methionine. Improving dietary habits to decrease estrogen sources, increasing fiber, and consuming low-fat foods also are therapeutic.

Balch and Balch recommend daily dosages of vitamin E, and further suggest that coenzyme Q10 (an antioxidant similar to vitamin E in action but more potent), and vitamins A, B-complex, and C be taken.

Michael Murray and Joseph Pizzorno recommend vitamin A supplements. They cite a study in which five out of twelve women had complete or partial remission of their FBD after three months of vitamin A supplementation. However, some patients developed mild side effects, resulting in two of the original twelve women withdrawing because of headaches (an early sign of vitamin A toxicity), and one patient having her dosage reduced.

Health Guidelines for Women

- Stop smoking. One of every four American women currently smokes cigarettes, a primary risk factor for lung and breast cancer and the leading cause of cancer mortality among women.
- Maintain good nutrition by reducing fat in the diet and taking calcium supplements to prevent osteoporosis.
- Get an annual pap smear to test for cervical cancer.
- Get a yearly clinical breast examination in a doctor's office, combined with self examination of the breasts each month.
- If over the age of 50, get an annual mammogram.
- Protect against sexually transmitted diseases.

Menopause

Menopause occurs when a woman no longer menstruates (because she no longer ovulates) and, as a result, can no longer bear children. The average age at which American women undergo menopause varies between 48 and 52, although it is not abnormal for it to occur several years earlier or later. Even after menopause, a woman's body continues to produce estrogen, but far less of the hormone is made in the ovaries. Some women undergoing menopause report experiencing sudden and severe hot flashes, their vaginal walls may become thinner and lose moisture, and intercourse may cause bleeding and pain. Vaginal itching and burning can occur, and women are more susceptible to yeast and bacterial infections, due to menopausal hormone changes that disrupt the delicate pH of the vagina. In addition, menopause can be accompanied by a loss of muscle tone in the pelvic region, resulting in stress incontinence (urine leakage when coughing, laughing, or exercising vigorously), and a drop of pelvic organs. As estrogen production declines, the relative increase in testosterone (also produced in the ovaries) may result in growth of facial hair and thinning of scalp hair.

The National Institute on Aging warns in *The Menopausal Time of Life* that mood changes may occur during menopause. Other common symptoms include fatigue, nervousness, excess sweating, breathlessness, headaches, sleeplessness, joint pain, depression, irritability, and impatience. These symptoms may be due to shifting hormonal balances or other factors such as heredity, general health, nutrition, medications, exercise, stressful life events (such as grown children leaving home or the need to care for parents who are ill), and attitude. The institute counsels women to develop a positive attitude toward menopause, regarding it as a normal life change (instead of as the end of a useful life) and continuing to participate in satisfying activities.

Treatments for Menopause

Botanical Medicines. Botanicals regarded as uterine tonics and recommended for menopause by Murray and Pizzorno include dong quai, licorice, unicorn root, black cohosh, fennel, and false unicorn root. The Chinese regard dong quai as the most important herb for the female hormonal system before, during, and after pregnancy. Hoffman also suggests that red raspberry leaves, sarsaparilla, wild yam, sassafras, and ginseng help lower blood pressure and increase energy in menopausal women.

Balch and Balch state that black cohosh, damiana, licorice (which stimulates estrogen production), raspberry, sage, Siberian ginseng (which helps relieve depression and stimulates estrogen production), and squaw vine are helpful in treating menopausal symptoms. They also claim that gotu kola and dong quai relieve hot flashes, vaginal dryness, and depression.

Deep Breathing. One study reported by Greg Gutfeld in the March 1993 issue of *Prevention* suggests that slow, deep breathing can relieve some of the symptoms of menopause, including hot flashes. A group of 33 women experiencing frequent hot flashes practiced one of three options: slow, deep breathing; muscle relaxation; or brainwave (EEG) biofeedback. Muscle relaxation and biofeedback had no effect, while deep breathing was linked to 50 percent fewer hot flashes. Slow, deep abdominal breathing probably reduces hot flashes by diminishing the arousal of the central nervous system that normally occurs in the initiation of hot flashes. This technique may be useful for women with hot flashes who cannot receive hormone replacement therapy due to other health reasons.

Estrogen Replacement Therapies (ERT). Conventional physicians sometimes prescribe synthetic estrogen to help alleviate hot flashes, nausea, bone loss, mood swings, a decline in vaginal lubrication, and other symptoms associated with menopause. Synthetic estrogen can be prescribed in several forms: pill, cream or ointment, or as a skin patch. The effectiveness of different forms of estrogen varies, and both synthetic and natural estrogens may pose a health risk. To minimize ERT's degree of risk, the lowest possible of doses of estrogen that are still effective are prescribed, and a synthetic form of the hormone progesterone is added. As ERT is still controversial, women considering long-term estrogen use should discuss the benefits (such as a lower risk of cardiovascular disease, stroke, and Alzheimer's disease, as well as reduction of postmenopausal bone loss) with their physician or gynecologist.

An option to using synthetic progesterone is a natural form of this female hormone found in wild yam (not to be confused with the tuberous sweet potato yam) which, according to herbalist Rosemary Goldstar in *Herbal Healing for Women,* is "the most widely used herb in the world today." More than 200 million prescriptions that contain its derivatives are sold each year.

New York City obstetrician Neils Lauersen, author of *PMS: Premenstrual Syndrome and You,* advocates the use of wild yam as well, claiming that—unlike synthetic progesterone—"natural progesterone (from the wild yam) does not cause masculinization and is known to reduce sodium and fluid retention." Wild yam progesterone is available as a cream, oil, tablet, or capsule through physicians or over the counter in pharmacies.

Holistic physicians use natural estrogenic substances from plants (so-called phytoestrogens) instead of synthetic estrogen. Phytoestrogens include dong quai, licorice, unicorn root, black cohosh, fennel, and false unicorn root.

Exercise. For women who do not wish to use estrogen replacement therapy (ERT), exercise may help reduce the symptoms of menopause. A University of Illinois trial reported in the April 1994 issue of *American Health* studied the effects of exercise on 279 women aged 37 to 64. Over the course of a year, participants filled out questionnaires describing their menopausal status and level of physical activity. They monitored symptoms of hot flashes and night sweats, fatigue, irritability, depression, vaginal dryness, urinary incontinence, loss of sex drive, and general health. Women who spent the most time

in exercise activities, such as ballroom dancing and tennis, reported fewer of all symptoms. Dr. JoEllen Wilbur, a family nurse practitioner who conducted the study, concludes that exercise may prove an effective substitute for ERT. She cautions that although ERT may help prevent heart disease and osteoporosis in women, it may also increase the risk of breast and endometrial cancer. Dr. Ernst Bartisch, an obstetrician/gynecologist at New York City's New York Hospital–Cornell Medical Center, in commenting on Wilbur's study, suggests that active menopausal women may not have to take estrogen as soon as inactive women, or may be able to take less of it.

Nutritional Therapies. According to Murray and Pizzorno, women who experience continual unpleasant symptoms of menopause, including hot flashes, will benefit from adopting a diet high in vegetables and fruits and low in fat and animal products. Balch and Balch agree, and claim that dairy products, sugar, and meat cause most hot flashes. They suggest that menopausal women should consume at least 50 percent raw foods and protein supplements (to avoid low blood sugar). Refined carbohydrate and alcohol intake should be minimal, and caffeine should be eliminated. Blackstrap molasses, broccoli, dandelion greens, kelp, salmon with bones, sardines, and low-fat yogurt should be added to the diet.

Vitamin and Mineral Therapies. There is not unanimity on which vitamins and minerals will help women with menopausal symptoms. Balch and Balch claim that vitamin E may relieve hot flashes. Calcium and magnesium chelate help alleviate nervousness and irritability accompanying menopause. Germanium, L-arginine, and L-lysine relieve the symptoms as well. Vitamin C and potassium may prevent severe hot flashes and heavy perspiration. Evening primrose oil, an excellent source of essential fatty acids, also is recommended.

Menstruation

Each month, from puberty until menopause, a woman's body prepares to conceive, nurture, and give birth to a new human being. The ovaries begin to make estrogen, which triggers the thickening of the lining of the uterus (the endometrium) with blood vessels, glands, and cells in anticipation of fertilization. Simultaneously, an egg begins to develop in the ovaries. Within ten days to three weeks, the lining and the egg are ready for conception, and the egg is released in a process called ovulation (which is when pregnancy can occur). After ovulation, the ovaries increase production of a second hormone, progesterone, which stimulates the uterine lining to complete its development in anticipation of the egg's fertilization by the sperm. If conception does not occur, hormone levels drop, and some of the endometrial layer is released or shed (menstruation). The cycle then starts over.

Although a normal menstrual cycle traditionally has been defined as 28 days, the length of the lunar cycle, Janet Shepherd claims in the March–April 1990 *Vibrant Life* that only one out of six women has a 28-day cycle. Anywhere between 23 and 35 days is considered normal, even if the cycle is irregular. During the average menstrual period, a woman loses two tablespoons to one-half cup of blood. The rest of the discharge (almost two-thirds) is fluid released from cells that shrink or die as the lining of the uterus breaks down.

Dysmenorrhea

According to the American College of Obstetricians and Gynecologists, as many as 70 percent of women experience some form of menstrual cramps during their period, and 15 percent have cramps severe enough to be disabling. This discomfort, dysmenorrhea, results primarily from hormones called prostaglandins that cause contractions of the uterus. Other symptoms of dysmenorrhea, in addition to cramping pelvic pain, include nausea, vomiting, diarrhea, headaches, dizziness, and fatigue. Most women who have menstrual cramps do not have any underlying illness.

For mild cramps, the best therapy may be aspirin, over-the-counter medications containing ibuprofen, or acetaminophen. Low-dose antiprostaglandin pain relievers also are available without a prescription. Felicia Stewart reports in *Understanding Your Body: Every Woman's Guide to a Lifetime of Health* that at least 80 percent of women treated for cramps with antiprostaglandin medication experience good results. Several closely related drugs called prostaglandin synthetase inhibitors have similar effects. All of them decrease production of the prostaglandin hormone within normal body cells, including the cells lining the uterus.

Treatments for Dysmenorrhea

Botanical Medicines. Herbal tonics for both menstrual cramps and heavy bleeding are widely available in natural food stores. In *Alternative Medicine: The Definitive Guide,* Hoffman recommends combining tinctures of skullcap, black haw, and black cohosh in equal parts and taking this mixture as needed. If a woman suffers from excess water retention, Hoffman suggests taking a tincture of dandelion or drinking dandelion tea. Dr. Susan Lark, in her book *PMS Self-Help Book: A Woman's Guide,* recommends ginger, white willow bark, red raspberry leaf, cramp bark, chamomile, hops, ginkgo biloba, and chaste tree berry. Bromelain extract from the pineapple plant has been documented as relieving menstrual cramping by decreasing spasms of the contracted cervix.

Consultation with an herbalist or a naturopathic physician can help determine which herbs are most appropriate. Herbalists normally use herb treatments for a minimum of three months. However, if a woman has suffered from hormonal imbalances for a long time, treatment may take six months or more to achieve results.

Nutritional Therapies. Menstrual cramps are caused by a variety of nutritional, vitamin, mineral, and hormonal factors. Generally, the nutritional therapies recommended by Murray and Pizzorno for PMS symptoms also may prove helpful for women with dysmenorrhea. They advise women to limit consumption of refined carbohydrates (sugar, honey, and white flour) and other concentrated carbohydrates such as maple syrup, dried fruit, and fruit juice. Milk and dairy products also should be decreased, along with natural and synthetically saturated fats. Vegetable oils rich in linoleic and linolenic acids should be substituted. Protein intake from vegetable sources such as legumes should be increased, with green leafy vegetables (except cabbage, brussels sprouts, and cauliflower) and fish replacing red meats. Alcohol, tobacco, coffee, tea, chocolate, and other caffeine-containing foods and beverages should be restricted.

Osteopathic Therapy. Dysmenorrhea can produce low-back pain and an electromyographic (EMG) pattern typical of trauma-induced low-back pain. Dr. D. Boesler reports on one trial in a February 1993 monograph published by the Health Sciences College of Osteopathic Medicine in Des Moines, Iowa. Twelve dysmenorrheic subjects were assigned to a group receiving osteopathic treatment, to a group not receiving osteopathic treatment, or both. Eight women participated in both groups, the other four women being equally distributed between groups. Osteopathic

manipulative treatment significantly decreased EMG activity during extension of the lumbar spinae erector muscles, abolished the spontaneous EMG activity, and alleviated low-back pain and menstrual cramping.

Traditional Chinese Medicine (TCM). Honora Lee Wolfe, a TCM practitioner in Boulder, Colorado, states in *Alternative Medicine: The Definitive Guide* that menstrual cramps usually are due to chi stagnation (when the vital energy is unable to move freely through the body) in the lower abdomen, blood stasis, or a combination of both. She claims that acupuncture and Chinese herbs can restore a balanced chi flow to the lower abdomen.

Premenstrual Syndrome

Premenstrual syndrome (PMS) is the term used to describe physical or behavioral changes that many women undergo seven to ten days before their monthly periods begin. About 7 million American women experience some symptoms of PMS, while 3 to 5 percent are affected by "premenstrual dysphoric disorder (PDD)," the most severe PMS, which is classified by the American Psychiatric Association as a depressive disorder in its *Diagnostic Manual of Mental Illness.* Although there is no unanimous agreement on what causes PMS, it is believed to be related to the change in hormone levels that occurs in a woman's body before menstruation.

The principal physical and emotional symptoms of PMS include water retention (edema), weight gain, abdominal bloating, breast tenderness, headaches, swollen hands and feet, constipation, feelings of depression, irritability, tension and anxiety, mood swings, a change in sex drive, and inability to concentrate. The symptoms, which reappear at about the same time each month, usually disappear once a woman's menstrual period begins.

How Exercise Relieves PMS Symptoms

- Exercise boosts metabolism and helps burn fuel (food) more effectively.
- Exercise stimulates the smooth muscle of the intestines to contract and relax more efficiently, preventing or relieving a sluggish bowel, constipation, and a bloated abdomen.
- Exercise decreases psychological tension and relieves some forms of anxiety.

- Exercise increases muscle density (the ratio of muscle to fatty tissue), which enhances energy and stamina.
- Exercise produces biochemical changes that relax muscles and elevate mood.
- Exercise prevents the build-up of lactic acid in the muscles that can make them feel tender or painful.

Treatments for Premenstrual Syndrome

Botanical Medicines. Balch and Balch report that dong quai relieves PMS symptoms, particularly bloating, vaginal dryness, and depression. Siberian ginseng (for those who are not hypoglycemic), cayenne, blessed thistle, kelp, raspberry leaves, squaw vine, and sarsaparilla also may be good for PMS, but should be taken only after consulting a physician or herbalist.

Good botanical sources of essential fatty acids (EFAs) obtainable in supplement form, according to the July/August 1993 issue of *Natural Health,* include borage oil, black currant oil, and evening primrose oil. However, high amounts of these supplements should be taken only under professional supervision. Unicorn root has been used in folk medicine for women with poor ovarian function and its estrogen-like activity may be useful in treating PMS.

Exercise. In one clinical trial conducted by exercise physiologist Jody Weizman at George Washington University, and reported in the September/October 1994 issue of *Fitness,* 14 women with chronic PMS worked

out on treadmills, bikes, stair-climbers, and rowing machines for 45-minute sessions three times a week for three months. The women kept daily diaries to chart their moods. By the end of the experiment, the PMS symptoms (specifically anxiety and depression) were on average only half as severe as before the women began exercising.

A larger study by the University of Kansas involving 968 women over the age of 30 found that exercise greatly benefits menstrual cycle function. The study, cited in the December 1993 issue of *New Body,* showed that women who worked out at least three times a week reported fewer negative symptoms—such as bloating, food cravings, irritability, and breast tenderness—than those who exercised infrequently or not at all.

Regular sexual intercourse also may help relieve the symptoms of PMS. Dr. Alfred Franger, associate professor at the Medical College of Wisconsin in Milwaukee, states in the February 8, 1994, issue of *Your Health* that the bloating feeling that can accompany PMS is caused by an increased blood flow to the pelvis five to seven days before a woman's period. Muscle contractions during orgasm force the blood to flow rapidly away from the pelvic region. According to Franger,

MENSTRUATION

Nutritional Guidelines for Relieving PMS

- Avoid caffeine and alcohol, which cause abnormal increases and decreases in blood sugar levels. Also avoid sugar, citrus juices, fructose, white flour, white rice, candy, cake, soft drinks, pastries, ice cream, sherbet, artificial sweeteners, and highly refined foods.

- Avoid simple carbohydrates such as refined sugars and flours, which raise glucose levels in the blood too rapidly.

- Eat complex carbohydrate and high protein products that provide the body with a constant supply of glucose to the bloodstream.

- Eat magnesium-rich foods such as whole grain breads and cereals, fresh green vegetables, and peanut butter.
- Eat potassium-rich foods including fresh fruits (not juices), especially bananas, tomatoes, oranges, and apricots.
- Eat calcium-rich foods such as dairy products (skim milk and low-sodium cheeses) and dark green and yellow vegetables, including zucchini, broccoli, and asparagus.
- Most importantly, do not fast or skip meals, or go longer than three hours without eating a small amount of complex carbohydrates such as grains or pasta; consume low-fat foods.

regular sexual activity before a menstrual period may be a more effective treatment for PMS than diet or hormone therapies.

Homeopathic Remedies. In *Discovering Homeopathy,* Dana Ullman lists the following homeopathic therapies that have been used successfully to treat women with occasional acute symptoms of PMS: deadly night shade (belladonna), phosphate of magnesia (magnesia phosphorica), bitter cucumber (colocynthis), black snake root (cimicifuga), chamomile (chamomilla), blue cohosh (caulophyllum), windflower (pulsatilla), cuttlefish (sepia), and salt (natrum mur).

Hot Baths. Taking a hot bath can be helpful in relieving PMS symptoms, as it temporarily raises the body temperature, increasing drowsiness. For prolonged pain, natural sedatives such as chamomile tea can be taken.

Nutritional Therapies. Nutritionists generally advise PMS patients to limit their con-

sumption of refined carbohydrates (sugar, honey, and white flour) and other concentrated carbohydrates such as maple syrup, dried fruit, and fruit juice. Murray and Pizzorno recommend in the *Encyclopedia of Natural Medicine* that women with PMS increase their protein intake, particularly from vegetable sources such as legumes. Milk and honey fats (especially natural and synthetically saturated fats) should be decreased and vegetable oils rich in linoleic and linolenic acids substituted. Women with PMS also should decrease salt intake, and restrict their use of alcohol and tobacco, as well as coffee, tea, chocolate, and other caffeine-containing foods and beverages.

Hudson recommends in *Alternative Medicine: The Definitive Guide* that women suffering from PMS adopt a diet that includes fresh fruits, whole grains, legumes, nuts, fish, seeds, and vegetables. She suggests that foods containing refined sugars and high amounts of protein or fat be avoided, along with dairy products, caffeine, and tobacco.

Balch and Balch recommend in *Prescription for Nutritional Healing* a diet of fresh fruits and vegetables, cereals and breads, whole grains, beans, peas, lentils, nuts and seeds, and broiled chicken, turkey, and fish. They also advise that drinking one quart of distilled water daily, starting one week before the menstrual period and ending one week after, also provide relief.

Essential fatty acids (EFAs), which cannot be made by the body and must be obtained from food sources or supplements, are helpful in the treatment of PMS symptoms. The July/August 1993 issue of *Natural Health* cites research studies in Europe and Canada that have shown that women taking supplements of EFAs report up to a two-thirds reduction in PMS symptoms. Food sources include walnuts, pumpkin, flax, sesame and sunflower seeds, soybeans, and fish such as salmon, trout, and sardines.

David Zimmerman, in *Zimmerman's Complete Guide to Nonprescription Drugs,* suggests that women who experience water retention may be able to relieve this condition by decreasing fluid consumption in the week before menstruation. He also recommends avoiding salt- and sodium-rich foods such as potato chips, pickles, sodas, and table salt, since salt and sodium hold water in the body tissues.

Progesterone Therapy. Conventional physicians often use progesterone to alleviate severe PMS symptoms such as migraine headaches and depression, although this treatment has not been shown to help all women. Side effects may include blood clotting and cancer. Although progesterone is the most widely used treatment for PMS, studies have not proven it is more effective than a placebo, according to the February 8, 1994, issue of *Your Health.*

Vitamin and Mineral Therapies. According to *Alternative Medicine: The Definitive Guide,* vitamin A relieves bloating (it is a diuretic) and is beneficial in reducing PMS symptoms in the second half of the menstrual cycle. Vitamin B6 helps combat depression and also relieves bloating. Vitamin E relieves nervous tension, headaches, fatigue, depression, and insomnia. Joseph Martorano reports in the December 1993 issue of *New Body* that taking magnesium supplements may relieve cravings for certain foods, such as chocolate, which are common in PMS sufferers.

Spotting Between Periods

Dr. Mona Shangold, professor of obstetrics and gynecology at Hahnemann University in Philadelphia and co-author of *The Complete Sports Medicine Book for Women,* warns that between-period spotting—even after strenuous exercise—is not normal and should be discussed with a gynecologist. Spotting could signal polyps, fibroids, infections, hormonal problems, or cancer. She suggests women use a calendar to record every episode of spotting to help determine whether they are spotting at certain times during each of their menstrual cycles.

Vaginitis (Yeast Infections)

Vaginitis, or yeast infection, is one of the most common reasons women visit a physician. More than 20 million American women report this inconvenience each year and, according to an article in the September 1990 *Redbook,* it is a recurring problem for an estimated 10 percent of women.

The symptoms of vaginitis include frequent moist vaginal discharges; vaginal odor;

vulval or vaginal itching, burning, or irritation; and painful urination after intercourse. The skin around the vagina may become sore and red. Women with these symptoms should see a physician because untreated vaginal infections have been linked to endometritis (inflammation of the uterus), inflammation of the pelvis (pelvic inflammatory disease), and cancer.

Several factors increase a woman's susceptibility to vaginitis. These include the use of antibiotics (which eliminate certain protective bacteria) and oral contraceptives, diabetes, pregnancy, obesity, excessive improper douching, a vitamin B deficiency, menopausal thinning of the vaginal wall, and cuts or abrasions in the genital area.

Yeast infections traditionally have been treated with prescription antifungal medications inserted into the vagina, including suppositories, tablets, creams, and gels. However, in mid-1993, two new antifungal drugs, Gyne-Lotrimin and Monistat 7, were introduced as over-the-counter treatments. No side effect or toxicity has been reported. However, an article in the March 1991 *Glamour* urges women who are pregnant (or think they may be pregnant), or who have had more than four yeast infections in the past year, to use the product under a doctor's supervision.

Treatments for Vaginitis

Acidophilus. Various prescription drugs, especially antibiotics, can destroy the natural intestinal flora and can cause constipation, diarrhea, and vaginitis. The intestinal tract of normal, healthy adults contains approximately three-and-one-half pounds of bacteria. Lactobacillus acidophilus accounts for most of the friendly bacteria found in the small intestine. These are critical for proper nutrient absorption, help prevent bacterial and yeast overgrowth, and also produce B-complex vitamins and vitamin K.

According to *Zimmerman's Complete Guide to Nonprescription Drugs,* Dr. Eileen Hilton and colleagues at the Long Island Jewish Medical Center in New York put 33 women with recurring yeast infections on one of two diets—with yogurt containing acidophilus, or without—for six months. Women on the yogurt diet had only a third (0.4 attacks per six months) as many yeast infections as those who did not consume yogurt (2.5 attacks per six months). Hilton and her colleagues concluded that eight ounces of lactobacillus acidophilus-rich yogurt daily "decreased candidal colonization and infection."

Women with yeast infections need to increase lactobacillus acidophilus in the bowels, intestines, and vagina. Lactobacillus acidophilus may be eaten in yogurt form, swallowed in capsules or tablets, or applied externally as a topical treatment. Douches that include apple cider vinegar, acidophilus, and garlic may relieve some symptoms, although

VAGINITIS

there is no clinical evidence that douches are effective.

Botanical Medicines. Botanical medicines can both prevent the spread of candida albicans and soothe the vaginal membranes. Balch and Balch suggest that black walnut and tea tree oil combined with pau d'arco may be effective. One botanical douche described in *Alternative Medicine: The Definitive Guide* includes antiseptic herbs, such as St. John's wort, goldenseal, echinacea, fresh plantain, and garlic, which strengthen the immune system to suppress the infection. The douche also includes comfrey leaves that soothe the membranes. The douche may be alternated with one of acidophilus, and is most effective when patients avoid eating fats, sugars, and refined foods.

Hudson has developed a botanical capsule for yeast infections, as described in *Alternative Medicine: The Definitive Guide.* Her formula consists of powdered boric acid mixed with berberis, hydrastis, and calendula. Calendula neutralizes the infection and heals the vaginal membranes. According to Hudson, "This works so well that I no longer prescribe douches for this condition."

Homeopathic Remedies. Ullman in *Discovering Homeopathy* suggests that homeopaths have successfully treated vaginitis using pulsatilla, sepia, and natrum mur. Rather than use medicines that attack a specific microorganism that may be causing the infection, Ullman suggests homeopaths prescribe remedies that stimulate the woman's immune system to eliminate the infectious agent. Homeopathic medicines are individually prescribed based on an assessment of the woman's nutritional, physical, and mental state.

Nutritional Therapies. In *Textbook of Natural Medicine,* Murray and Pizzorno advise women with yeast infections to test for possible allergies. They recommend a basic diet low in fats, sugars, and refined foods. Hudson suggests in *Alternative Medicine: The Definitive Guide* that women follow a yeast-free diet, avoid fermented foods and sugar that feed yeast growth, and increase their intake of acidophilus yogurt and garlic, both of which control the spread of the yeastlike fungus candida albicans.

Vitamin and Mineral Therapies. Depending on the patient's symptoms, holistic physicians may prescribe vitamins A, B-complex, C, and E; beta-carotene; the bioflavonoids; lithium; lysine; acidophilus; and iodine.

Balch and Balch warn women to avoid zinc and iron supplements until the infection disappears, as bacterial infections require iron for growth. They claim that the body actually stores iron in compartments of the liver, spleen, and bone marrow when a bacterial infection is present, to prevent further growth of bacteria. To relieve the itching that accompanies vaginitis, they suggest opening vitamin E capsules and applying them to the inflamed area, or using vitamin E or enzyme cream.

Summary

Women have unique hormonal response patterns that can make them vulnerable to sexual organ disorders and infections of the genitourinary tract. As more women enter the obstetrics and gynecology professions, new clinical programs will increasingly focus on safe, long-lasting, noninvasive, nutritional, botanical, and hormonal therapies to prevent, treat, and reverse common female health problems. The alternative approach to female health challenges women to be well informed and to form an equal partnership with health care professionals in exploring a variety of therapeutic approaches.

Resources

References

American College of Obstetricians and Gynecologists. *Gynecological Problems: Dysmenorrhea.* Washington, DC: American College of Obstetricians and Gynecologists, 1985.

American Psychiatric Association. *Diagnostic and Statistical Manual of Mental Disorders* (DSM-IIIR). Washington, DC: American Psychiatric Association, 1993.

Balch, James F., and Phyllis Balch. *Prescription for Nutritional Healing.* Garden City Park, NY: Avery Publishing Group, 1993.

Beil, Laura. "New Brain Drug that Beats PMS." *Your Health* (February 8, 1994): 18–19.

Boesler, D. "Efficacy of High-Velocity Low-Amplitude Manipulative Technique in Subjects with Low-Back Pain During Menstrual Cramping." *Monograph,* (February 1993): 213–14.

The Burton Goldberg Group. *Alternative Medicine: The Definitive Guide.* Puyallup, WA: Future Medicine Publishing, Inc., 1993.

"Drugs Used to Treat PMS Found Ineffective." *Health Facts* (August 1990): 5.

Edlin, Gordon, and Eric Golanty. *Health and Wellness: A Holistic Approach.* Boston, MA: Jones and Bartlett Publishers, Inc., 1992.

"EFA For PMS." *Natural Health* (July/August 1993): 3.

"Exercise and Menstrual Cycle." *New Body* (December 1993): 13.

Gilman, Eleanor. "Waltzing Through Menopause." *American Health* (April 1994): 98.

Goldstar, Rosemary. *Herbal Healing for Women.* New York, NY: Simon & Schuster, Inc., 1993.

Gutfeld, Greg. "Relax the Flash." *Prevention* (March 1993): 18.

Hudson, Tori. "Fibrocystic Breast Disease...Or Is It?" *Townsend Letter for Doctors* (May 1994): 549.

Lark, Susan. *PMS Self-Help Book: A Woman's Guide.* Berkeley, CA: Celestial Arts, 1984.

Lauersen, Neils. *PMS: Premenstrual Syndrome and You.* New York, NY: Simon & Schuster, Inc., 1983.

Martorano, Joseph. "Overcoming PMS." *New Body* (December 1993): 30–31.

McVeigh, Gloria. "Mastering Menopause: A Plan of Action for Every Symptom and Side Effect." *Prevention* (April 1990): 51–52.

Murray, Michael, and Joseph Pizzorno. *Encyclopedia of Natural Medicine.* Rocklin, CA: Prima Publishing, 1991.

———. *Textbook of Natural Medicine, Volumes 1–2.* Seattle, WA: John Bastyr College Publications, 1989.

National Institute on Aging. *The Menopausal Time of Life.* Bethesda, MD: National Institute on Aging. NIH Pub. No. 86-2461. July 1986: 13–15.

"Prescription Drug for Yeast Infections Goes Over the Counter." *Glamour* 89, no. 3 (March 1991): 76.

Rubin, Sylvia. "Women's Health Goes Mainstream." *San Francisco Chronicle* (March 21, 1994): E9.

Shangold, Mona. *The Complete Sports Medicine Book for Women.* New York, NY: Simon & Schuster, Inc., 1992.

Shepherd, Janet E. "Your Menstrual Period: As Unique as You Are." *Vibrant Life* (March–April 1990): 22–23.

Stewart, Felicia. *Understanding Your Body: Every Woman's Guide to a Lifetime of Health*. New York, NY: Bantam Books, 1987.

Ullman, Dana. *Discovering Homeopathy*. Berkeley, CA: North Atlantic Books, 1988.

"Working Off the PMS Blues." *Fitness* (September/October 1993): 45.

"Yogurt Fights Yeast Infections." *Redbook* (September 1990): 32.

Zimmerman, David. *Zimmerman's Complete Guide to Nonprescription Drugs*. Detroit, MI: Gale Research Inc. and Visible Ink Press, 1993.

Organizations

National Institute of Allergy and Infectious Diseases
9000 Rockville Pke., Bethesda, MD 20205.

National Women's Health Network
1325 G St. NW, Washington, DC 20005.

Planned Parenthood Foundation of America
810 7th Ave., New York, NY 10014.

Additional Reading

American College of Obstetricians and Gynecologists. *Estrogen Use*. Washington, DC: American College of Obstetricians and Gynecologists, 1988.

————. *Gynecological Problems: Dysmenorrhea*. Washington, DC: American College of Obstetricians and Gynecologists, 1985.

————. *Premenstrual Syndrome*. Washington, DC: American College of Obstetricians and Gynecologists, 1985.

————. *Vaginitis: Causes and Treatments*. Washington, DC: American College of Obstetricians and Gynecologists, 1984.

Bender, Stephanie, and Kathleen Kelleher. *PMS: A Positive Program to Gain Control*. Tucson, AZ: The Body Press, 1986.

Brody, Jane. *Jane Brody's The New York Times Guide to Personal Health*. New York, NY: Avon Books, 1982.

Burnett, Raymond. *Menopause: All Your Questions Answered*. Chicago, IL: Contemporary Books, 1987.

Hoffman, David. *The New Holistic Herbal*. Rockport, MA: Element Books, Inc., 1992.

Love, Susan. *Doctor Susan Love's Breast Book*. Reading, MA: Addison-Wesley Longman, 1990.

Ody, Penelope. *The Complete Medicinal Herbal*. London, England: Dorling Kindersley, 1993.

Stein, Diane. *The Natural Remedy Book for Women*. Freedom, CA: The Crossing Press, 1992.

Chapter 14

PREGNANCY, CHILDBIRTH, AND INFANT CARE

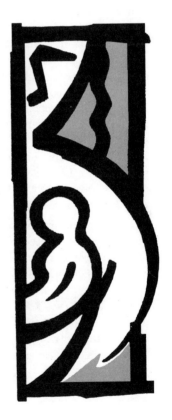

The entire process by which a women conceives, nurtures, and delivers her baby is certainly one of the most complex biological experiences a human body undergoes. Until the moment of birth, the woman and fetus are one organism and everything she does during her pregnancy impacts not only her health, but that of her baby as well.

This chapter provides a general outline of the alternative approach to pregnancy, birthing, and infant care. It attempts to answer the questions many pregnant women ask about foods, vitamin and mineral supplements, and exercise. Additional sources that discuss these topics in considerably more detail are listed in the Resources at the end of this chapter.

Pregnancy

Birth Defects

More than twenty-five hundred babies are born each year in the U.S. with neural tube defects, according to the Centers for Disease Control and Prevention (CDC). In addition, fifteen hundred fetuses are aborted in the second trimester because neural tube defects have been diagnosed. A neural tube defect occurs when the spinal column of the fetus fails to close early in pregnancy and the baby is born with an open spine (a condition known as spina bifida) or, in some cases, with most of its brain missing (anencephaly).

The most effective way to prevent neural tube defects is to take vitamins, especially folic acid, one of the eight vitamins that make up the B-complex. In 1993, the U.S. Public Health Service began advising pregnant women to take at least 0.4 milligrams of folic acid a day, the amount contained in an ordinary multivitamin. Its research indicated that half of all neural tube defects can be prevented with folic acid supplements. These recommendations were based, in part, on a study of 4,753 pregnant women in Hungary conducted by the National Institute of Hygiene in Budapest. That study found thirteen major birth defects per thousand births among women who took daily multivitamins that contained 0.8 milligram of folic acid, compared with twenty-three major defects per thousand births among those who consumed only trace elements. Folic acid can be taken in vitamin form or consumed in foods, especially green leafy vegetables, dried beans, liver, and orange and grapefruit juice. Like vitamin C, folic acid is water soluble and excess amounts are easily eliminated by the expectant mother's body, according to a report in the December 25, 1992, *San Francisco Examiner* by Daniel Haney.

It is important to note that to prevent neural tube birth defects, women must take adequate amounts of folic acid during the first month of their pregnancy, when the fetus's spine is being formed. However, since most women do not even know that they are pregnant at this point, the federal guidelines recommend that all women in their childbearing years obtain adequate amounts.

Testing for Fetal Birth Defects. Detecting genetic defects in the fetus used to involve a potentially dangerous procedure called amniocentesis in which a physician inserts a needle into the womb during the fourth month of pregnancy and extracts a small amount of the amniotic fluid that surrounds the fetus. After the procedure, expectant parents must

wait up to four weeks for the fetal cells to be grown in culture and analyzed. Although amniocentesis has a very small chance of causing a spontaneous abortion, some pregnant women are reluctant to risk it.

Physicians now have other methods they can use to predict genetic defects. As the March of Dimes Birth Defects Foundation reports in the January 1991 Public Health Information Sheet *AlphaFetoprotein Screening,* the Maternal Serum Alpha-Fetoprotein (MSAFP) test is a simple procedure, that normally is performed between the fourteenth and sixteenth week of pregnancy. The test measures the maternal blood level of alpha-fetoprotein (AFP), a protein produced by the fetus. Between 40 and 50 percent of expectant mothers with high AFP readings develop toxemia or experience premature labor, poor fetal growth, or stillbirth. They are also at risk of delivering stillborn babies or ones with retarded growth. A high AFP level can indicate a neural tube defect in which either the brain or the spinal cord of the fetus fails to form correctly. In some cases, high AFP levels may result in abdominal wall defects. The AFP test is as safe as any other blood test.

The March of Dimes Foundation goes on to describe ultrasound, another test which is normally administered between the eighteenth and nineteenth week of pregnancy. "The woman lies on her back and the doctor moves a transducer, a microphone-like device, over her abdomen. Sound waves produced by the transducer are bounced off of fetal bones and tissue, and are then converted into images on a television monitor." The test is reasonably safe, inexpensive, and can effectively detect abnormalities such as hereditary diseases.

Chorionic-villus sample (CVS) testing, which is similar to amniocentesis, allows an earlier diagnosis—usually between the ninth and twelfth week of pregnancy. A surgeon, guided by ultrasound, inserts a catheter

The Importance of Prenatal Testing

Prenatal testing can detect the following defects in fetuses.

Cystic Fibrosis. One in two thousand babies develops fibrosis of the pancreas, respiratory system, and sweat glands.

Down's Syndrome. One in fifty pregnancies occurring in women over the age of forty results in mongoloidism, mental retardation, or heart defects.

Duchenne's Muscular Dystrophy. This is a gene-related disease that causes paralysis, muscular degeneration, and early death.

Neural Tube Defects. Some fetuses have spinal cords that fail to close during embryonic development—causing them to be born without brains or bladders; some may suffer leg paralysis and lack bowel control.

Sickle-Cell Anemia. Babies with this disease may be anemic, be low in weight, or have infections and pain requiring hospitalization. It is found primarily in babies whose parents are black and who both carry the gene.

Tay-Sachs Disease. This disease is caused by a nonsymptomatic gene that can result in retardation, blindness, and early death.

---

through the cervix into the uterus and removes a small amount of chorionic villi (a part of the placenta). The tissue is subsequently examined to determine whether the fetus has any prenatal defects. As with amniocentesis, the procedure carries up to a 2 percent risk of miscarriage, according to Paula Adams Hilliard's article in the July 1989 issue of *Parent's Magazine.*

A relatively new technique, reported in the October 8, 1993, *Dallas Morning News,* involves taking blood samples from the pregnant woman and sifting out fetal cells that have leaked through the placenta. Such an early diagnosis could be especially valuable if therapies become available to correct genetic disorders before birth. Although routine use of this procedure is still several years away, blood tests of this type may eventually become a quicker and less risky substitute for amniocentesis.

Infertility

In order to conceive a child, of course, both the man and woman must be fertile. Unfortunately, approximately 15 percent of couples in the U.S. who wish to have children cannot. Infertility can result from genetic factors, venereal diseases, and many types of physical impairments. Venereal diseases, particularly gonorrhea, account for nearly 10 percent of infertility cases. If gonorrhea is not treated early enough, it can damage the body's tubes that carry the sperm or eggs. A small percentage of women also become infertile after they stop using birth control pills and devices.

According to Gordon Edlin and Eric Golanty in *Health and Wellness: A Holistic Approach,* forty percent of infertility cases are due to the inability of the male to produce or deliver into the vagina a sufficient number of viable sperm cells. This difficulty usually results from the man's inability to maintain an

INFERTILITY

erection or ejaculate into the vagina. Women who cannot conceive often have benign growths or tumors in the uterus that block the male sperm from moving to the fallopian tubes. There also are several hormonal imbalances in women that can prevent the development or release of reproductive female ova.

Twenty years ago, many infertile couples had to forego having children. Today more than half of all such couples in the U.S. can reverse their infertility through drugs or surgery. Several new drugs can stimulate ovulation, and surgical procedures have been developed to repair a woman's damaged fallopian tubes and to reconnect the sperm ducts of men who have had vasectomies. In addition, there now are operations to correct male vein disorders that impair sperm production.

In cases where the man has difficulty ejaculating in the vagina, a couple can try artificial insemination. In this procedure, his active sperm are deposited into the woman's cervix with a syringe. When the man cannot produce sufficient numbers of healthy sperm for this type of artificial insemination, the woman may be able to become pregnant by using semen from a donor.

Another method is in vitro fertilization (IVF), in which several eggs from an ovary are fertilized with active sperm in a laboratory dish. The resultant embryo is then placed into the woman's uterus, and a normal pregnancy may follow. Typically, IVF is used when a woman's fallopian tubes are blocked or fail to function correctly.

Prenatal Care

Once a woman becomes pregnant, holistic health habits are very important, including proper nutrition, exercise, and abstaining from nicotine products, alcohol, and other drugs. The first twenty-eight days of a woman's pregnancy are critical, because during this period the fetus is most sensitive and vulnerable to harm. Every pregnant woman should

consult an obstetrician within this time frame to prevent later complications. The obstetrician can run tests to monitor both the woman's and the fetus's health. This is also an ideal time for the woman to discuss the foods she should eat, whether she will need to take vitamin and mineral supplements, and whether she would like to have a home birth.

An expectant mother may want to consult a holistic nurse-midwife at this time, a trained professional whom she feels will guarantee the whole body health of herself and her baby. The midwife can assist the obstetrician in monitoring the growth of the fetus and be available for any emergencies. The midwife also can provide the companionship and moment-to-moment support that contribute to a short and successful delivery. Midwives usually are at the woman's side throughout her labor, and can help instruct the mother in breastfeeding and early infant care.

Experts agree that better prenatal care can reduce the number of babies who weigh less than 5½ pounds at birth. Newborns weighing less than 5½ pounds are forty times more likely to die within the first four weeks of life. If they survive, low-birth-weight babies are also far more likely to have a permanent disability, according to the *San Jose Mercury News* article.

Aspirin and High Blood Pressure. Several earlier studies seemed to suggest that aspirin could forestall high blood pressure (a serious complication of pregnancy) among certain women who were already at high risk of the condition, known as pre-eclampsia, an abnormal condition of very high blood pressure after the sixth month of pregnancy. As a result, some obstetricians began recommending low doses of aspirin to patients at moderate or low risk on the theory that it might help and probably was not harmful.

A 1993 study, however, found little benefit in routinely giving aspirin to healthy pregnant women as a way of preventing high blood pressure. Minuscule daily doses were given to 3,135 expectant mothers. An October 21, 1993, Associated Press story said the study found that the advantages of aspirin were slight and did not significantly improve the health of newborns.

Caffeine. Many holistic physicians now recommend pregnant women stop drinking coffee, although it is not clear that coffee has any serious side effects. Research findings on the effects of caffeine on pregnancy have been contradictory. The National Institutes of Health (NIH), for example, studied the caffeine consumption of 431 pregnant women. After ruling out other risk factors such as smoking, the researchers found that pregnant women who consumed as many as three 8-ounce cups of coffee, seven and a half 8-ounce cups of tea, or five 12-ounce cans of cola did not have a greater risk of miscarriage or of delivering a low-birth-weight baby than those who avoided caffeine, according to an article by Eileen Springer in the September 1993 issue of *American Health.* Despite the lack of scientific evidence, however, holistic physicians still counsel expectant mothers not to consume any caffeine, or to limit caffeine intake as an added safety measure, Springer reports.

Exercise. Regular exercise, as explained in Chapter 6, provides numerous physiological benefits to the human body. Moderate, safe exercise is even more important for pregnant women. Clinical studies cited by Robert W. Jarski and Diane L. Trippett in the February 1990 *Journal of Family Practice* have shown that expectant mothers who exercise have faster, easier deliveries. Physically conditioned pregnant women also typically have stronger abdominal muscles and, as a result, their second stage of labor is much shorter.

A pregnant woman will add to her normal weight, which can exert severe pressure on her legs and feet. This additional weight can be accommodated without severe side effects by exercises that improve circulation, reduce swelling, and help prevent the formation of varicose veins. The ideal amount and type of exercise will depend on each woman's health and how much weight she gains during pregnancy. Obstetricians suggest that one way pregnant women can decide how much they should exercise is the exercise-talk test. If they use a treadmill, for example, they should be able to exercise and talk comfortably. If they cannot, they need to reduce their level of exertion. In all cases, an expectant mother should never increase her heart rate to more than 60 to 70 percent of the maximum range for her age. Heart and respiration rates should return to normal ranges within fifteen minutes after exercising, according to Jarski and Trippett in the February 1990 *Journal of Family Practice.*

According to a recent two-year study of 463 women, conducted at the Columbia School of Public Health in New York City, expectant mothers who worked out for thirty minutes, five days a week, gave birth to bigger, healthier babies. Regular exercisers who burned up to a thousand calories a week doing both high- and low-impact activities, including stationary biking, aerobics, jogging, and strength training, delivered babies who weighed approximately 5 percent more than infants born to sedentary women. Birth weight jumped 10 percent when the women burned two thousand calories a week exercising. The researchers felt the study should reassure women who want to exercise more vigorously or even start exercising during pregnancy, although they cautioned that women who have not exercised before should be careful to build gradually up to a full routine, reported Denise Brodey in *American Health,* November 1993. Other studies also have shown that pregnant women who exercise have a heightened sense of well-being and seem to experience fewer complications and less pain during labor.

Swimming, walking, and abdominal exercises such as sit-ups are especially good for maintaining circulation and muscle suppleness, and relieving back pain. There may be reasons why some women should not continue the same exercise routine which they enjoyed before pregnancy, however. All expectant mothers who exercise should be careful not to fall, especially in the last three months. Also, very intense exercise may deprive the fetus of some blood flow and nutrients and should be avoided. Female athletes who compete during pregnancy should consult their physician because certain strenuous sports activities may cause birth complications.

Yoga and tai chi are both excellent forms of exercise. Pregnant women who practice yoga have even claimed that they have been able to do headstands several hours before going into labor. Exercise, as long as it is gentle and does not put pressure on the fetus, is highly recommended.

Hydrotherapy, which can help expectant mothers gently exercise their bodies without gravity, tones and relaxes the body at the same time. Immersion in water puts pressure on the arms and legs, thus pushing fluids into the bloodstream and helping to relieve edema, the normal but uncomfortable swelling that results from water retention during pregnancy. These baths, however, should not be hotter than 97 degrees Fahrenheit, as the fetus may suffer brain and nerve complications.

Dr. Dean Edell, writing in the July 22, 1993, *San Jose Mercury News,* reported that doctors at the University of North Carolina at Chapel Hill, found hydrotherapy particularly good for women in the last stage of pregnancy. They tested eleven healthy pregnant women in their third trimesters by submerging them shoulder-deep in 92-degree water for fifty minutes a day over the course of five days. As a result of the hydrotherapy, all the women urinated more—which is one way the body eliminates excess water—and each experienced a safe drop in heart rate and blood pressure.

Nutrition. When a woman becomes pregnant, she soon becomes aware that she is eating and living for two people. Indeed, the fetus obtains all of its nutrients directly from the woman via the placenta until the moment of birth. What the expectant mother should eat and what supplements she will need depend on her age, her health history, and the physiological characteristics of her pregnancy. The Recommended Dietary Allowances for essential vitamins and minerals for pregnant and lactating women are listed in Chapters 3 and 4.

Calcium is often the most important mineral for expectant mothers, because it helps prevent high blood pressure. Approximately 10 percent of American women develop high blood pressure during pregnancy, usually in the last trimester. In most cases, the elevation is mild and produces no adverse symptoms. However, if untreated or uncontrolled, it can progress to kidney failure, liver damage, seizures, and, rarely, death. According to an article by Elizabeth Rosenthal in the September 13, 1993, *New York Times,* six hundred Argentinean women were given 2,000 milligrams of calcium a day in pill form in the second half of pregnancy, almost twice the total intake currently recommended during childbearing. Less than 10 percent of the women had developed high blood pressure by the time they gave birth, compared to 14.8 percent who took a placebo that contained no calcium. Calcium also may reduce hypertension that can cause premature deliveries and low-birth-weight babies.

Women who are pregnant should take calcium supplements only with the advice of their physician as supplements can have several side effects, including constipation.

Normally obstetricians advise expectant mothers to consume as much calcium as possible through a natural diet, and to use supplements only if the diet does not provide sufficient amounts, Rosenthal reports.

Smoking. Most research strongly recommends that pregnant women not smoke during pregnancy. The National Center for Health Statistics reports that pregnant women who smoke are much more likely to have problem pregnancies and low-birth-weight babies.

Toxins. Pregnant women should avoid any prescription drugs that have been linked to birth defects and mental retardation. Tranquilizers such as Valium, Librium, and meprobamate, for example, can cause several types of brain defects in the fetus. Pregnant women also should discuss with their physicians the potential toxic effects of even mild nonprescription drugs that they may have taken in the past, including ointments and other topical drugs, cough and cold medicines, laxatives, sedatives, pain killers, antihistamines, and antacids.

All types of recreational drugs should be avoided. Alcohol, heroin, anticancer and anticonvulsant drugs such as methadone, testosterone, and steroids, as well as excessive doses of vitamins A and D, may be harmful to the fetus, according to Kurt Butler and Lynn Rayner in *The Best Medicine: The Complete Health and Preventive Medicine Handbook.*

The most hazardous environmental toxins are gases and heavy metals, including benzene, cadmium, lead, and insecticides. If possible, pregnant women should get an air humidifier and a water purifier to decontaminate their drinking water and the air in the home. X-rays, especially to the kidneys, bowel, or lower back, also may cause fetal defects and should be avoided unless prescribed for emergency reasons by the woman's health practitioner.

Expectant mothers are at a slightly greater risk of contracting infectious diseases while they are pregnant. Sexually transmitted viruses, such as cytomegalovirus, herpes virus, and AIDS, are particularly dangerous for both the woman and the fetus, and the woman and her sexual partner should be tested for these viruses and treated if they are present. The expectant mother should also avoid eating undercooked meat, which might be contaminated with bacteria. Viruses, liver infections, kidney damage, and malnutrition can all put the fetus at risk and can cause eclampsia. Symptoms of eclampsia include high blood pressure, high levels of protein in the urine, and excessive swelling (edema) of the hands, feet, and face. A holistic physician will carefully monitor for these complications throughout the pregnancy.

Symptoms During Pregnancy

Abdominal cramping and spotting are common in the early months of pregnancy. A slight increase in bleeding during the first trimester is not unusual, although continued or heavy bleeding should be discussed with a physician. Headaches, insomnia, depression, and fatigue also are common. Holistic physicians usually help expectant mothers avoid these symptoms with exercise and nutrition programs. They may prescribe a natural pain reliever, such as ginger or chamomile tea, in cases where a woman experiences persistent pain. Prescription drugs should be avoided as they may have toxic effects on both the expectant mother and the fetus.

Abnormal Heart Rate. The weight of the fetus and hormonal changes may accelerate a pregnant woman's heart rate. She may also experience periodic palpitations, nosebleeds, and dizziness. Normally, these are not serious unless persistent, in which case the woman should consult her physician.

Constipation, Hemorrhoids, and Varicose Veins. The growing pressure of the uterus against the bowels and intestines often increases constipation, hemorrhoids, and varicose veins. Holistic physicians usually will prescribe a diet with adequate fiber and water to help ease elimination. Adequate exercise, especially walking, is also important. If symptoms persist, the physician may prescribe a natural laxative.

Morning Sickness. More than 50 percent of pregnant women complain of morning sickness at some time during their pregnancy, usually in the first few months. Typical symptoms include nausea and vomiting, especially early in the day. Most physicians now think that the condition occurs as a result of liver imbalance. The liver is responsible for detoxifying the hormones produced during pregnancy, and if it does not function properly, toxic substances can circulate in the blood and eventually stimulate the symptoms of morning sickness, according to Murray and Pizzorno's *Encyclopedia of Natural Medicine*.

Vitamin B6 supplements have been used to reduce nausea and vomiting during pregnancy. Clinical trials have found vitamins K and C, used together, to be helpful, Murray and Pizzorno report. In one study, 91 percent of patients showed complete remission within 72 hours. The mechanism for this result is unknown, and either vitamin administered alone has little effect.

In some cases, eating a small amount of ginger helps to ease morning sickness. Ginger promotes the elimination of intestinal gas, soothes the intestinal tract, and forestalls the symptoms of motion sickness, especially seasickness. In one study, ginger was shown to be far more effective than Dramamine, a popular over-the-counter drug used to alleviate nausea and vomiting.

Spicy and gas-producing foods contribute to morning sickness. Because the expectant mother's stomach cannot hold as much food as before her pregnancy, heartburn and belching often occur. According to Butler and Rayner, some hormonal effects also may cause stomach juices to back up into the esophagus, which then becomes irritated. A health practitioner can test whether a pregnant woman is secreting adequate amounts of hydrochloric acid. Expectant mothers should ask their physician to recommend a diet that is gentle and that can be eaten in small amounts, while still providing the essential nutrients she and her baby need.

Urinary Tract Infections. Some pregnant women develop infections in their urinary tract because of hormonal or immune system reactions. If these become serious, they can lead to slowed fetal growth, serious kidney infection, and premature delivery. Most expectant mothers will urinate more frequently because of the pressure the uterus places on the bladder. This is normal and not necessarily a sign of infection. If fever or itching develops, however, a physician should be consulted.

Childbirth

Many women prefer to give birth without the use of anesthesia or pain-relieving drugs that may have side effects. More importantly, if a woman is fully conscious during delivery, especially with a midwife present, she is able to bond with the baby during the entire birthing process. Every woman differs in her pain threshold, and in some cases birthing may be facilitated with mild sedatives. If drugs are necessary, however, they should be given only by the physician in attendance.

General anesthesia usually is not necessary in a normal delivery. Most obstetricians prefer not to sedate the woman, because if she is asleep or sedated with anesthetics, she cannot consciously push or help the labor as effectively. The anesthesia also may put the baby to sleep and depress its breathing and heart rate, thereby reducing the oxygen supply to the brain.

Analgesics and tranquilizers, when needed, usually are given by injection or inhalation (nitrous oxide) and can ease the delivery pain enough to permit the woman to relax between contractions while remaining alert and attentive. The key factor is the amount and type of drug used. Excessive sedation in some cases can lengthen the early phase of labor.

Certified Nurse-Midwives (CNMs)

Whatever site is chosen for a baby's birth, be it a hospital, birth center, or at home, many expectant mothers are now choosing certified nurse-midwives to aid in the delivery. According to the American College of Nurse-Midwives (ACNM), the use of CNMs in American hospitals increased 700 percent between 1975 and 1990. The National Center for Health Statistics further reports that 3.6 percent of all births in the U.S. were attended by CNMs in 1990. Ninety-four percent of those births took place in hospitals, 3.8 percent at birth centers, and 2.3 percent at homes. The ACNM expects that the number of midwife-attended births will continue to climb, with CNMs attending 10 percent of all births by the year 2000, reports Susan Kushner Resnick in the November/December 1993 issue of *Natural Health.*

A CNM is a registered nurse who has two years of graduate-level midwifery training and has passed a national examination. They are extensively trained in routine gynecological and prenatal care and are familiar with the entire process of pregnancy and birthing. The majority are female and likely to be mothers. They stay with the woman during the entire labor period, whereas many physicians may be present only during the last stages and for the actual birth.

Wherever a baby is delivered, most certified nurse-midwives work in conjunction with the attending obstetrician. Today, there are almost 4,000 nurse-midwives in the U.S., and it should not be difficult for any pregnant woman to find a compatible one.

Research also indicates that when midwives assist in the delivery of a baby, women are more relaxed, their labors are shorter, and they need fewer drugs or medical procedures. An article in the November/December 1993 issue of *Natural Health* reported an ongoing five-year study sponsored by the NIH in which the birth records of approximately eight hundred women who delivered at the University of Michigan Hospital were examined. Some were attended by nurse-midwives and some by physicians. Among the preliminary results: 13 percent of CNM patients used epidural anesthesia during labor, compared to 41 percent of medical doctors (M.D.) patients; 36 percent of CNM patients received continuous electronic fetal monitoring compared to 74 percent of M.D. patients; 32 percent of CNM patients versus 59 percent of M.D. patients received episiotomies; and only 8 percent of CNM patients required Cesarean sections, whereas 19 percent of M.D. patients needed them.

This NIH study also shows that women cared for by CNMs were significantly less likely to experience postpartum hemorrhage, infection, and major perineal damage than doctors' patients. A 1987 study by the same researchers revealed that women assisted by nurse-midwives fared as well as doctors' patients and were less likely to have intravenous fluids, artificially ruptured membranes, painkillers or sedatives, or anesthesia, according to the *Natural Health* article.

CERTIFIED NURSE-MIDWIVES

Cesarean Deliveries

In a Cesarean section, the baby is delivered surgically by cutting through the woman's abdominal and uterine walls. In some emergencies, a Cesarean delivery is the only alternative, but it should be used only as a last resort because there is a risk of maternal complications. Women should insist their obstetrician perform the procedure only if it is absolutely necessary. According to J. Aylsworth in the spring 1990 *Priorities,* half of the 934,000 Cesarean sections performed in the U.S. in 1987 were not needed, costing the public an extra $1 billion and increasing maternal morbidity to an unknown degree. Women selecting an obstetrician should ask about the percentage of Cesarean deliveries performed in the doctor's practice. Some authorities calculate that, on average, Cesarean are necessary in only 12 to 14 percent of deliveries.

Postpartum Recovery

Immediately after childbirth the mother undergoes a two-week recovery period, usually called puerperium, which involves complex physiological and psychological changes. Her muscles, especially the vaginal ones, must first recover from the pain of delivery. Equally important, the mother's estrogen and progesterone (hormones), which were high during pregnancy, drop rapidly until they are no longer detectable seventy-two hours after birthing. Fatigue, mood shifts, and post-delivery depression can accompany these changes.

These first two weeks following birth can be critical to both the mother's and baby's health. Holistic obstetricians focus on ensuring that the mother bonds immediately with her newborn baby, eats a balanced diet, and exercises regularly. They often work with the mother using a variety of exercise and relaxation therapy techniques to reduce anxiety and depression and increase self-esteem during the postpartum period.

Infant Care

Baby Formulas

Virtually all pediatricians agree that breast milk is a baby's best food source. Yet despite the popularity of breast-feeding, most babies drink baby formulas—either exclusively or as a supplement—at some point during the first year of life. Infant formulas are available in ready-to-use, liquid-concentrate, and powdered forms. Ready-to-use formula offers the advantage of convenience, but it is significantly more expensive than concentrate or

Benefits of Breast-Feeding for the Baby

- Breast-feeding promotes the development of the baby's digestive system.

- Breast-fed babies have lower rates of childhood disease, ear infections, respiratory infections, and meningitis than do bottle-fed infants.

- Breast-fed babies have fewer allergies and less diarrhea, colic, stomach aches, and dental problems.

- Breast-feeding strengthens the bonding process between the mother and baby.

- Breast-feeding stimulates the release of hormones that help the uterus return to its normal size, and decreases painful postpartum contractions in the uterus.

powder alternatives. Water must be added to formula concentrate, and care should be taken so that the formula given to the baby is neither too strong nor too diluted. Once opened, it is perishable. Powdered formula also is mixed with water and should be used within two weeks to retain its full potency.

Most formula directions call for adding only sterilized water as a precaution, although this not necessary as the baby gets older. To better match the chemistry and milk sugar content of breast milk, some manufacturers of milk-based formulas dilute the proteins and add vegetable oils and lactose. Parents who bottle-feed their baby must be careful to regularly boil both the bottles and the rubber nipples to reduce the level of carcinogenic substances in the rubber.

Babies who develop frequent diarrhea usually are sensitive or allergic to cow's milk. Soy-based formulas that contain vegetable proteins and nonlactose are a good substitute. Other signs of sensitivities include hives, a runny nose, and rashes. Parents who suspect that their baby has a problem with cow's milk should ask their pediatrician to recommend a substitute.

Breast-Feeding

The many advantages of breast-feeding an infant have been extensively documented in clinical trials. Breast-feeding appears to protect both the mother and baby against infection, while nursing stimulates the development of the baby's own immune system.

Breast-feeding is extremely important for the development of healthy teeth. A Johns Hopkins study of ten thousand babies, for example, found that babies who were breast-fed for more than one year had fewer crooked teeth than those who were bottle-fed. As reported in the October 12, 1993, *San Jose Mercury News,* the researchers postulated that breast-feeding requires babies to suck more vigorously to draw in milk, thus strengthening the development of the infant's teeth.

Breast-feeding is also beneficial for new mothers who want to lose post-baby weight. In a two-year study at the University of California at Davis, women who breast-fed during their child's first year lost an average of 4¼ pounds more than those who formula-fed. There was little weight loss, however, during the second year. According to Kathryn Dewedy, professor of nutrition at UC-Davis, women who breast feed secrete more of the lactation-regulating hormone prolactin, which helps burn calories, the *Los Angeles Times* reported on November 11, 1992.

There is a slight risk that women who breast-feed their babies in the six months after giving birth may suffer bone loss of as much as 5 percent. Researchers at the University of Michigan studied ninety-five white and three Asian women, twenty to forty years old, for a year. All the women ate adequate amounts of calcium. After six months, women still breast-feeding had mineral loss averaging 5.1 percent from the spine and 4.8 percent from the thigh bone. A year after giving birth, however, the women who weaned their babies at nine months or earlier had regained normal bone density. To regain bone mass, holistic physicians usually recommend that breast-feeding women take calcium supplements. Researchers also claim that bone loss poses few concerns for most American women because their generally good diets should be sufficient to rebuild their bones. The majority of American women who breast-feed their babies do so for only three months, and therefore do not appear to suffer bone loss, according to an article by Fran Sowers in the June 23, 1993, *Chicago Tribune.*

The findings of new bone loss research are especially important for teenager mothers and women who are poorly nourished or who become pregnant often. The bones store calcium in the body and, according to one report, women who lose bone density before menopause may be at greater risk for fractures and osteoporosis in later years. A woman's bone loss also can affect her children. If a mother's calcium is severely depleted while nursing one child, it may reduce the amount of calcium available to infants born later. A nursing woman, according to the *Chicago Tribune* report, should consume approximately 1,250 milligrams of calcium daily, including supplements, to meet her own and her infant's need for calcium.

Circumcision

Traditionally, many male babies born in Western countries are circumcised—that is, they have the foreskin of the penis cut back at birth or shortly thereafter. However, obstetricians now disagree on the value of this procedure. While circumcision is usually a painless procedure without side effects or complications, some physicians caution that pain, hemorrhaging, and surgical trauma can occur, reports the February 1990 *Journal of Family Practice.* However, some studies suggest that urinary tract infections can be as much as ten times more common in uncircumcised boys than in circumcised ones. As a result, the American Academy of Pediatrics now advises that circumcision may reduce the incidence of urinary tract infection.

Massage

Infant massage accentuates the bonding between mother and child, both physically and psychologically. The technique involves a series of firm but light pressure strokes especially designed to soothe the baby's delicate limbs and torso. When it is performed gently and correctly, studies show infant massage helps circulation, digestion, and sinus congestion, and is deeply relaxing for the baby. These studies also claim that the more children are touched as infants, the healthier they will be as adults, according to Yamil Berard in the October 24, 1993, *Long Beach Press Telegram.*

Respiratory Disorders

Although many infant deaths occur during the first year of life, infant death rates in the U.S. have declined since 1989. A report by the National Center for Health Statistics estimates that the overall infant mortality rate decreased in the U.S. from 9.7 deaths per thousand live births in 1989 to 9.1 deaths per

Feed a Crying Baby

One of the first things a new mother learns is that crying babies often calm down once they are fed. Scientists have long wondered if the babies are comforted by being held, by the act of suckling, or by the food itself. Researchers at McGill University in Montreal selected fifty-three healthy bottle-and-breast-fed newborns and randomly assigned each to receive either an extra feeding of water, water-diluted lactose (the sugar present in milk), or commercially available infant formula. The lactose and the formula both provided nutrients that the babies would receive from a typical meal of formula or breast milk.

While infants in all three groups were alert and calm for ten minutes after their meal—suggesting that cuddling or suckling or both had soothed them—babies fed formula or lactose were then much more likely to fall asleep. The babies who got only water fretted and cried and needed more soothing. The study supports what most mothers have known for ages: a good meal will calm babies and help them sleep.

thousand live births in 1990. That decrease represents the largest single-year reduction in the nation's infant mortality rate since 1981. According to the center, this success rate was due to the development of a new drug used to treat infant respiratory disorders, the *San Jose Mercury News* reported on May 2, 1991.

In the U.S., approximately fifty thousand babies develop respiratory distress syndrome annually; in 1989, about thirty-four hundred babies died of the disease. Death results from an infant's inability to breathe naturally. A baby's lungs are one of the last organs to develop before birth, and many premature babies are born without a surfactant, the natural internal liquid coating that keeps the lungs from collapsing when the infants exhale. Premature babies can be put on respirators to keep their lungs inflated, but this can result in other serious consequences, ranging from cerebral palsy to blindness.

Exsosurf, a white, foamy liquid drug, has proven the most successful way of treating infant respiratory disorders caused by a lack of surfactant in a baby's lungs. An artificial form of surfactant, Exsosurf is administered by inserting a tube down an infant's airway soon after birth and squirting the liquid into its lungs. Some babies show immediate and dramatic improvement.

Starting Solid Foods

There is no hard and fast rule as to when a baby should start eating solid foods. However, early solid food feeding may increase the likelihood of allergies. Most physicians stress that solid food should be used when the mother either has to return to work or, for other reasons, can no longer breast-feed. It is best to begin by introducing the baby to small amounts of plain, nonacidic organic foods. Most women start with unprocessed organic baby foods. Regular organic foods that the family eats can also be fed to the baby, as long as they are unsalted, are not strongly seasoned, and are pureed.

One advantage of starting solid foods within six months after birth is that they encourage the baby's teeth to develop. Early tests should be taken to determine if the baby has any allergies to foods such as dairy products, citrus fruits and juices, or wheat.

Teething

When a several-months-old infant suddenly becomes fussier than usual, the baby is probably cutting a tooth. Teething babies typically need to "work" their gums, and do so by chewing on crib edges, teething rings, bottle nipples, their parents' fingers, or their own fingers. Several anesthetics have been approved for use to relieve teething pain in infants from four months to two years of age. These contain alcohol, however, and are not recommended by holistic physicians.

One safe way of relieving teething pain is to give the baby a pacifier that contains crushed ice, or a bottle containing a few ounces of cool water, to cool the gums. This soothes most cases of teething, although if the baby continues to be uncomfortable, it may suffer from sore gums and parents should consult their doctor or dentist.

Sudden Infant Death Syndrome (SIDS)

SIDS is the leading cause of death in infants between one month and twelve months old in the U.S. One to two infants per thousand live births die of SIDS annually. Overall, between five thousand and six thousand babies die each year, reports the California Medical Association in the November 1990 Health Tips.

The peak age for SIDS is two to four months, and more deaths also occur in winter. Premature babies, siblings of SIDS victims, and infants born to substance-abusing women are at high risk for developing the syndrome.

Less than 10 percent of SIDS victims have manifested any life-threatening symptoms. Parents should be alert for several signs

which do, however, predict SIDS: cessation of breathing, change of skin color, irregular heartbeats, choking, or gagging.

As SIDS most often occurs during sleep, the syndrome increasingly has been linked with a baby's sleeping position. Infants who are put to sleep on their stomachs, for example, are at higher risk of SIDS. Several studies conducted by Dr. Warren Guntheroth at the University of Washington Medical Center found that the incidence of SIDS is substantially lower when babies are placed on their backs to sleep. Other SIDS studies conducted in England, Australia, Hong Kong, and the Netherlands showed the same results, according to the September/October 1993 issue of Natural Health.

The link between sleeping positions and SIDS comes from the fact that babies experience pauses (known as apneas) in breathing while asleep. After a prolonged apnea, an infant will usually arouse itself with a gasp that fills the lungs with air. If the infant lies on its stomach, the gasp response is less effective, which can result in SIDS. Parents are commonly advised to place babies on their stomachs to guard against choking, in case the infant should vomit. However, the University of Washington's study also shows that the rate of choking was lower for babies who slept on their backs.

According to Sandra Blakeslee in the February 14, 1989, New York Times, many experts believe that SIDS babies have a subtle brain abnormality, either in the brain stem that controls breathing and heart rates or in brain areas controlling sleep patterns and learning processes. Recent insights into brain chemistry and advanced imaging techniques now make it possible to test for SIDS-related abnormalities. Also, babies can be fitted with monitoring devices that sound an alarm when their breathing becomes irregular during sleep.

Summary

Becoming a parent is truly one of life's magical moments, and it should be approached with a plan to do everything possible to ensure that the new infant is healthy and will enjoy a natural, peaceful development. The expectant mother and child are one biological organism until the moment of birth, and whatever the woman puts into her body will most likely be passed to her baby. Therefore, it is extremely important that the pregnant woman eat properly and avoid consuming any drugs or toxins that could harm the fetus. Starting and maintaining an exercise routine has been strongly linked in several studies with good health during pregnancy, an easier delivery, and larger, healthier babies. Childbirth should be a natural process except in cases of emergency, and the baby should be bonded to the mother as soon as possible. Women who breast-feed significantly increase the chances that their babies will enjoy healthy physiological and psychological development. The most important factor in ensuring a safe and successful pregnancy is a woman's confidence in her obstetrician and nurse-midwife and her awareness of her own body.

Resources

References

Aylsworth, J. "Unnecessary Cesarean Operations." *Priorities* (spring 1990): 19–20.

Berard, Yamil. "Massage Rubs in the Baby Bond." *Long Beach Press Telegram* (October 24, 1993).

Blakeslee, Sandra. "Crib Death: Suspicion Turns to the Brain." *New York Times* (February 14, 1989): 17.

"Breast Feeding May Mean Straighter Teeth." *San Jose Mercury News* (October 12, 1993).

Brodey, Denise. "Building Bigger Babies." *American Health* (November 1993): 11.

Butler, Kurt, and Lynn Rayner. *The Best Medicine: The Complete Health and Preventive Medicine Handbook.* New York, NY: Harper & Row Publishers, Inc., 1985.

California Medical Association. "Sudden Infant Death Syndrome." *Health Tips* index 305 (November 1990): 1–2.

Castelman, Michael. "Even Breast-Fed Babies are Liable to be Fed Some Formula." *Los Angeles Times* (November 11, 1992): 8.

"Childbirth." *Natural Health* (November/ December 1993): 127.

Edell, Dean, M.D. "Medical Journal." *San Jose Mercury News* (July 22, 1993).

Edlin, Gordon, and Eric Golanty. *Health and Wellness: A Holistic Approach.* Boston, MA: Jones and Bartlett Publishers, Inc., 1992.

Haney, Daniel. "Aspirin of Little Help to Pregnant Women." Associated Press (October 21, 1993).

———. "Evidence That Folic Acid Can Block Birth Defects." *San Francisco Examiner* (December 25, 1992): 87.

Jarski, Robert W., and Diane L. Trippett. "The Risks and Benefits of Exercise During Pregnancy." *The Journal of Family Practice* (February 1990): 187–88.

March of Dimes Birth Defects Foundation. *AlphaFetoprotein Screening* (January 1991): 1.

Murray, Michael, and Joseph Pizzorno. *Encyclopedia of Natural Medicine.* Rocklin, CA: Prima Publishing, 1991.

RESOURCES

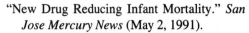

"New Drug Reducing Infant Mortality." *San Jose Mercury News* (May 2, 1991).

"Preventing Sudden Infant Death Syndrome." *Natural Health* (September/October 1993).

Resnick, Susan Kushner. "My Baby: Childbirth that Blends Tradition and Technology." *Natural Health* (November/December 1993): 86.

Rosenthal, Elisabeth. "Study Says Calcium Helps High Blood Pressure in Pregnancy." *New York Times* (September 13, 1993).

Rubin, Rita. "Testing Genetic Disorders." *Dallas Morning News* (October 8, 1993).

Sowers, Fran. "Nursing Mothers May Risk Bone Loss." *Chicago Tribune* (June 23, 1993).

Springer, Eileen. "Caffeine and Pregnancy." *American Health* (September 1993): 86.

Taxel, Laura. "Doulas Help Deliver Health Babies." *Natural Health* (July/August 1993): 44–48.

Organizations

Alan Guttmacher Institute
11 5th Ave., New York, NY 10003.

American College of Obstetricians and Gynecologists
409 12th St. SW, Washington, DC 20024.

American Sudden Infant Death Syndrome Institute
275 Carpenter Dr., Atlanta, GA 30328.

Association for Voluntary Sterilization, Inc.
112 E. 42nd St., New York, NY 10168.

Health Research Group
2000 P St. NW, Washington, DC 20036.

National Association of Childbirth Assistants (NACA)
205 Copco Ln., San Jose, CA 95123.

National Sudden Infant Death Foundation
8200 Professional Place, Ste. 104, Landover, MD 20784.

National Women's Health Network
1325 G St. NW, Washington, DC 20005.

Planned Parenthood Foundation of America
810 7th Ave., New York, NY 10014.

Additional Reading

American College of Obstetricians and Gynecologists. *Barrier Methods Familiar, Safe.* Washington, DC: American College of Obstetricians and Gynecologists, Patient Education Pamphlets, n.d.

Kahan, Barbara. *Healthier Children.* New Canaan, CT: Keats Publishing, Inc., 1990.

Leach, P. *Your Baby and Child.* New York, NY: Knopf, 1993.

Public Health Service. *Fact Sheet: What Is SIDS?* Public Health Service, Sudden Infant Death Syndrome Program, n.d.

Schneider, Vimala. *Infant Massage: A Handbook for Loving Parents.* New York, NY: Bantam Books, 1989.

Shapiro, H. *The New Birth Control Book: A Complete Guide for Women and Men.* Englewood Cliffs, NJ: Prentice-Hall, 1988.

RESOURCES

Chapter 15

DENTAL CARE

Until recently dental care was considered peripheral to general health, and cavities and eventual tooth loss were regarded as inevitable. However, recent advances in conventional and unconventional dental treatment now make it possible for people to maintain healthy teeth and prevent virtually all dental and oral infections. In fact, dentists are often the first to diagnose many types of diseases, not just those in the mouth. A recent survey revealed that 52 percent of the dentists said they had been the first to uncover oral cancer, 28 percent were the first to diagnose bulimia, and 26 percent first detected diabetes. This survey clearly suggests that dentists are increasingly concerned with the whole body health of their patients. As an example, nearly half of the 603 dentists surveyed said they ask patients about tobacco use and counsel smokers on how to quit, according to an article by Gannett News Services that was published in the *Marin Independent Journal* on November 28, 1993.

Healthy teeth and gums, like other parts of the body, depend on a strong immune system, and if this system is weakened, the teeth and gums are more likely to become infected. For this reason, a holistic approach to dental care should include eating natural whole foods that both strengthen the immune system and prevent the formation of bacteria and acids that corrode the teeth and cause gum disease and infections.

Teeth, like other bones, are affected by the foods a woman eats during her pregnancy. Dental care should encourage pregnant women to consume sufficient amounts of vitamins A, B, C, and D, as well as calcium, phosphorous, and fluoride. Vitamin A is essential because a deficiency in the fetus (or during infancy) can cause abnormal tooth development, poor calcification, and

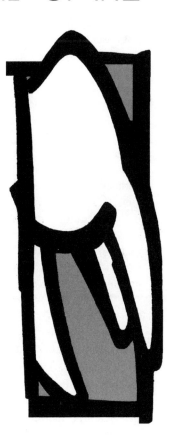

reduced enamel formation. Vitamin C is important because a deficiency can weaken the connective tissue of the gums and decrease the formation of dentin, the bone-like bulk of the tooth. A deficiency of vitamin D, calcium, or phosphorous can cause poor tooth positioning, decreased dentine and enamel, and increased susceptibility to decay. And a mild deficiency of the B vitamins, especially folate, has been shown to weaken the soft tissues and tooth-supporting structures and to increase their vulnerability to infection.

The primary teeth (sometimes called the baby teeth) are already formed when a baby is born, while the permanent teeth begin developing immediately after birth. The primary teeth usually appear through the gums by the seventh month. By the age of two or three years, most babies have all twenty primary teeth, and a full set of permanent teeth is usually formed by the age of five. Oral hygiene, fluorides, and diet are the main factors that affect the health of the primary teeth. If the primary teeth are not brushed regularly and monitored by a dentist for straightness, the permanent teeth are likely to develop problems. Oral hygiene practices for primary teeth include regularly cleaning the baby's teeth with a cotton or gauze pad, rinsing the baby's mouth daily with water, and adding fluoride liquids to the baby's food if fluoride is not present in the drinking water, according to Jane Brody in *Jane Brody's The New York Times Guide to Personal Health*. Fluoride supplements should be added only upon the advice of a dentist, and are not necessary in areas with fluoridated water.

Infant tooth decay can occur when a baby is given a bottle filled with milk, formula, or fruit juice at bedtime, naptime, or for long periods during the day. Extended exposure to the sugar in these liquids can cause teeth to discolor and decay. Since breast milk also contains sugar, decay can occur if a baby falls asleep when breast-feeding. To prevent damage, a child's teeth should be cleaned after each feeding, and, if necessary, the infant be given a bedtime or naptime bottle filled only with water.

Cavities

It has been estimated that half of all American children have at least one cavity by the age of two. Cavities are caused by bacteria that adhere to the teeth and excrete a sticky transparent film of dextran called plaque. When the plaque becomes thick enough, it produces acids that can eat away the enamel covering a tooth and eventually erode (decalcify) the underlying bone, leaving a hole in the tooth. Once this occurs, the bacteria that created the defective tooth structure must be removed, restored, and filled.

Several factors determine whether a young child will develop cavities. First, genetic structure will affect how well teeth resist the bacteria that form on them. Some people are actually genetically immune to tooth decay. What a person eats is also a factor, because sugar and honey left on the surface of teeth produce acids that damage tooth enamel. Sweet snacks, particularly sticky foods containing caramel, cause significant damage. Sweet drinks also produce cavities, especially colas that contain tannic acids.

Despite the role of genetic or nutritional factors in causing cavities, the American Dental Association (ADA) claims that virtually all cavities can be prevented by proper oral hygiene. Even if teeth are inherently weak and exposed to sweet substances that can cause cavities, proper brushing will neutralize and eliminate most sugars through the saliva. Even if brushing after a snack is not possible, chewing sugarless gum helps neutralize the acid environment.

Preventing Tooth Decay

The following guidelines are recommended by the American Dental Association (ADA).

- **Brushing.** A toothbrush should be replaced often, ideally once every three months or when the bristles show wear. A worn-out toothbrush will not clean teeth properly. Change the position of the toothbrush frequently, as it will clean only one or two teeth at a time. Brush gently and with very short strokes, but use enough pressure so that the bristles can be felt against the gum. Only the tips of the bristles clean, so do not squash them. Be sure to brush at least twice a day to help prevent plaque damage.

- **Toothpaste.** Some fluoride toothpastes prevent 25 to 30 percent of the decay a child might otherwise develop. However, not all fluorides are effective. The seal of the ADA Council on Dental Therapeutics guarantees the most effective products.

- **Mouthwashes.** A mouthwash can temporarily freshen breath or sweeten the mouth, but none remove plaque or prevent tooth decay. However, mouthwashes with fluoride provide minor protection against some tooth diseases. Do not rely on mouthwashes to relieve pain or other symptoms of gum disease.

- **Flossing.** Floss regularly, preferably after every meal.

- **Dental Visits.** Regular checkups and professional cleanings are essential.

The ADA recommends using a toothbrush with soft, rounded bristles and a flat brush surface. The head of the brush should be small enough to reach all sides of the teeth, and should be held against the teeth with the bristles at a forty-five-degree angle facing into the gum. The tongue also should be brushed to remove bacteria and to freshen breath. Gum stimulators, pointed rubber tips at the end of toothbrushes, are useful for massaging gum tissue. The ADA now endorses the use of electric toothbrushes and specifically urges people to avoid abrasive toothpastes or powders. Water Piks can replace toothbrushes and are useful for people with bridgework or braces. Because there are many developments in this area, San Francisco holistic dentist Gary Lindsey suggests following recommendations for a product made by a dental professional rather than a manufacturer's advertisement.

Dental floss, either waxed or unwaxed, should be used twice a day to clean under the gumline and between the teeth. An eighteen-inch piece of floss, held between the thumbs and forefingers of each hand, should be eased between the teeth and curved into a C shape around each tooth at the gumline. When it is moved up and down gently between the tooth and gum, the floss scrapes against the side of the tooth and removes bacteria. Flossing should be followed by a thorough rinsing of the mouth to wash out loosened bacteria. The ADA also recommends that people regularly monitor the effectiveness of their brushing by using a solution or tablets containing a vegetable dye that stains plaque.

Dental Chewing Gums

For the last twenty years, chewing gums containing sugar were thought to cause cavities. But nonsugar gum, especially chewing gums with xylitol (a sweetener extracted from corn stalks), may help prevent cavities. In one recent clinical trial, reported in the July/August 1993 issue of *Health,* University of Michigan researchers asked a thousand children in Belize to chew gum containing either xylitol, sugar, or sorbitol (a natural sweetener) three to five times a day. Another 140 children chewed no gum at all. After twenty-eight months, children who chewed sugared gum had an average of 50 percent more cavities than when the study began—about the same as those who did not chew any gum. Those who chewed sorbitol gum had only slightly more cavities than at first. The children who chewed xylitol gum, however, had a third fewer cavities than they did before the study began. The researchers believe that the xylitol gum generated minerals that filled shallow cavities and caused the cavities to harden. Chewing gum stimulates saliva, which washes away some cavity-causing bacteria, and reduces the acidic environment. Regular sugar gum feeds the bacteria and neutralizes the effect of saliva. Xylitol, on the other hand, slows bacterial growth, allowing saliva to break down and eliminate the bacteria (acid).

Dental Sealants

Dental sealants were invented in the early 1980s but are still not widely used in the United States. While the ADA promotes sealants, for example, only 17 percent of American eight-year-olds have had their permanent teeth sealed. In Finland, the figure is 85 percent, according to Steven Shepherd in *FDA Consumer Reports,* May 1990.

While some dentists seal baby teeth, most sealants are applied only to the chewing surfaces of permanent teeth to create a barrier against food and bacteria that can cause decay. Most dental sealants are applied to molars, whose deep grooves make them difficult to brush and most vulnerable to cavities. After the molars are etched with an acidic solution to help the sealant adhere, the sealant—which can be milky white or colorless—is applied and hardened with a bonding light. Chewing and brushing eventually wear away sealants, but they give the teeth enough time to resist decay, especially if they are used in conjunction with regular brushing. Sealants do not eliminate the need to brush and floss, because cavities still can develop between teeth. Regular dental care also is necessary, because sealants must be checked for wear and occasionally touched up. Sealants currently cost $25 to $50 per tooth, a cost covered by many dental insurance plans. They are nearly 100 percent effective in preventing decay on back teeth, according to Shepherd.

Fluorides

Ninety-eight percent of all Americans have at least one cavity, and virtually all of these can be prevented by fluoride, and proper oral hygiene, according to the ADA. When infants and young children swallow fluoride, it is incorporated into the teeth as hard, insoluble crystals called fluorapatite. Fluorapatite replaces some of the natural outer-tooth enamel and penetrates into the deeper layers of the teeth. Fluoride in the saliva also helps to remineralize enamel by retaining calcium and phosphate. These crystals inhibit the ability of bacteria to become attached to teeth and to produce the acids that contribute to the onset of decay.

The best sources of fluoride include natural drinking water, drinking water fortified with fluoride supplements, and fluoride products available over the counter in mouth rinses and treatment gels. The most common source of fluoride in the U.S. is drinking water. Of 133 million Americans who live in communities where the public water supply contains 0.7 parts per million (ppm) of fluoride, 9 million drink naturally fluoridated water, while 124 million use water that contains fluoride supplements. Most ground, river, and lake waters contain some natural fluoride, according to David Zimmerman, in *Zimmerman's Complete Guide to Nonprescription Drugs.*

While the use of fluoride in drinking water and in supplement forms is still controversial, it is quite clear that fluoride effectively prevents cavities. Zimmerman reports in an article in the December 22, 1989, *Journal of the American Medical Association,* which reviewed all the literature on fluoride and concluded that community water fluoridation "yields a 50 to 65 percent reduction in cavities, while fluoride drops or tablets, mouth rinses, toothpaste and dental applications yield from 20 to 65 percent reduction in cavities."

People who are reluctant to take fluoride supplements should consider substituting cardamom, an aromatic seed often used in curries, stews, and pastries. The Academy of General Dentistry reports that cardamom, a natural spice, contains more than ten compounds that have varying degrees of cavity-fighting potential. According to Paul Stephens, D.D.S., president of the academy, as quoted in the winter 1993 *Healthy Woman,* "The trend of society is to go back to nature. So we can expect natural substances such as cardamom to be used instead of chemicals in toothpastes and mouthwashes to fight cavities and bad breath."

Another natural spice, oil of cloves, extracted from the spice commonly used to flavor apple cider and pumpkin pie, can be used to temporarily ease tooth pain. For emergency relief, depending on what causes the pain, holistic dentists sometimes recommend

Benefits of Fluoride

These sources of fluoride reduce cavities by the following percentages:

- Fluoride in drinking water: 50 to 65 percent.
- Fluoride in school drinking water: 40 percent.
- Fluoride drops or tablets taken at home: 50 to 65 percent.
- Fluoride mouth rinses: 30 to 40 percent.
- Fluoride toothpastes yield: 20 to 40 percent.
- Annual fluoride applications by dentists: 30 to 40 percent.

an application, which will temporarily numb the nerves in the tooth that is signaling pain. Available at natural food stores and many pharmacies, oil of cloves can be used to soak a cotton ball or swab, which is then rubbed on the painful tooth and surrounding gums. An alternative is to soak several whole cloves in a small amount of hot water in a covered pot to activate the essential oils. The cloves should then be held next to the affected tooth with the tongue or cheek until pain subsides.

Fillings

Once a tooth develops a cavity, it must be restored. The type of filling a dentist recommends depends on the cost, the size of the cavity, its location, and cosmetic considerations. Fillings vary in hardness, endurance, and cost. Most dentists prefer to use gold or porcelain fillings because they are the strongest and last the longest. Porcelain also has the same whiteness as natural teeth, and is one choice for cosmetic reasons. Composite fillings are made from several materials, including small amounts of metal oxide that dries as hard as glass. According to Lindsey, "composite fillings are very technique sensitive and are not the easiest and fastest to apply. But when composite fillings are done by an expert practitioner, they wear better and polish better than amalgam fillings."

Amalgam fillings (sometimes called silver fillings) are permanent, easy to install, and fill holes in teeth quite adequately. Most Americans with fillings have had at least one that is amalgam. They last a significant period of time and are less expensive than gold. Most contain approximately 40 to 54 percent mercury, 35 percent silver, small amounts of tin mixed with copper, and a trace of zinc.

Many holistic dentists believe that the small amounts of mercury contained in amalgam fillings may gradually leach into the body (either as part of the saliva or as a gas), and may subsequently pass along nerve roots directly to the brain. Most crowns also have amalgam fillings under them, and the mercury can leak out through the root of the tooth and into the bloodstream. Mercury has been shown to affect the nervous system, sometimes resulting in numbness, extreme fatigue, mental incapacity, or even paralysis. As a result of the potential danger of mercury toxicity, several countries, including Sweden and Austria, have or soon will ban amalgam fillings in pregnant women, according to the *CDA Journal*, February 1985.

The ADA's official position is that the small amount of mercury that may get into a person's system from amalgam fillings does not present a health threat. However, many dentists are switching to a composite material made from particles of silica with a plastic matrix binder.

A new technique is now being used instead of drilling to treat tiny cavities before they destroy larger areas of the tooth. The technique, called kinetic cavity preparation (KCP), uses a high-speed stream of particles that sandblasts away superficial decay and stains. Although dentists tend to ignore discolored pits on teeth, decay can often be present, particularly on the back teeth. If a cavity has not yet developed, the stain alone is removed and a sealant applied to the tooth to prevent further trouble and discomfort. Treating these areas with KCP prevents more serious damage. And, because the sandblasting device provides greater control than conventional drilling, it also removes less of the tooth's enamel. However, it does not replace drilling for more extensive work. The Academy of General Dentistry claims that anesthesia is not necessary when the KCP technique is used, because of the lack of pain, heat, and vibration, reports Diana Reese in the November 1993 *American Health.*

Gingivitis and Periodontal Disease

Periodontal disease is any form of disease affecting the periodontium, or the tissues that surround and support the teeth. These include diseases of the gums (gingivitis), the bone of the tooth socket, and the periodontal ligament (the thin layer of connective tissue that holds the tooth in its socket and acts as a cushion between tooth and bone).

Gingivitis is an inflammation of the gum tissue caused by bacterial infection. A nationwide survey by the National Institute of Dental Research found that 40 to 50 percent of U.S. adults studied had at least one spot on their gums with inflammation that was prone to bleeding, according to Shepherd in the May 1990 issue of *FDA Consumer Reports.* Since gingivitis is painless in the early stages, many people do not know until it is too late that their gums have developed this potentially serious infection.

Plaque is a major contributor to gum disease. Plaque bacteria produce toxins that inflame the gums, which then become swollen and start to pull away from the teeth. Plaque that causes gingivitis starts first above the gum line (it is referred to as supragingival plaque). Over time, as Shepherd explains, areas of supragingival plaque become covered by swollen gum tissue or spread below the gum line, and in this airless environment the harmful bacteria within the plaque proliferate. Pockets of pus and cell debris may form between the teeth under the gum line, allowing the toxins to move down along the roots of the teeth to the bones which support them. Hundreds of bacterial species may thrive in the spaces between the teeth and the gums, and at least seven or eight can generate serious infections. Eventually the bone retreats, the fibers that hold the teeth to the bone are eaten away, and the teeth loosen and fall out. Proper and frequent flossing, however, can play an important role in preventing the formation of plaque and eventual gum disease.

Tartar is the yellow mineral deposit that forms on teeth. It provides a surface for additional plaque to adhere and grow and is a major contributor to gingivitis. Without proper brushing and flossing, plaque and tartar can build up and extend below the gumline, accelerating the development of periodontal disease. Once tartar develops, only a dental hygienist or dentist can remove it by either scraping the crown and root of the tooth or by laser incision.

In their early stages, both gingivitis and periodontal disease are preventable and reversible. Dentists can remove plaque and tartar from the crowns and roots of teeth by scaling. Scaling is usually performed with root planing, in which the rough surfaces of the root are smoothed, allowing the gum to heal. The key to preventing and treating gum disease in its early stages is to recognize the symptoms: red, puffy, tender, or easily bleeding gums; signs of pus at the gumline; evidence that gums seem to be shrinking away from the teeth; teeth that have shifted or loosened; or persistent bad breath. People with any of these symptoms should immediately visit their dentist or oral health care professional.

Scientists are developing new procedures for early detection of these destructive infections. One of them, nearing final approval by the FDA, is a test to detect an enzyme in the mouth that is released only by cells that are dead or are dying. The enzyme, called amino aspartate transferase, has long been used to uncover evidence of dying cells in heart vessels during coronary disease. Also nearing approval are new gene probe techniques that can identify genetic material in the bacteria principally responsible for periodontal infections. One such test can be completed in a dentist's office while the patient is undergoing routine cleaning. Dentists now can also detect the first signs of gum disease by noting the existence of pockets and analyzing the bacteria found in them. Using periodontal screening and recording (PSR), a dentist can probe the patient's gumline with a tool that measures the depth of any existing pockets and signs of bleeding at six areas around each tooth. The result is a scorecard that helps the dentist decide whether gum therapy is necessary, according to David Perlman in his report of a San Francisco dental conference, published in the November 9, 1993, *San Francisco Chronicle.*

In severe cases, gum surgery may be required to remove shallow pockets around the teeth. When this surgery (called flap surgery) is performed, the gum is lifted from the tooth and bone so that the infection can be removed. The infected bone also may be reshaped. After surgery, the gum is repositioned and sutured to hold it in place until it heals. Advanced periodontal disease may require grafting of bone and gum transplants. Treatment may involve grinding or capping teeth to correct abnormal pressure points, or the use of splints to control harmful mouth habits and reduce movement of loose teeth. Conventional periodontal disease treatment can take six to eight months or longer, and cost several thousand dollars.

A prescription product called Peridex, which contains the antimicrobial chlorhexidine, was approved by the FDA in 1986 based on studies showing that it reduced gingivitis by up to 41 percent. Chlorhexidine mouthwashes have long been used in Europe, and chlorhexidine is now approved for use in mouthwashes in the U.S. Listerine has also received approval by the FDA and ADA as a plaque-deterrent, Shepherd reports.

Treatments for Gingivitis

Studies at the National Institute of Dental Research tentatively suggest that holistic treatments for gingivitis may be effective. Dental scientists have experimented with treating gingivitis patients with daily solutions of salt, baking soda, and hydrogen peroxide.

Using an electric toothbrush and pulse-water irrigator (which delivers an antiseptic solution directly into the pockets between teeth and gums), along with frequent dental cleanings and antibiotic treatments, also has been successful. The ADA has suggested that further research is required to confirm whether this treatment can slow down irreversible periodontal disease, according to Zimmerman.

Malocclusion (Crooked Teeth)

Nearly 50 percent of American children aged six through eleven have a normal bite with only slight abnormalities in tooth formation. However, 25 percent have definitely crooked teeth, a condition known as malocclusion—literally, "bad bite." At one time, crooked teeth were thought to be primarily inherited from the parents with little recourse to prevent them. Today, Zimmerman reports, the American Academy of Periodontics estimates that 50 to 80 percent of orthodontics can be avoided if problems are detected early enough. More than 15 percent of orthodontic patients in the U.S. are adults who have their teeth straightened to improve their appearance and to prevent the tooth loss that is fostered by malocclusion.

Treatments for crooked teeth vary, but in most cases the teeth are straightened by the use of orthodontic braces. *Jane Brody's The New York Times Guide to Personal Health* identifies several types of braces. Some braces are removable, some can be worn part of the time outside the mouth, and others are attached to the teeth for several years. Most braces consist of wire-connected brackets that are fitted across the teeth. Increasingly, permanent braces are constructed of plastic that blends more naturally with the color of the teeth. Facial bones, as well as teeth, can be realigned to improve both bite and appearance.

All forms of braces pressure the teeth to reposition themselves inside the bone socket in which they sit. In children whose bones are softer and still growing, the process of reshaping the bone through pressure is faster than in an adult, claims Brody. Direct pressure on facial bones can have a similar effect, with the amount and direction of pressure determining the shape the bone will assume.

The American Association of Orthodontics reports that tiny magnets implanted in a person's teeth can correct many common orthodontic disorders without using braces or surgery. Although magnets have been used to correct certain dental problems since the mid-1980s, only recently has the procedure gained widespread popularity.

The tiny magnets, only three to four millimeters in diameter, are made of materials such as neodymium-iron-boron and are essentially the same type of magnets used in stereo equipment and other electronics. Depending on the type of problem being treated, magnets are used to pull teeth in a certain direction or push them apart, which can be particularly effective in treating children who traditionally

required braces to correct misaligned teeth. The magnets can be bonded directly onto teeth, eliminating the possibility of losing them or not wearing them correctly. They often work more quickly than ordinary braces, according to Don Vaughan in *Your Health,* October 19, 1993.

Dentures

According to a 1985–86 survey conducted by the National Institute for Dental Research, Americans sixty-five years or older have lost an average of ten teeth, and those thirty-four to sixty-four years old have an average of nine teeth missing. Four out of ten (42 percent) of Americans aged sixty-five or older have lost all their teeth, as have 4 percent of those thirty-four to sixty-four years of age, according to an article by Vern Modeland in the December 1988–January 1989 *FDA Consumer Reports.*

Dentures are one way to replace missing teeth. Ordinary dentures are generally made of plastic and tailored to each patient's mouth. They are normally fitted to match and adhere to the upper or lower jaw or made to clamp on to remaining teeth with metal supports or bridges. Difficulties with dentures can result from a failure to initially detect such problems as cysts, tumors, inflammation, bone loss, tooth roots that are lodged in the jaw, and distorted positions of the jaw, according to Modeland.

Dentists sometimes are able to save a portion of damaged teeth, which serve as anchors for a partial denture. When a full denture (upper, lower, or both) is needed, the muscles of the cheeks and the tongue must be relied upon to keep it in place. Careful measurements must be made to ensure that the dentures fit correctly. An ill-fitting denture may put undue tension on the jaw muscles, irritate the gums and cheeks, and cause loss of underlying bone.

Dental Implants

For people considering dental implants, the ADA suggests the following guidelines:

- First determine if it is possible to save the natural teeth.
- Make sure the schedule for required implant surgery and follow-up is feasible. Some implants require many visits and a second stage of surgery.

- Find out in advance what pain, soreness, and long-term restriction to diet are involved. Temporary devices may have to be worn.
- Ask the dentist whether the implant is likely to be rejected by the body after several months or years.

To prevent staining of dentures, dentists recommend daily cleaning with special brushes and dental aids (not ordinary toothpastes). Dentures should be placed in water or a cleansing solution when they are out of the mouth. In addition, the mouth should be rinsed each morning, after every meal, and before bed to clean out harmful bacteria and food particles. The dentist should exam the dentures once each year to monitor and refit them, if necessary.

Dental Implants

In the U.S., forty million people wear dentures and another sixty million Americans are missing one or more teeth, according to the *FDA Consumer Reports* for December 1988–January 1989. To avoid the problems and inconvenience of dentures, and to utilize the bone of teeth which are still in place, dental researchers have begun experimenting with new methods of implanting artificial tooth supports surgically set directly and permanently to the jaw bone. The advantage of dental implants is that they are permanent and there is no need to remove them, as with dentures.

The first dental implant was developed in Sweden in 1965 by Dr. Per-Ingvar Branewmark. His method involved drilling a hole in living bone at the implant site and inserting a tiny fixture made of titanium, which was screwed or pressed into place in the jawbone. After three to six months, when the bone had grown around the implant, the gum was reopened and an abutment attached to the titanium fixture. The new tooth, several teeth, or an entire row of teeth was then attached to the abutment. A clear plastic healing cap prevented the gum from growing into the abutment.

Today, there are four different types of dental implant procedures. According to the FDA's Center for Devices and Radiological Health, the two most frequently used are one- and two-stage cylindrical implants and blade implants. The former is very similar to the method developed by Branewmark, and features channels that are cut lengthwise into the jaw bone. The blades have openings that can accept bone regrowth through their framework, Modeland reports.

In 1992, the FDA claims that more than one hundred thousand Americans underwent surgery to be fitted with titanium dental implants. Titanium's advantage is that bone tissue fuses to it. For reasons that are not fully understood, titanium seems to bond with successive generations of bone cells while other materials lose their bonding power over time.

In general, the chances for dental implant success are much higher in the lower jaw—about 95 percent—because it is a thicker bone. People considering this type of surgery should consult a specialist who will recommend the appropriate implant design. The ADA has cautioned that there is no substitute for natural teeth, and that implants will never function as well as real teeth. With today's technology, dentists can salvage even badly damaged teeth, and the ADA advises that people first try everything possible to restore their own teeth.

There are risks associated with dental implants, including inadvertent perforation of the nasal sinus, infection, and nerve injury. The dental implant surgery may also result in pain and swelling and gingivitis. A holistic dentist will normally conduct a complete medical history of the patient before performing dental implant surgery. The use of tobacco, alcohol, and most drugs must be discontinued during dental implant surgery and post-surgery recovery. The same is also true for cosmetic surgery, according to Lindsey. He counsels that it is always best to avoid harmful substances which may compromise healing.

New Dental Technologies

Many dental procedures, such as the conventional means of removing diseased gum tissue, are extremely painful. However, new laser surgical techniques developed for use in gum surgery cause no apparent pain because they vaporize only a few layers of cells at a time, and the body can easily repair the minimal damage to surrounding healthy tissue. According to the Michael Castelman in the

January 10, 1993, *West,* lasers have now been used in more than one hundred thousand dental procedures in twelve countries, including Canada, England, Japan, Mexico, and Australia. With laser surgery, dentists can clean out diseased pockets of gum tissue to the point where the body can heal itself. They can also make the teeth more resistant to future decay by sterilizing the deep crevices toothbrushes cannot reach.

However, since lasers cannot cut through the healthy enamel of teeth, dentists still need to use a drill to enlarge or modify a hole in a tooth to get at a cavity or to shape a tooth to receive a restoration. Some reports have documented using the laser in place of a needle to anesthetize a tooth which needs to be drilled. The advantage of this procedure is that, unlike a drill, the laser exerts no pressure and does not cause stress. With laser surgery, there usually is very little pain and swelling. An increasing number of holistic dentists routinely use laser surgery because there is less trauma, bleeding, infection, and need for anesthesia, and teeth can be saved in ways that are impossible with conventional surgery. Within several years, lasers may painlessly drill cavities as well.

Dental X-rays are a critical component in a dentist's analysis of the bone and gum structure of teeth. A disadvantage of X-ray machines is that they emit a very slight amount of radiation. With the advent of computers, inventors have experimented with forms of digital radiography that eliminate the need for X-ray films and film processing. Direct digital radiography can deliver instantaneous computer-enhanced X-ray images with less radiation. The newest radiographic systems depend upon a charged-couple device (CCD), a small cassette-style intraoral silicon receptor with a solid-state electronic circuit embedded in the silicon that captures the X-ray signal. The X-rays strike the silicon, and electrons are released and stored as a digital

Guidelines for Choosing a Holistic Dentist

- **Prevention.** Because tooth decay and tooth loss are not inevitable, the dentist should stress the importance of diet and daily home care (proper brushing and flossing) as well as periodic cleanings. The dentist should be sensitive to the health of a person's entire body, provide counseling to minimize any pain associated with surgery (if needed), and recommend using natural preventive measures and therapies whenever possible.

- **Examination.** The dentist should conduct a thorough evaluation, including a visual examination of the soft tissue of the mouth (cheeks, tongue, throat, gums, and bite) and a periodontal examination to measure the depth of pockets that have formed between gums and teeth. A full set of X-rays should be taken, and head and neck examinations performed to test for clinically observable pathology.

- **Treatment.** The dentist should discuss what treatment is needed and why, how long it will take, how much it will cost, and what nontraditional alternatives might be available. If extensive work is recommended, obtain a second opinion from another dentist. For serious gum disease, the dentist should make a referral to a periodontist.

image that can be sent immediately to a computer monitor for viewing. The dose of radiation using digital radiography is 90 percent less than from conventional X-ray machines,

according to D. Reis in the October 1993 issue of *Dental Products Report.*

Summary

Dental health affects the whole body, because the mouth cavity is a primary site of many different types of infection and dental abnormalities often reflect immune disorders. For both these reasons, it is important to eat a diet of natural whole foods that help prevent tooth decay and significantly enhance the maintenance of healthy teeth throughout life. Poor nutrition can result in weakening of the microstructure of the calcified tissues and vulnerability to tooth decay. Proper and frequent brushing and flossing also can play an important role in preventing cavities and the formation of plaque that can lead to gum disease and tooth loss.

Resources

References

Brody, Jane. *Jane Brody's The New York Times Guide to Personal Health.* New York, NY: Avon Books, 1982: 282.

Castelman, Michael. "Dentistry." *West* (January 10, 1993): 10–17.

"Chewing Away Tooth Decay." *Health* (July/August 1993).

Gannett News Services. "Dentists Report a More Holistic Approach." *Marin Independent Journal* (November 28, 1993).

"Kaleidoscope." *Healthy Woman* (winter 1993).

Liles, Alan. "Mercury Free Dentistry." *Shared Guide* (1993): 16.

"Mercury Breath...How Much is Too Much?" *CDA Journal* (February 1985): 42.

Modeland, Vern. "Dental Implants." *FDA Consumer Reports* (December 1988–January 1989): 13.

Perlman, David. "S.F. Dental Conference Gives Gum Disease High-Tech Treatment." *San Francisco Chronicle* (November 9, 1993): A19.

Reese, Diana. "Sandblasting Cavities." *American Health* (November 1993): 20.

Reis, D. "Direct Digital Intraoral Radiography Systems." *Dental Products Report.* (October 1993): 22.

Shepherd, Steven. "Anti-Plaque Mouth-washes." *FDA Consumer Reports* (May 1990): 14.

———. "Brushing Up on Gum Disease." *FDA Consumer Reports* (May 1990): 9–10.

Vaughan, Don. "No More Braces!" *Your Health* (October 19, 1993): 19.

Zimmerman, David. *Zimmerman's Complete Guide to Nonprescription Drugs.* Detroit, MI: Gale Research Inc. and Visible Ink Press, 1993.

Organizations

American Academy of Implant Dentistry
6900 Grove Rd., Thorofare, NJ 08086.

American Academy of Periodontology
211 E. Chicago Ave., #114, Chicago, IL 60611.

American Dental Association
211 E. Chicago Ave., Chicago, IL 60611.

National Institute of Allergy and Infectious Diseases
9000 Rockville Pke., Bethesda, MD 20205.

National Institute of Dental Research
NIH Building 30, Bethesda, MD 20892.

National Women's Health Network
1325 G St. NW, Washington DC 20005.

Additional Reading

American Academy of Periodontology. *Dental Implants: Are They Right for You?* Chicago, IL: American Academy of Periodontology, 1989.

"Combating Periodontal (Gum) Disease." *Health News* (June 1989).

"Dental Implants: How Good They Are, How Long They Last." *Johns Hopkins Medical Letter* (March 1989).

Holland, Lisa. "Dental Implants." *Good Housekeeping* (January 1990).

Langer, Burton. "Dental Implants Used for Periodontal Patients." *Journal of the American Dental Association* (October 1990): 505–08.

McVeigh, Gloria. "High-Tech Tooth Savers from the American Academy of Periodontology." *Prevention* (May 1990).

Williams, Ray. "Periodontal Disease." *New England Journal of Medicine* (February 8, 1990).

Chapter 16

EYE, EAR, NOSE, AND THROAT DISORDERS

The eyes, ears, nose, and throat, along with the skin and mucous membranes, serve as the body's first line of defense against external toxins and infectious organisms. They are often the first organs to decline with aging, which many people assume is natural. However, physical, mental, and emotional stress, along with poor nutrition and vitamin deficiencies, can accelerate the process. This chapter focuses on alternative approaches to keeping these organs healthy and preventing chronic disorders.

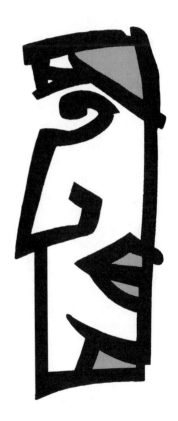

Eyes

Virtually 80 percent of what people perceive and know about the world around them comes from the eyes. Like a camera, the eye has a single lens that focuses on objects and projects an image of those objects onto the retina, the light-sensitive region at the back of the eyeball. A normal clear lens allows light to pass through unobstructed. For a number of reasons, however, the lens, cornea, iris, or eye muscle may develop problems, and vision can become impaired.

Most common eye defects, if detected early enough, can be treated by an ophthalmologist, a specialist in diagnosing and treating eye diseases. Diagnosis normally consists of a vision test during which an ophthalmologist tests the patient's ability to focus on near and far objects. At the same time, the physician will check for signs of blood vessel damage, blank spots, and weakness of the eye muscles, which can cause the retina to become detached.

Preventing Eye Damage

- **Annual examinations:** Adults over the age of 40 should have their eyes examined annually by a specialist.

- **Sunglasses:** Always wear sunglasses with polarized lenses when out in the bright sunlight. These glasses block 95 percent of the sun's harmful rays, especially at the beach or in snow areas.

- **Avoid dangerous chemicals:** Wear protective eyewear whenever handling dangerous chemicals or doing household or shop work that raises dirt or debris. Heavy polycarbonate lenses offer more protection than regular glasses and should be worn when playing racquet sports or high-impact sports such as hockey and football.

- **Be careful with makeup and facial creams:** Cosmetics can cause eye irrita-

tion and possible infection. Mascara and eyeliner should be replaced with new supplies every three to six months to prevent bacterial buildup. Never share makeup or applicators with others.

- **Contact lenses:** Contact lens wearers should use makeup designated as safe for contact lenses. It also is advisable to insert lenses before applying makeup and to take them out before using makeup remover. The hands should be washed thoroughly before lenses are handled. Follow all cleaning and storage instructions exactly.

- **Eye drops:** A variety of eye drops and other lubricating preparations are available to relieve occasional discomfort caused by common allergens such as pollen, dust, or pet dander, as well as smog and pollution.

A recent Gallup poll indicated that 75 percent of Americans value their eyesight above all other senses. Yet 85 percent admitted that they are not as careful in caring for their eyes as they should be. Virtually all eye injuries and half of the 50,000 cases of blindness that occur annually could be prevented, according to experts, with simple, common-sense precautions.

Cataracts

Cataracts are the leading cause of impaired vision and blindness in the United States. Approximately 4 million Americans have some degree of vision-impairing cataract, and at least 40,000 people in the U.S. become blind each year as a result. A cataract is any clouding of the normally clear and transparent lens of the eye. It is not a tumor or a new growth of skin or tissue over the eye, but a yellow fogging of the lens itself. The lens, located behind the pupil, focuses light on the retina at the back of the eye to produce a sharp image. When a cataract forms, the lens becomes so opaque that light cannot be transmitted easily to the retina. If only a small part of the lens is involved, sight is not greatly impaired, and there may be no need to remove the cataract. If a large portion of the lens becomes cloudy, however, sight can be partially or completely impaired, and the cataract must be removed.

Many factors contribute to the progression of cataracts, including other eye disorders, injury, systemic diseases (such as diabetes mellitus or galactosemia), toxins, hereditary diseases, and ultraviolet and near-ultraviolet light or radiation exposure. Cataracts usually occur in elderly persons, although people of any age can develop them as well. Cataracts that appear in children generally are hereditary, or are caused by infection or inflammation that the pregnant mother transmits to her baby.

Prevention and Treatment of Cataracts

Cataracts develop slowly and often do not reach the point of interfering with a person's normal vision. The most important ways to prevent cataracts are to consume nutritional foods and supplements that maintain the integrity of the central nucleus and soft outer cortex of the lens, and to keep the lens from being damaged by chemical toxins and the sun's ultraviolet rays. The Food and Drug Administration (FDA) is considering regulations to require all new sunglasses to block 99 percent of ultraviolet B radiation.

Botanical Medicines. The Chinese herbal formula hachimijiogan has been shown to increase the glutathione content of the lens and has been used in the clinical treatment of cataracts in China and Japan. In one Japanese clinical study, 60 percent of the subjects who used hachimijiogan did not develop cataracts, while 20 percent showed no progression and 20 percent developed cataracts. An extract of ginkgo biloba produced in Austria also may help prevent the formation of cataracts. It is known for its antiaging properties, and is being tested as a treatment for degenerative eye disorders.

Nutritional Therapies. Dr. Glen Swartwout, an optometrist in Hilo, Hawaii, reports in a 1986 issue of The Holistic Optometrist that cataracts in many of his patients result directly from nutritional imbalances and are further aggravated by smoking, drinking alcohol, and the use of some pre-

scription drugs (especially cortisone and other steroids). Two-thirds of the patients in one study he conducted showed improved vision within four weeks after changing their diet and adding nutritional supplements.

To prevent cataracts, Swartwout advises his patients to restrict consumption of processed, high-fat foods, along with alcohol, caffeine, sugar, and nicotine. He recommends eating more legumes (which are high in sulphur-containing amino acids), yellow vegetables (carotenes), and foods rich in vitamins E and C (particularly fresh fruits and vegetables).

Surgery. Severe cataracts that impair vision are normally treated with surgery. Modern cataract surgery typically takes less than an hour and involves making a small incision through the cornea and sclera that permits removal of the cloudy lens, leaving the lens capsule in place. In 90 percent of cases, according to Jane Brody, writing in the July 21, 1993, edition of the *New York Times,* an artificial lens can be slipped in to replace the one that was removed. Most patients are able to go home the same day.

Traditional Chinese Medicine (TCM). According to Dr. Maoshing Ni, vice-president of Yo San University of Traditional Chinese Medicine in Santa Monica, California, acupuncture and herbs can relieve both cataracts and glaucoma. He suggests in *Alternative Medicine: The Definitive Guide* that dietary changes combined with acupuncture, Chinese herbs, and stress management can reverse the growth of cataracts in some patients.

Vitamin and Mineral Therapies. Several studies have shown a link between deficiencies of vitamins A, E, and C and the development of cataracts. Preliminary research suggests that vitamin C can prevent changes in proteins in the eye associated with cataracts.

In one study reported in the July 1992 issue of *Environmental Nutrition,* people who took several vitamin supplements, including vitamin C, had four times less risk of developing cataracts than those who took no supplements. Research on vitamin C's role in preventing cataracts is inconclusive, however, as other antioxidant nutrients such as vitamin E and beta-carotene also help prevent cataracts.

A Finnish study reported in the July 13, 1993, issue of *Your Health,* for example, found a strong link between low nutrient levels of vitamins A and E and the likelihood of needing cataract surgery. The study collected blood samples from 1,419 people between 1966 and 1972, and concluded that people with low levels of vitamins A and E were nearly "twice as likely to need cataract surgery compared to those with high levels." The investigation concluded that "free radicals contributed to the growth of cataracts and vitamins A and E appeared to neutralize free radicals." Similar results, according to the *Your Health* article, were reported in a study of 660 people in Baltimore, Maryland. Those with the most vitamin E in their blood were least likely to develop the most common form of cataracts.

Many holistic physicians believe that cataracts are caused by free radical damage to some of the sulfur-containing proteins in the lens. The lens is dependent on adequate levels of superoxide dismutase (SOD), catalase, and glutathione (GSH). When a cataract begins to form, these protective nutrients are damaged by free radicals. Glutathione levels can be increased by taking cysteine, glutamine, or glycine supplements that have proven beneficial in cataract treatment.

Zinc supplements also may be helpful in treating cataracts. Zinc is a well-known antioxidant believed to be essential for normal lens functioning. In addition, beta-carotene may act as a filter, protecting against light-induced damage to the fiber portion of the lens. People with cataracts also have far lower selenium levels than people who do not have cataracts, which suggests that taking selenium supplements may retard the progression of cataracts.

Glaucoma

According to the May 1994 issue of *The Johns Hopkins Medical Letter,* more than 3 million Americans are visually impaired because of glaucoma. Several different types of glaucoma have been identified, including chronic open-angle glaucoma, congenital glaucoma, acute angle-closure glaucoma, and secondary glaucoma, which is caused by secondary conditions such as hemorrhages, tumors, and inflammations. People with glaucoma usually experience hazy vision, eye and head pains, nausea, and rapid loss of vision. Glaucoma can occur in people of all ages; but is more likely to develop in people over the age of 35 years who are very nearsighted or diabetic.

Causes of Glaucoma

Glaucoma occurs when extra fluid builds up inside an eye and presses against the optic nerve at the back of the eye. The buildup usually results from genetic factors or as part of the aging process. Normally, a clear, transparent liquid called aqueous humor flows continually through the structures of the inner eye. If this flow becomes blocked, liquid pressure can build up against the optic nerves, which impairs their ability to transmit visual images to the brain.

In chronic open-angle glaucoma, the drainage channels of the aqueous humor become smaller with age and clogged with deposits that gradually increase pressure against the optic nerves. This is the most common type of glaucoma in adults, and many do not realize they have the condition because they assume it is a natural part of aging. This type of glaucoma causes a loss of peripheral vision, and, if it is detected early by an ophthalmologist, can be treated with eye drops that decrease fluid buildups in the aqueous humor.

Congenital glaucoma is caused by genetic abnormalities in the drainage openings of the eye. It is quite rare and can be reversed only by surgery. Acute angle-closure glaucoma is caused by the iris pressing against the drainage canals in the inner eye. Fluid backs up and increases eye pressure, which results in blurred vision, severe pain, and nausea. Patients with these symptoms should see an eye physician immediately as blindness can result within several days. Secondary glaucoma is caused by hemorrhages, tumors, or inflammations in the inner eye that block the drainage channels.

Prevention and Treatment of Glaucoma

If diagnosed promptly, the eye pressure that causes glaucoma can be stabilized, and future glaucoma attacks can be prevented. An important aspect of alternative treatment is testing patients to determine what type of glaucoma they have and whether prescription medications they take for other disorders are increasing their risk for glaucoma. According to *Alternative Medicine: The Definitive Guide,* more than 90 medications, including antihypertensives, steroids, and antidepressants, can lead to glaucoma if used over a prolonged period of time.

Biofeedback. Dr. Steve Fahrion, director of the Center for Applied Psychophysiology at the Menninger Clinic in Topeka, Kansas, cites several studies in *Alternative Medicine: The Definitive Guide* that suggest that biofeedback can relax the forehead muscles and help reduce the pressure on the eyeball caused by glaucoma. One technique involves placing electrodes on the forehead, which allow

patients to monitor their own stress levels and stimulate the relaxation response.

Botanical Medicines. James F. Balch and Phyllis Balch cite several botanical medicines in *Prescription for Nutritional Healing* that they say effectively relieve glaucoma. They suggest that rutin helps reduce inner-eye pressure when used in conjunction with standard drugs. They also recommend warm fennel herb eye baths, alternated with chamomile and eyebright, as helpful in relieving the pain that accompanies glaucoma. No clinical trials on the effectiveness of these botanical medicines have yet been reported.

Eye Drops. Although the eye damage caused by glaucoma usually cannot be reversed, it can be controlled with eye drops, pills, and surgery to prevent further damage. Patients with minor chronic open-angle glaucoma can recover some visual abilities if their condition is detected early enough and they begin using eye drops. Eye drops prescribed by an ophthalmologist usually are administered two to four times daily along with prescription pills. These medications decrease eye pressure either by assisting the flow of fluid out of the eye or by decreasing the amount of fluid entering the eye.

Surgery. Simeon Margolis and Hamilton Moses III state in *The Johns Hopkins Medical Handbook* that surgery is the sole treatment for acute angle-closure and congenital glaucoma, because it is the only way to open up blocked or incorrectly formed drainage canals of the eye. Laser surgery, the least painful and invasive surgical procedure, uses a laser beam of light to burn an opening in the iris and open the eye's drainage canals.

Traditional Chinese Medicine (TCM). Ni reports in *Alternative Medicine: The Definitive Guide* that acupuncture and herbs can relieve both cataracts and glaucoma. Acupuncture and Chinese herbs can signifi-

GLAUCOMA

cantly decrease the interocular pressure associated with glaucoma, allowing patients to reduce the amount of medications they are taking or even to postpone surgery. Ni also notes that Forskolin, a drug extracted from the coleus plant, has been used successfully at Yale University to relieve glaucoma without side effects.

Vitamin and Mineral Therapies. Vitamin C supplements and foods that contain bioflavonoid compounds may help prevent glaucoma by protecting the optic nerves from free radical damage. Vitamin, mineral, or botanical treatments have not been shown to be effective in treating acute forms of glaucoma, however, and eye damage caused by glaucoma usually cannot be reversed.

Macular Degeneration

The macula is the point of the retina in back of the eye responsible for fine vision. When the macula is damaged, images are either blocked or blurred. The condition that results, macular degeneration, is the leading cause of difficulty with reading or closeup vision in the U.S., according to the American Academy of Ophthalmology's *Macular Degeneration: Major Cause of Central Vision Loss.*

Approximately 70 percent of macular degeneration cases occur in elderly people, and are caused by a breakdown or thinning of the tissues in the macula. Another 10 percent are due to blood vessels that burst and leak fluid that damages the macula. In both instances, vision becomes distorted and blurred as dense scar tissue develops, blocking a person's central vision. Other types of macular degeneration are genetic or are caused by injury, infection, or inflammation of the macular. There are no noninvasive treatments for macular degeneration. Alternative therapies focus on preventing the condition through early detection and taking vitamin supplements that maintain the integrity of the macular tissue.

Treatments for Macular Degeneration

Biofeedback. Trachtman claims that he has helped patients suffering macular degeneration with biofeedback treatments. Using his Accomotrac Vision Trainer machine, patients have been trained to use a part of the eye other than the deteriorating macula.

Nutritional Therapies. According to an article in the April 1988 issue of *Health Facts,* blueberry extract, bilberry, ginkgo biloba extract, and zinc sulfate have been shown in several preliminary clinical trials to be effective in retarding severe visual loss due to macular degeneration. However, patients are advised to consult an eye specialist before taking any supplements. Antioxidants such as vitamin C, selenium, and vitamin E also may be beneficial.

Surgery. Advanced macular degeneration can be treated only by laser surgery. Such surgery, however, according to Margolis and Moses, can damage small parts of the retina and leave blind spots. Researchers at Johns Hopkins University have developed a new prototype laser treatment that effectively seals blood leaks in wide areas of the retina without damaging it. Tests are under way to further improve the technique.

Refractive Eye Disorders

Myopia (nearsightedness), hyperopia (farsightedness), and astigmatism (distorted vision) are caused by differences in the length or shape of the eye. Presbyopia (aging eye) occurs when the lens inside the eye loses its focusing ability for near vision.

Common Refractive Eye Defects

- **Amblyopia.** A slightly crossed or drifting eye (called lazy eye) that can lead to permanent loss of vision.

- **Astigmatism.** Vision is partially blurred because of irregularities in the curvature of the cornea, causing haphazard focusing on the retina of both near and far images.

- **Farsightedness** (hyperopia). People can adjust their eyes to see distant objects clearly, but develop eyestrain when trying to see things nearby.

- **Nearsightedness** (myopia). Nearby objects can be focused on the retina, but

the image of distant objects focuses in front of the retina, causing blurred vision. A nearsighted person needs to squint to bring distant objects into focus.

- **Presbyopia.** With aging, people find it more difficult to focus on close objects. This is caused by weakening of the eye muscles that adjust the lens, as well as a loss of elasticity in the lens itself.

- **Strabismus.** Found mostly in children, in this condition crossed or drifting eyes cannot focus together on the same object.

Treatments for Refractive Eye Disorders

Biofeedback. Biofeedback can correct refractive problems. Joseph Trachtman, a New York-based optometric physician, reports in *Alternative Medicine: The Definitive Guide* that he has helped people with extremely poor vision to eliminate or reduce their need for eyeglasses. Trachtman uses a machine that he invented, called the Accomotrac Vision Trainer, to help patients retrain their eye muscles to overcome refractive problems.

Surgery. Acute refractive eye problems that cannot be treated with noninvasive treatments normally require corrective eye surgery. Radial keratotomy is the most common corrective eye surgery technique. During the procedure, a surgeon makes a series of spoke-like microscopic incisions with a knife that reshape the surface of the cornea. When the cuts heal, the cornea is slightly flattened,

so that light rays focus directly on the retina, not in front of it. This type of surgery works best with patients who have moderate myopia. As reported by David Holzman in the January 22, 1990, issue of *Insight,* 90 percent of patients who undergo surgery for myopia achieve vision of 20/40 or better, which enables them to pass the vision test for a driver's license without glasses. Photoreflective keratotomy, another surgical procedure, uses a new laser device to reshape the cornea. The procedure is being tested by the FDA and is not yet available.

Retinopathy

Retinopathy (RP) is a disease in which capillaries that nourish the retina leak fluid or blood that damages the rod and cone cells of the eye. At least 60 percent of patients suffering from diabetes for 15 years or more have some form of RP. Diabetic RP affects approximately 7 million people in the U.S., and causes blindness in about 7,000 Americans

Other Common Eye Problems

- **Spots Before the Eyes.** This condition, in which people see spots (or "floaters"), is believed to be caused by a clear gel-like fluid inside the eye that increases with age. The spots seldom interfere with vision, however, and usually disappear on their own. If they suddenly increase in number or size, especially if accompanied by pain in the retina, people should be treated by an ophthalmologist.

- **Twitching.** Some people experience frequent twitchings in their lower eyelids. These twitches usually disappear spontaneously over time and require no treatment. If they persist, consult a neurologist.

annually, according to the National Eye Institute. Patients with diabetes should have regular eye examinations to detect the onset of RP, because laser surgery to seal leaking blood vessels can prevent loss of vision.

A new form of intensive therapy developed for diabetics corrects elevations in their blood sugar levels. Dr. Ping Wang, director of a research study at the Joslin Diabetes Center in Boston, reported in the May 23, 1993, edition of the *New York Times* that this therapy significantly prevents the long-term consequences of diabetes-related eye diseases such as RP.

Treatments for Retinopathy

Vitamin and Mineral Therapies. In a controlled study involving 601 patients with common forms of RP, Dr. Eliot Berson, professor of ophthalmology at Harvard Medical School, found that high doses of vitamin A can slow the loss of remaining eyesight by approximately 20 percent per year. In the study, reported by David Tenenbaum in the September 1993 issue of *American Health,* a typical 32-year-old embarking on this therapy, for example, could retain vision until age 70 instead of losing it at age 63. However,

people taking vitamin supplements to prevent RP should be careful not to combine vitamins A and E. While high daily doses of vitamin A appeared to be effective in Berson's trials, large doses of vitamin E (400 IU) seemed to worsen the disease. Berson urges people with RP to consult an eye specialist before beginning any treatment. He also suggests that people who take large doses of vitamin E consult an ophthalmologist to ensure they are not developing RP.

Ears

The ear consists of three important components: the outer ear, including the ear canal leading to the tympanic membrane (eardrum); the middle ear, consisting of three bones connected to the throat by the eustachian tube; and the inner ear, where mechanical vibrations are converted to nerve impulses.

Deafness (Total Hearing Loss)

Hearing involves a complex process by which sounds outside the ear are transmitted as auditory signals through the middle and inner ear and to auditory centers in the brain.

Some infants, due to genetic factors or birth abnormalities, are born deaf—that is, they are born with structural abnormalities of the three middle-ear bones. Other causes of deafness include impairments of the eight nerve fibers concerned with hearing. As Margolis and Moses report in *The Johns Hopkins Medical Handbook,* more than 4,000 infants are born deaf every year in the United States. Approximately half of these cases are due to hereditary disorders.

Deaf patients with structural abnormalities can never recover full hearing. They can, however, be given cochlear implants that stimulate partial hearing. Cochlear implants—tiny microphones placed behind the ear—pick up sound signals and relay them to a speech processor the patient wears in a pocket. Gillian Weiss reports in the November 1990 issue of *American Health* that the implants eventually may become common treatment for total deafness.

People with partial deafness can benefit from using hearing aids that amplify sound signals, stimulating the cochlear hair cells. However, hearing aids can only help people who still have some hearing abilities. Their effectiveness varies according to their design and how well the aid matches the individual's needs.

Ear Blockages

Small children frequently push objects into the ear that either block sound or cause an outer-ear infection. If an adult decides to try to remove the object, caution should be taken not to push the object deeper into the ear canal.

For minor buildups of wax, physicians recommend that adults remove the wax themselves by gently pushing warm water into the ear. In *Alternative Medicine: The Definitive Guide,* nutritionist Katie Data of Fife, Washington, recommends gently washing the

inner ear with lukewarm water and a few drops of vinegar or hydrogen peroxide. Virender Sodhi, M.D., an Ayurvedic physician, suggests in the same book washing the inner ear with warm herbal oils such as garlic or mullein combined with olive oil. Earwax that cannot be removed using heated water generally has to be removed by a physician.

Earwax occasionally can interfere with hearing. The buildup often is caused by food or mold allergies. Ear specialist Dr. Constantine A. Kotsanis reports in *Alternative Medicine: The Definitive Guide* that excessive earwax in children may result from allergies to cow's milk.

Ear Disorders

According to the American Speech and Hearing Association (ASHA), more than 2.1 million Americans develop hearing impairment annually in the U.S. Ear disorders are extremely difficult for people to diagnose themselves and usually require medical attention by an ear specialist—either an otologist or an otolaryngologist. According to ASHA, the three most common hearing impairments in the U.S. are those that involve conductive hearing loss, ear nerve loss, or both.

In conductive hearing loss, sound waves are blocked as they travel through the auditory canal of the middle ear and cannot reach the inner ear. Common causes include wax blocking the ear canal, infection, or a punctured eardrum. Most problems of this nature can be easily treated.

Otosclerosis, the second most common hearing disorder, is a condition in which the bones of the middle ear soften, do not vibrate well, and eventually calcify. Once this problem occurs, it can be corrected only by surgery.

"Nerve deafness" involves either temporary or permanent damage to the hair cells or nerve fibers of the inner ear. Causes of nerve deafness include high fevers, heredity, excess noise, adverse reactions to drugs, diseases such as meningitis, and head injuries.

Treatments for Ear Disorders

Nutritional Therapies. Toxins such as caffeine, tobacco, aspirin, some diuretics, and chemotherapy can cause sensory hearing loss and benign tumors or ulcers in the ear. In some cases, these conditions can be prevented and treated with balanced diets low in saturated fats and cholesterol, wheat, diary products, sugar, alcohol, and yeast. A study reported by J. Spencer in the October 1981 issue of the *Southern Medical Journal* showed that 1,400 patients with inner-ear symptoms who reduced lipoprotein (proteins that carry fat) blood levels decreased pressure in their ears and improved their hearing. A small study reported by M. Strome in the February 1993 issue of *Laryngoscope* found that when several children with "fluctuating hearing loss" were placed on a low fat diet, their hearing returned.

Exercise and Inner-Ear Disorders

Dr. Michael Weintraub, clinical professor of neurology at New York Medical College in Valhalla, reports in the April 6, 1994, edition of the *New York Times* that 20 to 25 percent of people who regularly do high-impact aerobics may eventually develop inner-ear problems. Weintraub has found in preliminary clinical studies that 80 percent of those with symptoms suffered damage to the parts of the inner ear involved with balance. He warns that the repeated jarring of some forms of exercise such as aerobic dancing and running may loosen tiny stone-like structures called otoliths, jamming them down among the hair cells that transmit information to the brain about the body's position in space. Once

otoliths are unbalanced, they send the wrong signals to the brain, which can result in a persistent off-balance sensation, dizziness, a feeling of disorientation, and difficulty in navigating. Many people with these symptoms experience motion sickness and vertigo. According to Weintraub, 67 percent also had ringing in their ears (tinnitus), or a sensation of ear muffling or fullness. Eighty-seven percent of the aerobics instructors studied and 67 percent of enthusiasts also had high-frequency hearing loss. These symptoms indicate damage to the hair cells of the cochlea, the organ that transmits nerve impulses for sound to the brain. To prevent problems, Weintraub urges aerobic exercisers to wear good shoes that absorb the impact of dancing and to avoid using loud music. Even better, he counsels, would be to switch to a less jarring activity such as low-impact or step aerobics.

Meniere's Disease

Meniere's disease (vertigo) is a disorder of the inner ear characterized by a sensation of whirling motion or ringing in the ear. Some people also experience a feeling of fullness in the ear, and fluctuating hearing loss. About 250,000 people develop Meniere's disease annually in the U.S.

The cause of Meniere's disease is not known, although it has been linked to brain tumors, high or low blood pressure, allergies, lack of oxygen circulation in the brain, anemia, infections, nutritional deficiencies, neurological disease, stress, excess earwax, and poor cerebral circulation. It also can occur when a person moves suddenly from a sitting to a standing position. Sometimes the disease results from a watery fluid buildup in the inner-ear, which clouds messages being sent to the brain. Dizziness, the most noticeable symptom, can be so severe that sufferers are unable to work or remain independent.

Treatments for Meniere's Disease

Ayurvedic Medicine.   In *Alternative Medicine: The Definitive Guide,* Sodhi describes an Ayurvedic treatment for Meniere's disease that uses albad oil in the ear to draw out excess fluid. He also internally administers albad oil in a solution with sesame oil and ghee (clarified butter), and prescribes rest and lymphatic drainage massage.

Helium-Neon (HN) Laser Treatments. Homeopath Dr. Arabinda Das of Merrillville, Indiana, reports in the May 1994 *Townsend Letter for Doctors* that he has successfully used helium-neon lasers to treat Meniere's disease. A one-time application of laser for 10 minutes can effectively remove mild symptoms, while two to five treatments are needed for patients with severe symptoms. Five-year followup studies show no recurrences of the symptoms. He suggests that laser treatments inhibit the DNA and RNA of bacteria that cause the disorder. According to Das, laser surgery is a noninvasive holistic treatment that constitutes the "fourth generation of homeopathic remedies."

Homeopathic Remedies.   Milne reports in *Alternative Medicine: The Definitive Guide* that many patients with Meniere's disease also complain of migraine headaches, which suggests that their hearing disorder is partly dietary in origin. Depending on a patient's specific symptoms, he treats Meniere's with homeopathic remedies such as carboneum sulphuratum and salicylicum acidum, in addition to ginkgo biloba. He also prescribes vitamin B6 to decrease fluid buildup and restricts sodium, caffeine, and chocolate. Finally, he determines whether the patient is sensitive to dental amalgams.

Nutritional Therapies.   Michael Glasscock, president of the Ear Foundation in Nashville, Tennessee, has found that 85 percent of his patients suffering from Meniere's disease can be treated with a low-salt diet and diuretics, both of which reduce the amount of fluid in the inner ear. Ear specialists at Sunnybrook Health Sciences Centre in Toronto eliminated vertigo in 89 percent of patients using several doses of gentamicin each day for four days. These findings were reported in the November 3, 1992, edition of the *San Jose Mercury News.*

Surgery.   Patients with Meniere's disease who do not respond to noninvasive treatments may need to undergo surgery (vestibular neurectomy), which generally involves spending five to six days in the hospital. Risks of postsurgical complications include some hearing loss, infections, headaches, and small leaks of brain or spinal fluid, as reported in an article that appeared in the *San Jose Mercury News* on November 3, 1992.

Vestibular Rehabilitation Therapy. According to Melinda Henneberger, writing in January 26, 1994, edition of the *New York Times,* a new type of exercise therapy has been used at approximately 50 vestibular rehabilitation centers to successfully treat some patients suffering from Meniere's disease and other forms of dizziness caused by inner-ear disorders. The therapy combines several home exercise programs custom-designed for each patient, including jumping on a mini-trampoline, sitting up and lying down rapidly, and turning in circles. Patients also do eye exercises at home to retrain the vestibular ocular reflex (a nerve reflex of the inner-ear), which allows the eyes to maintain a steady field of vision as a person moves. The eye exercises, in which patients repeatedly move their heads from side to side or up and down while focusing on specific objects, help patients steady their gaze and regain their equilibrium. Most inner-ear disorders such as Meniere's disease require between 6 weeks and 18 months of treatment. Studies show that 70 percent of patients with inner-ear problems achieve at least partial relief from the therapy, and 30 percent recover completely.

Vitamin, Mineral, and Botanical Therapies.

Balch and Balch report in *Prescription for Nutritional Healing* that patients with vertigo symptoms may benefit from vitamin and mineral supplements that increase circulation of oxygen in the brain, including vitamins B3, B12, C, and A. They also suggest that coenzyme Q10, calcium with magnesium, germanium, and kelp may be helpful. In addition, botanicals such as butcher's broom, cayenne, chaparral tea, dandelion extract or tea, and ginkgo biloba extract have been used effectively to treat vertigo. People who manifest the symptoms should also restrict their intake of nicotine, caffeine, salt, and fried foods.

Otitis Media (Infections of the Middle Ear)

The middle ear is the small space between the outer and inner ear that contains three delicate bones—the hammer, anvil, and stirrup—that are essential for hearing. Air pressure is kept constant by the eustachian, or auditory, tube, which leads into the middle ear from the back of the nasal cavity. If a virus or bacteria invades the middle ear, it can cause inflammation and a buildup of fluids, the two major symptoms of otitis media.

There are several types of otitis media, each defined by its causes. Secretory otitis media is an infection caused by an allergen that enters the middle ear through the eustachian tube. Acute serous otitis media results from a bacterial or viral infection in addition to fluid buildup. Acute purient otitis

media is caused by pus from a bacterial infection and may result in a ruptured eardrum. Chronic otitis media is caused by an untreated bacterial infection, infected adenoids, or structural deformities of the bones of the middle ear.

Symptoms of the four types of otitis media vary substantially. Most sufferers first experience sharp, stabbing, dull and/or throbbing pains in the ear. Some bleeding or discharge of pus may occur as well. These symptoms usually result from ruptures of the eardrum through which pus flows. Children with middle-ear infections may experience nausea and vomiting. People with chronic otitis media also experience constant swelling in the middle ear. Any indication of a middle-ear infection should be referred to an ear specialist. Such infections are not dangerous if they are treated before serious complications occur. If left untreated, otitis media can lead to severe complications such as mastoiditis, brain abscesses, or meningitis.

Treatments for Otitis Media

Ayurvedic Medicine.

Sodhi, as reported in *Alternative Medicine: The Definitive Guide*, uses neem oil to kill bacteria and fungus that cause some middle-ear infections. He also recommends combining neem oil with warm adardica indica oil and placing the solution in the ear. Sodhi employs lymphatic massage outside the ears to open the eustachian tube and facilitate draining. In addition, he prescribes the herb amla, an antibacterial and antiviral, which can be added to honey to help strengthen the immune system.

Botanical Medicines.

Murray and Pizzorno recommend taking goldenseal and licorice to reduce ear pain and help drain excess fluid of the inner ear. Echinacea and goldenseal also kill bacteria that may cause inflammation.

Homeopathic Remedies. Homeopath Randall Neustaedter, director of the Classical Medicine Center in Palo Alto, California, notes that acute ear infections are simple to treat with homeopathic remedies. Those he has used with success include deadly nightshade (belladonna), windflower (pulsatilla), phosphate of iron (ferrum phose), chamomile (chamomilla), and Hahnemann's calcium sulphide.

According to *Alternative Medicine: The Definitive Guide,* Robert Milne, M.D., a Las Vegas homeopath, has treated the early stages of middle-ear infections with two homeopathic remedies, aconit and ferrum phas. For later stages, he gives his patients chamomilla, lycopodium, pulsatilla, and silicea.

Nutritional Therapies. To treat ear infections caused by allergies, holistic physicians recommend diets that eliminate allergic foods, including milk and dairy products, eggs, wheat, corn, oranges, and peanut butter. These diets may also restrict concentrated simple carbohydrates (such as sugar, honey, dried fruit, and concentrated fruit juice) because they can weaken the immune system.

Garlic has been used successfully to treat ear infections caused by bacteria. Researchers at Boston University School of Medicine conducted tests in which garlic proved as effective as an antibiotic in killing 14 bacteria that cause recurrent ear infections in children. As cited in the April 1994 issue of *Your Health,* the garlic even killed some bacteria known to be resistant to common antibiotics.

Surgery. When ear infections cannot be cured by alternative treatments, a surgical procedure called myringotomy is necessary to drain excess fluids. The treatment involves placing a tiny plastic tube through the eardrum to assist drainage of fluid into the throat. Myringotomy is not a curative procedure, however, as demonstrated in a double-blind study published in the October 1981 issue of *The Lancet,* which found that children with tubes in their ears were more likely to have further problems with ear infections. The researchers recommended that natural antibiotics such as garlic be used first, because children not receiving chemical antibiotics had fewer recurrences of infection than those receiving antibiotics.

Vitamin and Mineral Therapies. In addition to eliminating allergens from the diet, Murray and Pizzorno suggest in the *Encyclopedia of Natural Medicine* that beta-carotene, vitamin C, zinc picolinate, bioflavonoids, and evening primrose oil have proved useful in preventing or alleviating ear infections. They also claim that some symptoms have been successfully treated with the herbs echinacea, goldenseal, and licorice.

Infections of the inner ear caused by the destruction of inner-ear hair cells may be treatable by a new procedure that uses chemicals made from vitamins. Dr. Thomas R. Van De Water of the Albert Einstein College of Medicine in New York City has found that retinoic acid, a derivative of vitamin A, can cause the inner ear to grow new auditory hair cells. The destruction or malfunction of auditory hair cells is believed to be the major cause of deafness for approximately 18 million Americans, according to an article entitled "Vitamin A May Be a Key Deafness Cure" that appeared in the May 4, 1993, edition of the *San Jose Mercury News.*

Other Treatments. Locally applied heat often is helpful in reducing the discomfort of an ear infection. It can be applied as a hot pack with warm oil (especially mullein oil), or by blowing hot air into the ear. Also of value is putting hygroscopic anhydrous glycerine into the ear, which helps pull out fluids, thus reducing pressure in the middle ear.

OTITIS MEDIA

Otosclerosis

Otosclerosis is a hereditary hearing problem that develops primarily in adults. Usually the disorder is caused by the tiny stirrup-shaped stapes bones in the middle ear. When the bones become overgrown, they impede the conduction of sound signals traveling through the middle ear.

There are no alternative treatments for acute otosclerosis. This hearing problem often can be completely remedied by surgery that removes the excess bone and replaces all or part of the stapes with an artificial part.

Tinnitus

When sound waves enter the ear, they travel down the ear canal and strike the eardrum, a skin-covered tympanic membrane. The drum is shaped like a broad flat cone approximately one half-inch across and less than one-fiftieth of an inch thick. Prolonged exposure to loud noises can harm the organ of the inner ear called Corti's arch, which converts vibrations to nerve impulses. Teenagers, for example, who listen to music at extremely loud levels often develop tinnitus, a condition in which they experience prolonged ringing or buzzing sounds in their ears. Their ability to enjoy music or any other sound in later years may be seriously impaired.

Treatments for Tinnitus

Botanical Medicines. Ginkgo biloba increases circulation in and around the ear and, according to Kotsanis, is commonly used to treat tinnitus. He reports in *Alternative Medicine: The Definitive Guide* of successfully restoring full hearing to a teenage girl who had lost her hearing in one ear. David Hoffman also reports in the same book that tinctures of black cohosh and ginkgo biloba in equal parts can restore hearing to tinnitus patients.

Homeopathic Remedies. Several homeopathic remedies help treat tinnitus, including salicylicum acidum, chenopodium, and cinchona officinalis. Dr. Robert Milne recommends that people suffering from the disorder see a homeopath who will prescribe a remedy based on the type of noise that initially damaged the ear.

Nutritional Therapies. Because the inner ear is supplied with blood, nutrient excesses or deficiencies can affect hearing. High levels of blood fats and cholesterol, for example, have been shown to cause poor circulation of blood in the ear, and restricting saturated fats in the diet has proved helpful. Vitamin A is highly concentrated in the inner ear, and vitamin A and B supplements have resulted in improved hearing, especially in cases of inner-ear circulation problems and ear infections, according to Kurt Butler and Lynn Rayner in *The Best Medicine: The Complete Health and Preventive Medicine Handbook.*

Nose

The nose is the body's main channel for breathing and performs several critical functions. The nasal membranes that line the nasal passages secrete liquid mucus containing lysozyme, a chemical that destroys bacteria. The nose also plays an important role in warming and humidifying the air that enters the lungs. In addition, the nose and the olfactory senses help create appetite.

Nasal Polyps

Nasal polyps are swollen sinus tissues that protrude into the nasal cavity. Polyps occur either singly or in grapelike clusters, and usually are caused by allergies. They can easily be removed by surgery, although the best treatment is to eliminate the allergens or bacteria that cause them, because polyps often reappear.

Treatments for Nasal Polyps

Nutritional Therapies. A diet that enhances the immune system is important, and animal fats should be reduced. As with all infections, the diet should include green vegetables and fiber and exclude fried and highly processed foods, caffeine, tobacco, and alcohol.

Vitamin and Mineral Therapies. Vitamin C has proved helpful for eliminating cervical polyps and may help relieve nasal polyps. Vitamin A, beta-carotene, and calcium also are recommended by Balch and Balch. Vitamin E may be effective as well, because the mucous membrane linings are more vulnerable to damage when a person has a vitamin E deficiency.

Sinusitis

The nose contains four large sinus cavities: two inside the cheekbones (the maxillary sinuses) and two above the eyes (frontal sinuses). The sinuses are lined with membranes that secrete antibody-containing mucus which protects the respiratory tract from toxins in the air.

Sinusitis is a disorder that occurs when the cavities become inflamed, or swollen. Acute bacterial sinusitis results from a viral infection in the upper respiratory tract (a common cold) which fills the sinus cavities with mucus. Chronic sinusitis is an inflammation of the sinuses caused by allergies—usually food allergies. Symptoms include swelling of the sinuses, a dull pain over the involved sinus, persistent nasal congestion and discharge, postnasal drip, and a diminished sense of smell. Richard Podell and Beth Weinhouse state in a February 1991 article in *Redbook* that sinusitis is the most common chronic nose disorder in the United States, affecting an estimated 14 percent of all Americans.

Chronic sinusitis is a circular process in which the sinuses first become inflamed and then become cracked, scarred, or swollen. Once they are scarred or cracked, they may be infected by bacteria and then become more sensitive to allergens and even more inflamed. If not treated in its early stages, sinusitis can progress to asthma, bronchitis, and inflammation of the brain.

Many people develop sinus problems because of dry-air heating systems (in winter) or air-conditioning systems (in summer). As a result, many holistic physicians advise sinusitis patients to use humidifiers in their homes and work places. Salt-water sprays inhaled through the nose five or six times a day also can help drain a temporary inflammation.

Treatments for Sinusitis

Acupuncture. William Cargile, chairman of research for the American Association of Acupuncture and Oriental Medicine, believes that acupuncture is one of the most effective alternative therapies for sinusitis. He states in *Alternative Medicine: The Definitive Guide* that sinus problems often are related to toxins in the bowels and intestines. Acupuncture treatments that stimulate the body to detoxify almost immediately detoxify the sinus membranes as well. In some cases, the relief lasts for weeks or the sinusitis is cleared up completely.

In severe cases, antibiotic medicines may be necessary. Prescription drugs for sinus problems, however, can be addictive and repeated use of drugs can lead to the development of tolerance by the bacteria, according to Podell and Weinhouse, writing in the February 1991 issue of *Redbook*. Podell and Weinhouse cite a number of studies that suggest that decongestants such as pseudoephedrine constrict blood vessels and may permanently shrink the sinus and nasal membranes. Those that contain antihistamines often cause drowsiness. Spray decongestants such as Afrin and Dristan are effective for only a few days, and are known to have a rebound effect: when patients stop their use, the sinuses become more congested and more spray is needed to provide relief. Prescription inhalers offer temporary relief, but do not fight bacteria directly and do not heal the inflamed sinus membranes. Antihistamines can relieve nasal itchiness and inflammation by blocking the action of histamines, but do not help drain the mucus, Podell and Weinhouse conclude.

Botanical Medicines. For some patients heat, volatile oils, and antibacterial botanicals are helpful in draining sinuses and preventing chronic infection. Intranasal douches with goldenseal tea provide relief, as does swabbing the nasal passages with oil of bitter orange. Murray and Pizzorno also suggest that menthol or eucalyptus packs held over the sinuses are sometimes helpful. Hot botanical liquids help the mucus flow and relieve congestion and sinus pressure. Balch and Balch suggest that mild sinusitis can be alleviated with the following herbs: anise and horehound, echinacea, fenugreek, lobelia, marshmallow, mullein, red clover, and rose hips.

Homeopathic Remedies. According to Dr. Stephen Cummings and Dana Ullman in *Everybody's Guide to Homeopathic Medicine,* homeopathic therapies have been used for several hundred years to treat sinus infections. Depending on the cause of sinus inflammation and the symptoms, arsenicum album, nux vomica, mercurius iodatus, and silicea have been used with some effectiveness. A trained homeopath can prescribe the right remedies according to the cause and symptoms of sinusitis and an individual's unique biochemistry.

Hydrotherapy. Dr. Richard Barrett of the National College of Naturopathic Medicine in

Portland, Oregon, states in *Alternative Medicine: The Definitive Guide* that the dry heat of a sauna or hydrotherapy is the most helpful treatment for relieving sinus congestion. In the early stages, nasal lavages of salt water and steam inhalations help loosen up sinus mucus for secretion. An alternative is applying a hot compress over the sinuses for three minutes, followed by a cold compress for thirty seconds.

Another method, according to Barrett, is to inhale hot steam. The patient can do this easily by boiling a quart of water, covering the head with a towel, and breathing in the steam. Small amounts of aromatic herbs such as mint or eucalyptus are sometimes added to the hot water.

Nutritional Therapies. If early inflammations are caused by food allergies (chronic sinusitis), a strict diet is implemented that eliminates common allergens such as milk, wheat, eggs, citrus fruits, corn, and peanut butter. Murray and Pizzorno describe several food allergy elimination diets that have proved effective in treating sinus disorders. Most sinusitis diets require that patients drink large amounts of fluids such as diluted vegetable juices, soups, and herb teas. Simple sugar consumption (including fruit sugars) also should be limited.

Vitamin and Mineral Therapies. According to Murray and Pizzorno, both types of sinusitis can be treated with vitamin and mineral supplements, including vitamins C and A, beta-carotene, bioflavonoids, and zinc lozenges. These should be taken only under the supervision of a physician, and Murray and Pizzorno do not recommend prolonged supplement treatments. They also suggest that thymus extract has helped some patients with sinusitis. Bee pollen and vitamin B-complex with extra vitamin B6 (pyrodoxine) and pantothenic acid (B5) help sufferers increase their immunity to new infections and may relieve mild sinus congestion.

Throat

The throat (pharynx) is the five-inch-long muscular tube through which food and air enter the body. It is composed of two divisions: the trachea (windpipe), which inhales air and sends it to the lungs, and the esophagus (food passage), which helps break down foods and transports them to the stomach. The throat also conducts air through the vocal cords (larynx), which allows people to speak and sing.

Sore Throats

Ninety percent of sore throats in adults are caused by viruses that are not serious, and the condition normally heals within two to three days. The other 10 percent are "strep throats" caused by streptococcal bacteria. Strep throats are more common in children than in adults and produce a variety of symptoms, including throat pain, fever, muscle aches, swollen lymph glands in the neck, and chills. Strep throats require immediate treatment because they can lead to kidney disease, rheumatic fever, and heart complications.

Treatments for Sore Throats

Antibiotics. Antibiotics such as penicillin should be given only to patients who do not respond to natural holistic treatments. The danger of prolonged use of penicillin is that the streptococcal bacteria develop a tolerance to it. In addition, penicillin fails in approximately 20 percent of cases to eliminate the streptococci. In all cases of sore throat, any treatment must eliminate the virus or bacteria by restrengthening the immune system through rest and drinking large amounts of fluids.

Botanical Medicines. According to Murray and Pizzorno, goldenseal and echinacea angustifolia are natural antibiotics that prevent the spread of streptococcal bacteria. They also suggest several other botanical therapies to treat infection, including osha root (ligusticum porteri). An infusion of lavender or hyssop can relieve sore throats caused by smoking or pollution. Slippery-elm tea and ginger also are reported to be beneficial.

Homeopathic Remedies. Cummings and Ullman, in *Everybody's Guide to Homeopathic Medicines,* list the following homeopathic remedies for sore throats: lachesis, ignatia, arnica, aconite, hydrastis, gelsemium, and phytolacca. They stress that homeopathic treatments must be individualized and that a licensed homeopath should be consulted.

Hydrotherapy. Heat compresses can provide relief and reduce swelling caused by infection. A warm, wet face cloth covered with a wool sock can be applied directly to the throat. Gargling several times a day with water and salt or with apple cider vinegar mixed with hot water, salt, lemon juice, and honey also can offer relief.

Vitamin and Mineral Therapies. The holistic treatment for sore throats employs diet, vitamins, and botanical medicines to treat the early stages of viral or bacterial infection. Patients with symptoms should increase their fluid intake, including filtered water, hot herbal teas, diluted fruit juices, and broths. One effective remedy is drinking warm water mixed with powdered vitamin C, along with lemon and honey. In addition, vitamin C-rich foods (especially orange juice), along with vitamin A and bioflavonoids, beta-carotene supplements, and zinc lozenges have been found effective in uncontrolled clinical trials.

Throat Cankers

Small mouth ulcers, or canker sores, may develop inside the mouth or along the throat channel. These can be caused by infections, skin burning (eating hot foods such as pizza, for example), or emotional stress. Alternative remedies focus on neutralizing the infecting organisms and healing the sores. Carbamide peroxide, which contains glycerin and peroxide, is available in over-the-counter medications and can provide temporary relief. Peroxide releases oxygen and kills the bacteria, while glycerin coats and protects the sore.

Treatments for Throat Cankers

Botanical Medicines. Dermatologists sometimes recommend applying a wet black-tea bag to a throat canker. Black tea, which contains tannin, has been used as an herbal astringent to relieve pain. Alum, the active ingredient in styptic pencils, is an antiseptic and pain reliever that can prevent a throat canker infection from worsening. Goldenseal, either as a tea or applied directly to a canker, mouthwashes made with sage and chamomile, or pastes made of echinacea tincture and myrrh gum also are reported by Balch and Balch and Murray and Pizzorno to provide relief.

Vitamin and Mineral Therapies. Cankers almost always develop when the immune system is weak. Vitamin C, vitamin B-complex lozenges, or vitamin B-complex tablets with folic acid and B12 taken with meals restrengthen the immune system. Lysine taken on an empty stomach also may prove helpful. Acidophilus will balance the intestinal flora, and zinc gluconate lozenges may provide relief as well.

Dentists sometimes recommend squeezing vitamin E oil from a capsule onto canker sores. This is a safe, natural treatment that usually is supplemented with vitamin C to restrengthen the immune system against infection. If the sores persist for more than several days, people should consult their doctor, who may in severe cases prescribe a topical steroid and/or oral antibiotic.

Summary

The eyes, ears, nose, and throat often are considered a single medical system because their functions overlap and, in the case of the ears, nose, and throat, they share the same nerve supply. An infection or imbalance in any one of the areas may manifest in the others. Because they function as the first line of defense against external infectious organisms and toxins, their disorders are often immune system-related. And, because they degenerate over time, it may be necessary for some people to take vitamin, mineral, and botanical supplements to help maintain the integrity of the immune system and to supply necessary nutrients to these tissues.

Resources

References

American Academy of Ophthalmology. *Macular Degeneration: Major Cause of Central Vision Loss.* April 1987: 1–6

Balch, James F., and Phyllis Balch. *Prescription for Nutritional Healing.* Garden City Park, NY: Avery Publishing Group, 1993.

Brody, Jane. "Personal Health." *New York Times* (July 21, 1993): B7.

The Burton Goldberg Group. *Alternative Medicine: The Definitive Guide.* Puyallup, WA: Future Medicine Publishing, Inc., 1993.

Butler, Kurt, and Lynn Rayner. *The Best Medicine: The Complete Health and*

Preventive Medicine Handbook. New York, NY: Harper & Row Publishers, Inc., 1985.

Cummings, Stephen, M.D., and Dana Ullman. *Everybody's Guide to Homeopathic Medicine*. New York, NY: St. Martin's Press, 1991.

"Garlic Kills Ear Infection Bacteria." *Your Health* (April 1994): 53.

"Glaucoma: Arresting this Thief of Sight." *The Johns Hopkins Medical Letter* (May 1994): 4–6.

Henneberger, Melinda. "Exercise Therapy Can Help Inner-Ear Dizziness." *New York Times* (January 26, 1994): D7.

Holzman, David. "Test Give a Better Vision of Future." *Insight* (January 22, 1990): 46.

Kasper, Rosemarie. "Hearing Loss and You: Hearing Impairment is One of the Most Prevalent Disabilities in the Country." *Independent Living* (August–September 1990): 59–60.

"Lasers Battle Blindness." *Consumer Reports Health Letter* (December 1990): 96.

Margolis, Simeon, and Hamilton Moses III. *The Johns Hopkins Medical Handbook*. New York, NY: Medletter Associates, Inc., 1992.

Murray, Michael, and Joseph Pizzorno. *Encyclopedia of Natural Medicine*. Rocklin, CA: Prima Publishing, 1991.

Podell, Richard N., and Beth Weinhouse. "The Cold That Won't Go Away— Sinusitis." *Redbook* (February 1991): 93–94.

"Surgery for Vertigo Carries Chance of Some Hearing Loss." *San Jose Mercury News* (November 3, 1992): 3C.

Swartwout, Glen. "Cataract Prevention: A Nutritional Approach." *The Holistic Optometrist* (1986).

Tennebaum, David. "Saving Sight." *American Health* (September 1993): 66–67.

Van Buchen, F. "Therapy of Acute Otitis Media: Myringotomy, Antibiotics, or Neither?" *The Lancet* (October 9, 1981): 883–87.

"Vitamin A May Be a Key Deafness Cure." *San Jose Mercury News* (May 4, 1993): 5.

"Vitamin C: A Secret to a Long Life and a Healthy Heart." *Environmental Nutrition* (July 1992): 3.

"Vitamin E and Cataracts." *Your Health* (July 13, 1993): 7.

"Warding Off Diabetes Complications." *American Health* (September 1993): 13.

Weintraub, Michael, M.D. "Inner-Ear Ailments Traced to High-Impact Aerobics." *San Jose Mercury News* (April 7, 1994): C1.

Weiss, Gillian. "New Hope for Deaf Children: Implant Gives Them Hearing and Speech." *American Health* (November 1990): 17.

"Zinc Retards Macular Degeneration." *Health Facts* 13 (April 1988): 5.

Organizations

National Eye Research Foundation
910 Skokie Blvd., Ste. 207A, Northbrook, IL 60062.

National Institute of Allergy and Infectious Diseases
9000 Rockville Pke., Bethesda, MD 20205.

Optometric Extension Program Foundation, Inc.
2912 Robeson, Fall River, MA 02720.

Sound, Listening and Learning Center
2701 E. Camelback, Ste. 205, Phoenix, AZ 85016.

Additional Reading

Maloney, William, Grindle Lincoln, and Donald Pearcy. *Consumer Guide to Modern Cataract Surgery.* Fallbrook, CA: Lasenda Publishers, 1986.

Public Citizen's Health Research Group. *Cataracts: A Consumer's Guide to Choosing the Best Treatment.* Washington, DC: Public Citizen's Health Research Group, 1981.

Schmidt, Michael. *Childhood Ear Infections (What Every Parent and Physician Should Know).* Berkeley, CA: North Atlantic Books, 1990.

RESOURCES

Chapter 17

CANCER

In 1993, more than 5 million Americans were diagnosed as having some type of cancer. Currently, one of every five Americans is likely to develop cancer during his or her lifetime, and in that group, one person in five is likely to die from it. Approximately one-third of all cancers are caused by cigarette smoking and other forms of tobacco use. It is estimated that 80 percent of all cancers could be prevented if people ate nutritious low-fat foods, did not smoke, and limited other unhealthy behaviors.

This chapter describes the causes and major types of cancer and outlines alternative methods of prevention and treatment. The holistic approach is ably summarized by Dr. Bernie Siegel in his book *Love, Medicine & Miracles:* "A vigorous immune system can overcome cancer if it is not interfered with, and emotional growth toward greater self-acceptance and fulfillment helps keep the immune system strong."

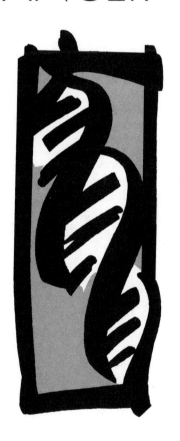

What Is Cancer?

Cancer is not one disease, but a group of diseases, all of which occur when healthy cells stop functioning and maturing properly. Normal, healthy cells grow, divide, and replace themselves in an orderly way. Sometimes, however, for reasons which still are not fully understood, cells lose their ability to control their growth, and begin to multiply abnormally. In the process, they can develop their own network of blood vessels that siphon nourishment away from the body's blood supply.

While every cell in the body has the ability to turn cancerous, normally the immune system is able to either destroy these cells or to reprogram them back to normal functioning. However, if the immune system is severely weakened (suppressed), it cannot destroy or reprogram the cells and they form tumors. Tumors are masses of abnormal cells (usually more than a billion before they become detectable). If the cancer cells do not spread beyond the tissue or organ where they originated, the cancer is considered to be localized. Benign tumors, such as warts and cysts, remain localized, can be removed by surgery, and are not life-threatening.

Malignant tumors, which can develop in any organ or tissue in the body, are composed of cells that multiply much faster than normal cells and usually have one or more abnormal chromosomes. The cells of malignant tumors do not remain localized. Instead, they enter the bloodstream and migrate to vital body organs where they can form new tumors. By diverting essential nutrients from normal cells and releasing toxins into the blood and organ systems, malignant tumors interfere with the functioning of those organs so that serious illness and death ensue. If fact, if left untreated, cancer is almost always fatal.

Cancers are defined according to the organ or kind of tissue in which the tumor is located. And, although there are more than 100 types of cancer, the five basic categories include carcinomas, sarcomas, myelomas, lymphomas, and leukemias. Carcinomas are tumors that form in tissues that cover or line internal organs; they are the most common type, accounting for 80 to 90 percent of all cancers. Cancers of the intestines, lung, breast, prostate, and skin are carcinomas.

Sarcomas originate in connective tissues and muscles, cartilage, or the lymph system. They represent the smallest number of cancer cases and are also the most likely to be fatal. Myelomas form in the plasma cells of bone marrow. Lymphomas are cancers of the lymph glands (or nodes) found in the neck, groin, armpits, and spleen. Hodgkin's disease and non-Hodgkin's lymphomas are the two most prevalent types in the United States. Leukemias are tumors that form in the tissues of the bone marrow, spleen, and lymph nodes. They are not solid, and are characterized by an overproduction of white blood cells.

Although scientists do not agree on the causes of cancer, there is consensus that all tumors share a common feature: they develop as a result of changes or rearrangement of information coded in the DNA within single cells. Four of the primary causes of cancer, scientists now concur, are environmental factors (including exposure to carcinogenic substances such as air pollution, tobacco smoke, and industrial chemicals), diet, heredity, and lifestyle.

Prevention of Cancer

Preventing cancer depends on avoiding the risk factors linked with cancer and maintaining a healthy immune system that efficiently eliminates abnormal cells from the body. This can be accomplished in a number of ways, including adopting a diet that ensures the optimal intake of immunoenhancing nutrients and decreases the intake of immunosuppressing foods—foods that weaken the immune system. Living a life free from continual emotional or mental stress is important, as is avoiding carcinogenic toxins in the home and in the environment.

Botanical Medicines. Several botanicals discussed in Chapter 5 have been shown to be effective preventive agents against cancer, including spirulina, aloe vera, green tea made from the leaves of camellia sinensis, echinacea, garlic, mistletoe, shiitake mushrooms (extract of lentinus edodes), and maitake mushrooms. Botanical therapies used to treat cancer are discussed later in this chapter.

Exercise. Several studies have indicated that men and women who are physically fit or physically active have lower death rates from cancer. As Michele Wolf reports in the October 1993 issue of *American Health,* a study of more than 10,000 men and 3,000 women examined at the Institute for Aerobics Research in Dallas found that those who were most fit on a treadmill test had much lower cancer death rates in the ensuing eight years. There was a fourfold difference in cancer deaths among the men and a sixteenfold difference among the women. The strongest evidence for exercise's protective effect involves colon cancer, a leading cause of cancer deaths among Americans.

Wolf goes on to report that exercise for women, particularly during teenage and young adult years, seems to be associated with lower rates of breast cancer and various hormone-related cancers of the reproductive tract. Dr. Rose Frisch of the Harvard School of Public Health found that among nearly 45,400 female college graduates, those who had been college athletes or who trained regularly had about half the risk of later developing breast cancer than did nonathletes. Nonathletes also had higher rates of cancers of the uterus, ovary, cervix, and vagina.

The main benefit of exercise in reducing cancer risk in women is believed to be a lower lifetime exposure to estrogen, which can stimulate growth of cells in the breasts and reproductive organs. Physical activity can change the hormone ratio and reduce body fat. A third of a woman's estrogen, before menopause, is produced by body fat; thus, leaner, fitter women will have less of this cancer-stimulating hormone.

Wolf adds that exercise also may help fight other forms of cancer because of its ability to boost the performance of two types of immune system cells—natural killer (NK) cells and macrophages. Although NK cells and macrophages seem to inhibit tumor

Symptoms of Cancer

According to the American Cancer Society, anyone with one or more of the following symptoms should be examined by a physician.

- A sore, especially in the mouth, that persists.
- A sore throat that does not heal.
- A nagging cough or hoarseness.
- A lump, white spot, or scaly area on the lip or in the mouth.
- A swollen lymph gland in the neck, armpit, or groin that last three weeks or more.
- Moles, freckles, or warts that have changed in color or shape, or that bleed.
- Unusual bleeding or discharge between periods, especially during or after menopause.
- A thickening of, or lumps in, the breast.
- A testicular lump or enlargement.
- Difficulty in swallowing or a lump on or near the thyroid gland.
- Rectal bleeding or changes in bowel habits, unexplained by dietary or other changes.
- Urinary difficulties such as pain, frequency, weak flow, or blood in the urine.

growth, once a tumor takes hold, working out will not help the immune system eliminate it. It may, however, prevent malignant cells from spreading. Exercise physiologists have not yet determined exactly how much exercise is needed to lower the risk of cancer.

Dietary Guidelines

Dr. Bernie Siegel, a leading holistic cancer specialist, recommends following the dietary guidelines prepared by the American Institute for Cancer Research and endorsed by the National Academy of Sciences:

1. Reduce intake of dietary fat—both saturated and unsaturated—to a maximum level of 30 percent of total calories. This can be done by limiting consumption of meat, trimming away its excess fat, avoiding fried foods, and eating limited amounts of butter, cream, and salad dressings.

2. Increase consumption of fresh fruits, vegetables, and whole-grain cereals. Siegel suggests increasing the intake of beta-carotene (a vegetable precursor of vitamin A), vitamins C and E, selenium, and dietary fiber—all of which, according to Siegel, are known to have a protective effect against cancer.

3. Consume salt-cured and charcoal-broiled foods only in moderation (or not at all).

4. Drink only moderate amounts of alcoholic beverages (or none at all).

In addition, Siegel recommends eliminating the following from the diet:

• Nearly all salt except that found in food itself.

• All stimulants such as coffee and tea.

• All refined sugar and flour.

• Hydrogenated fats.

• Pepper and other hot spices.

• Foods containing artificial additives or preservatives.

Nutritional Therapies. Cancer rates differ appreciably in various parts of the world, which suggests that diet may play a direct role in cancer. Diets that contain foods with high levels of carbohydrates and cholesterol are considered risk factors for cancer, while diets high in vitamin E, vitamin C, beta-carotene, fiber, and other substances may prevent certain cancers. A five-nation study of 802 patients with pancreatic cancer, reported by G. Howe in the May 1992 issue of *International Journal of Cancer,* for example, showed that cancer was directly related to intake of carbohydrates and cholesterol and inversely related to dietary fiber and vitamin C. Nevertheless, even with strong worldwide evidence supporting the view that certain cancers are caused by particular diets, many scientists argue that convincing clinical proof identifying the specific foods or substances is still lacking.

Vitamin and Mineral Therapies. Chapters 2 and 3 detail a number of clinical trials proving that vitamins and minerals have a protective effect against cancer. These include beta-carotene, vitamin A, vitamin C, vitamin E, selenium, and zinc.

Diagnosing Cancer

Physicians use a variety of diagnostic tests to determine if a symptom is cancer-related. The American Cancer Society recommends a Pap smear, a simple test for cervical cancer, every three years for women over 20. It recommends a pelvic exam every three years from the ages 20 to 40 and annually thereafter. The American College of Obstetricians and Gynecologists recommends an annual Pap swear. Women who have had genital warts or herpes should have Pap smears at least once a year. Women also should examine their breasts regularly by checking for any areas of thickening or for lumps. After the age of 50, women should have an annual mammogram. Those at high risk of breast cancer may need earlier and more frequent mammograms. Breast self-examinations should be done about one week after the menstrual period when temporary hormonally induced changes will be minimal. Men should regularly examine their testicles for unusual lumps as well, and be examined yearly by a physician to test for prostate cancer.

Early Detection of Cancer

The most recent research suggests that while cancer is partly a genetically caused disease, it is most importantly a disease of lifestyles. And, as with many other diseases, there is a great deal that people can do to reduce their risk of contracting it. The alternative approach to cancer focuses on prevention by identifying these risk factors and adopting lifestyles that minimize them Another crucial component of the holistic approach is detecting the early warning signs of cancer. Many cancers are curable by surgery, drugs, or other treatments if detected in the initial stages.

Conventional Cancer Treatments

Once a person is diagnosed with cancer, there are three conventional treatments: surgery, radiation therapy, and chemotherapy. The treatment recommended varies with the type of cancer, whether the cancer is localized or has begun to spread, and the general health of the patient. All three conventional treatments are invasive and have potentially severe side effects, but they do prevent the cancer from spreading, with varying success rates. Everyone who is diagnosed as having cancer should insist on a full discussion and understanding of the condition, and should ask the doctor to fully evaluate the risks and benefits of any recommended therapy.

Chemotherapy. Treatment with anticancer drugs, called chemotherapy, destroys cancer cells by disrupting their ability to multiply. Many different drugs are used to treat cancer, and are given to patients either orally or by injection into a muscle, vein, or artery. Some drugs are administered in cycles, followed by a rest period. Whether taken orally or by injection, chemotherapy drugs enter the bloodstream and are carried throughout the body. For this reason, the treatment is called systemic. Depending on the drugs a doctor prescribes, most patients undergo chemotherapy as outpatients at a hospital. Sometimes a hospital stay is needed in order to monitor side effects.

While chemotherapy primarily kills cancerous cells, it also affects other rapidly growing cells, including hair cells and cells that line the digestive tract. As a result, patients often experience hair loss, nausea, and vomiting. Most anticancer drugs also affect bone marrow, decreasing its ability to produce blood cells. Some chemotherapy patients develop weaker immune systems and are at a higher risk of infection. The side effects of chemotherapy vary depending on the drugs being given, the dosage, and the patient's age and general health. Patients should fully discuss all the advantages and disadvantages with their physician before undergoing treatment.

Radiation Therapy. In radiation therapy (also called X-ray therapy, radiotherapy, cobalt treatment, or irradiation), high-energy rays are used to damage cancer cells so they are unable to grow and multiply. Like surgery, radiation therapy is localized and affects only the cells in the treated area. For some cancers, such as leukemia and lymphoma, the whole body may be radiated. Radiation therapy may be used before surgery to shrink the tumor, or after surgery to destroy any cancer cells that remain in the area. The two most common types of radiation therapy are external radiation therapy and radiation implants.

In external radiation therapy, a machine directs high-energy rays at the cancer cells. Patients usually receive these treatments five days a week for several weeks as outpatients. Most patients receive either X-ray or cobalt gamma ray radiation, both of which gradually lose their energy as they pass through the body, damaging not only the tumorous cells but also the nearby healthy cells. However, radiation treatment is not always effective. Several forms of cancer, including gland and prostate cancer, have proven resistant to X-ray therapy.

Radiation implant treatment involves placing a small container of radioactive material in the affected body cavity or directly into a cancer cell. By using radiation implants, doctors are able to give patients higher doses of radiation than is possible with external therapy, while sparing most of the healthy tissue around the tumor. Dr. Gerald DeNardo of the University of California, Davis, has treated 58 B-cell lymphoma patients with radiation implants. About two-thirds of the patients, according to an article by J. Bishop in the October 21, 1993, edition of the *Wall Street Journal,* responded to the treatments and half of these are in complete remission.

Radiation therapy has strong side effects, including fatigue and skin reactions (such as rashes or red blotches) in the area being treated. It also may decrease the number of white blood cells, which help to protect the body against infection. The type and degree of side effects partially depend on the area of the body being treated.

Surgery. Surgery, the most common treatment for cancer, involves removing cancerous cells from the body. For cancers that develop in areas close to the surface of the body, surgery is usually recommended first. Sometimes healthy cells may have to be removed from the area surrounding the tumor in order to prevent the cancerous cells from spreading.

Alternative Cancer Treatments

Holistic physicians regard cancer as the manifestation of an unhealthy body whose defenses can no longer destroy or repair cells that turn cancerous. Alternative treatments therefore focus on strengthening the immune system of the cancer patient, using physiological and psychological therapies. The therapies summarized in the following sections have either proven effective for some types of cancer or offer promise for further investigation. People with cancer should discuss all of the available proven treatments for specific cancers with their physician or health professional and together choose the most appropriate treatment or combination of treatments.

Antineoplaston Therapy. Antineoplaston therapy was developed by Stanislaw Burzynski, a Polish physician who began practicing in the late 1960s in Houston, Texas, where he currently oversees the Burzynski Research Institute, a cancer treatment clinic. In an article entitled "Synthetic Antineoplastons and Analogs" appearing in a 1986 issue of *Drugs of the Future,* Burzynski explains that the therapy is based on his theory that the body has a parallel biochemical defense system (BDS), independent of the immune system, which helps reprogram defective cancer cells so they begin to function normally. According to Burzynski, the BDS consists of short-chain amino acids, known as polypeptides, that are able to inhibit the growth of cancer cells.

Burzynski claims that the body of a cancer patient has only about 2 or 3 percent of the amount of antineoplastons contained in a healthy person. As a result, the BDS becomes deficient against chemical and physical carcinogens, viruses, and other cancer-causing agents. To rebuild the BDS, Burzynski has given synthetic antineoplastons to more than 2,000 patients (most of them diagnosed with advanced or terminal cancer). According to *Alternative Medicine: The Definitive Guide,* the majority of patients have benefited from antineoplaston therapy, experiencing complete or partial remission, or stabilization of their conditions. In addition, few side effects have been observed. The cancers treated include lymphoma, leukemia, and cancers of the breast, bone, prostate, lung, and bladder.

From 1988 to 1990, Burzynski conducted clinical trials of different forms of antineoplaston treatment, such as capsules or injections, in groups of 15 to 35 patients diagnosed with specific types of cancer. The first trial involved patients with astrocytoma, a highly malignant form of brain tumor. Most of the patients had been unsuccessfully treated with surgery, radiation therapy, and/or chemotherapy. According to Burzynski, the majority of patients improved rapidly, and some of the adults were able to resume working part-time after only six weeks of treatment. Eighty percent experienced "objective response," which Burzynski defines as complete or partial remission or stabilization of their tumors. The National Cancer Institute subsequently issued its approval for Burzynski to undertake outside clinical trials involving brain tumors.

Dr. Dvorit Samid reported in the July–August 1990 issue of *Oncology News* that "AS2-1 (the antineoplaston) profoundly inhibits…the proliferation of malignant cells without exhibiting any toxicity toward normal cells…. Such a dramatic phenomenon is seldom seen," he noted.

Botanical Medicines. As noted in Chapter 5, Japanese physicians have used shiitake mushrooms (lentinus edodes) to shrink several types of tumors by as much as 80 percent. Nutritionist Dr. Donald Brown writes in the April 1994 *Townsend Letter for Doctors* that an extract of lentinus edodes has been shown to suppress viral oncogenesis and prevent cancer recurrence after surgery. Results of clinical trials indicate that shiitake mushrooms prolong the life span of patients with advanced and recurrent stomach, colorectal, and breast cancer, with minimal side effects. The active ingredient, lentinan, appears to increase production of T-lymphocyte (natural killer) cells.

Maitake mushrooms also may help treat cancer. Anthony Cichoke, writing in the May 1994 *Townsend Letter for Doctors,* claims that the compounds contained in maitake mushrooms stimulate immune function and inhibit tumor growth. Research is being conducted by Dr. Dennis Miller of the Cancer Treatment Centers of America on the effect of these mushrooms in stabilizing tumors. The double-blind study, designed to last six months, involves patients with stage IV (metastatic) colorectal cancer. Cichoke notes that Dr. Abram Ber, a homeopathic physician practicing in Phoenix, Arizona, has used maitake mushroom tablets to treat 12 patients with prostatic cancer. Not only were their symptoms ameliorated, but the patients reported improved urinary flow and a decreased need to urinate.

Shark cartilage may be an effective secondary cancer treatment. Tumors grow because they develop their own blood supply—a process known as angiogenesis. Cartilage, a tough, elastic, connective tissue found in sharks and humans, contains an "anti-angiogenic" substance that stops the blood supply from developing. Shark cartilage therapy is based on the premise that if the blood supply to tumors can be interrupted, they will stop growing and eventually die.

Dr. William Lane of New Jersey reports in *Sharks Don't Get Cancer* that the first study documenting the effectiveness of shark cartilage was conducted at the Hospital

Ernesto Contreras in Tijuana, Mexico. Eight patients chosen for the study suffered from a variety of cancers, including cervical, colon, and breast, and all had life expectancies of three to six months. Shark cartilage, administered via retention enemas, was the only form of cancer treatment the patients received. After one month of therapy, seven of the eight patients experienced tumor reductions ranging from 30 to 100 percent. Symptomatic improvement was observed in all eight patients, including weight gain, improved energy, and pain control.

In a Cuban clinical trial reported by D. Williams in the February 1993 issue of *Alternatives Newsletter,* 19 terminal cancer patients experienced shrinking of their tumors after 16 weeks of shark cartilage therapy, with rates varying between 15 and 58 percent. No toxic side effects were reported.

Dr. Charles B. Simone of Lawrenceville, New Jersey, a National Cancer Institute-trained oncologist and immunologist, monitored 20 patients with advanced cancers who were using shark cartilage as a food supplement. He reported to the June 24, 1993, U.S. Senate Subcommittee on Appropriations Special Hearing on Alternative Medicine that after eight weeks, tumors were eliminated in four patients and reduced in three others.

Shark liver oil is one of the best natural sources of alkoxyglycerols, natural alcohols that promote a generalized antibody response that may shrink cancer tumors. Judith Hooper, writing in the July 13, 1993, issue of *Your Health,* cites a study in Holland in which cervical cancer patients pretreated with shark liver oil before receiving radiation had far better survival rates than patients who did not receive the treatment. In many cases, tumors shrank significantly before radiation began, thereby rendering the radiation more effective.

Hooper also claims that shark fin soup (available in shark cartilage capsules) inhibits angiogenesis, the development of tiny blood vessels—or capillaries—through which tumors spread. She cites studies conducted at several Boston hospitals associated with Harvard Medical School that concluded that cancer tumors require angiogenesis to grow beyond approximately two millimeters; without new capillary networks in place, metastasis probably cannot occur.

An extract of mistletoe (iscador) has been used for 30 years in Europe as a potential anticancer agent. As reported by E. Kovacs in a 1991 issue of the *European Journal of Cancer* (Volume 12), Swiss scientists gave iscador to 14 patients with advanced breast cancer. Twelve of the 14 patients showed an improvement of DNA repair 2.7 times higher than before iscador was administered.

According to Hooper's *Your Health* article, carnivora, an extract of the meat-eating Venus's flytrap plant (dionaea muscipula), has been used on more than 2,000 patients since 1981 to treat cancer, AIDS, and other immune-suppressed diseases. In an initial clinical study conducted by German physician Dr. Helmut Keller of 210 patients with a variety of cancers, all of whom had undergone unsuccessful chemotherapy or radiation, 40 percent were stabilized by carnivora treatment and 16 percent went into remission. According to Keller, "Carnivora proved to be extremely nontoxic and non-mutagenic." Its effects included cytostatis (destruction of cancer cells), immune enhancement, mitotic (cancer-cell division) inhibition, viricidal (virus-killing) effects, and pain relief.

Hydrazine Sulfate. Dr. Joseph Gold, director of the Syracuse Cancer Research Institute in Syracuse, New York, began research in the late 1960s focused on controlling the weight loss (cachexia) that often accompanies cancer. He discovered that the chemical hydrazine sulfate could reverse cachexia, providing the body with extra strength to fight cancer. In addition to weight gain, the benefit of this therapy according to *Alternative Medicine: The Definitive Guide* is the documented ability of hydrazine sulfate to shrink tumors, and even cause them to disappear. It has been particularly effective in treating cancers of the rectum, colon, ovaries, prostate, thyroid, breast, and lung, as well as for Hodgkin's disease, melanoma, and lymphoma.

Although Gold's experiments in the U.S. were controversial, Soviet scientists at the Petrov Research Institute of Oncology in Leningrad began testing the effectiveness of hydrazine sulfate therapy in 1976. Dr. V. Filov subsequently reported in a 1990 issue of *Voprosy Onkologii* that 740 terminal cancer patients with a broad range of tumors were treated with hydrazine sulfate over a 15-year period. According to Filov, approximately 50 percent of these patients saw an improvement in their cachexia, 14 percent saw pronounced benefits, and all experienced a stabilization of the disease process.

Dr. Rowan T. Chlebowski of the University of California at Los Angeles, writing in the January 1990 issue of the *Journal of Clinical Oncology,* reported he and his colleagues at Harbor–UCLA Medical Center had found that hydrazine sulfate, used in conjunction with the best available conventional chemotherapeutic treatment, significantly increased survival in a controlled clinical trial of 65 patients with advanced inoperable, non-small-cell lung cancer (one of the most difficult of all cancers). Hydrazine therapy extended life to a median of 328 days, compared to a median of 209 days for patients who received chemotherapy alone.

Livingston Therapy. In the 1940s, an American physician named Virginia Livingston discovered a bacterium, progenitor cryptocides, which caused cancer in experimental animal studies. She contended it was present in virtually all human and animal cancers, and subsequently developed a vaccine derived from a culture of the patient's own bacteria—either from the tumor, urine, blood, or pleura (lung fluid). She also used the Bacillus Calmette–Guerin (BCG) vaccine, a mild tuberculin vaccine that stimulates white blood cells of the immune system to kill cancer cells. Because Livingston believed that certain foods such as beef, chicken, eggs, and milk can be contaminated with progenitor cryptocides (thereby providing a basis for the infectious transmission of cancer), her therapy to restore the immune system included a primarily vegetarian whole-foods diet, along with nutritional supplements.

In her book, *Conquest of Cancer: Vaccines and Diet,* Livingston analyzed the effectiveness of her combined vaccine and nutritional therapies for 62 patients (17 of them diagnosed as terminal) with breast, lung, uterine, ovarian, colon, prostate, kidney, pancreatic, pelvic, esophageal, or larynx cancer. Other patients were suffering from melanoma or skin basal cell cancer. According to Livingston, the success rate of therapy was 82 percent. However, as she did not conduct controlled clinical trails, her therapy has not been officially endorsed by the National Cancer Institute.

In another book, *Physician's Handbook: The Livingston-Wheeler Medical Clinic,* Livingston outlined her nutritional therapy, which included individualized dosages of vitamins A, B6, B12, C, and E; liver supplements; organic iodine (which she felt was essential to the metabolism of thyroid, the oxidative hormone); additional thyroid supplements (whenever tolerated); and hydrochloric acid.

Livingston's diet emphasized raw or lightly cooked fresh vegetables, fresh vegetable juices, whole grain breads and cereals, fresh fruits, nuts, baked or boiled potatoes, salads, and homemade soups. No sugar, refined flours, processed foods, or high-sodium foods were allowed, and few—if any—animal foods because of the likelihood of their being contaminated with progenitor cryptocides. Smoking, alcohol, and coffee also were prohibited.

Livingston's patients were given frequent baths in a hot tub with one cup of white vinegar to help eliminate toxins through the skin, along with purging and enemas. Her primary focus was instituting immunization, especially if patients were taking chemotherapy, because she believed patients could survive cancer only if they restrengthened their immune systems.

Livingston died in 1990. A group of cancer specialists continues to investigate the effectiveness of the vaccine she developed, including Dr. Neil Nathan, who currently carries on Livingston's work at the Livingston Foundation in San Diego, California. According to *Alternative Medicine: The Definitive Guide,* these physicians have noted shrinkage or disappearance of tumors, as well as complete remissions in patients with lymphocytic leukemia and malignant lymphoma.

Nutritional Therapies. As noted earlier, no conclusive clinical proof has been found for the theory that nutritional therapies can effectively prevent or reverse cancer. There is mounting evidence, however, that diet can play an important adjunctive role in treatment (as discussed later in this chapter).

Cancer specialist Dr. Keith Block of Evanston, Illinois, is described in a November 1988 monograph prepared for the Office of Technology Assessment (updated in 1990) as "one of the significant figures in the emerging 'middle ground' approach to integrated management of cancer."

Block believes that diet is a critical factor in health and that what people eat makes a significant difference in the body's ability to resist disease and maintain health. His diet for cancer patients consists of whole cereal grains, vegetables, legumes, fruits, nuts and seeds, soy foods, fish, and free-range poultry. Restricted or eliminated are most dairy products, eggs, red meat, refined sugar, caffeinated or alcoholic drinks, processed foods, some less healthy oils, and some vegetables in the nightshade family such as eggplant and green peppers. Block individualizes the diet based on the patient's physical condition, cultural background and tastes, climate and geographical location, activity level, and physical needs. Extensive exchange lists make it easy for a patient to "trade" different food or drinks from the same list. The Block diet provides 50 percent to 60 percent of nutrients in complex carbohydrates and restricts fat intake to between 12 and 25 percent (primarily from vegetable sources). The remainder of calories in the diet are derived from protein.

The Block diet is very similar to the diets the American Cancer Society, the National Cancer Institute, the American Academy of Sciences, and the American Heart Association have endorsed as having some preventive value in protecting against cancer and coronary disease.

Positive Mental Attitudes and Social Support. A number of studies have shown that positive mental states affect the outcome of cancer therapy, can assist the physician in making treatment more effective, minimize the negative side effects of medical treatments such as chemotherapy, and may even facilitate cures. As Siegel states in *Love, Medicine & Miracles,* "We don't yet understand all the ways in which brain chemicals are related to emotions and thoughts, but the salient point is that our state of mind has an immediate and direct effect on our state of body. We can change the body by dealing with how we feel. If we ignore our despair, the body receives a 'die' message. If we deal with our pain and seek help, then the message is 'living is difficult but desirable,' and the immune system works to keep us alive."

The therapy group Siegel founded, called Exceptional Cancer Patients (ECaP), is designed to help people mobilize their full resources—mental, emotional, physical, and spiritual—against their disease. Through regular group support meetings, nutritional counseling, exercise, meditation, visualization, and a trusting relationship with their physician (in which both take part in the decision-making process), patients "are accorded the conviction they can get well, no matter what the odds," Siegel explains. "If a person can turn from predicting illness to anticipating recovery," he continues, "the foundation for cure is laid."

Siegel, 1988 president of the American Holistic Medical Association, recommends that patients not reject standard medical techniques such as radiation, chemotherapy, and surgery—at least as one option. "Drugs and surgery buy time, and may cure, while patients work to change their lives. The most important thing is to pick a therapy you believe in and proceed with a positive attitude," viewing that therapy as energy that can heal, he says.

Dr. David Spiegel, a psychiatrist at the Stanford University Hospital, also has shown that psychosocial support can be of great benefit in coping with cancer. In a study with metastatic breast cancer patients, cited in the October 14, 1989, issue of *The Lancet,* women were randomly allocated into a control group that received standard medical therapy alone, or into one that attended weekly group therapy meetings and was taught self-hypnosis for pain. The patients who received therapy and learned hypnosis lived twice as long as the patients in the control group (36.6 months versus 18.9 months), and three of the women who received group therapy were still alive 10 years later.

Cancer patients now are offered a wide range of services to help them deal with the emotional and psychological aspects of the disease. Virtually every hospital serving cancer patients offers some form of psychosocial support, and many independent groups provide counseling, psychotherapy, and instruction in meditation, relaxation, and guided imagery or visualization. Biofeedback, hypnosis, and audiocassettes are other techniques. The common belief underlying these approaches is that patients' efforts to promote their emotional and spiritual well-being may affect biological states and help restore them to wellness.

Expressing the negative emotions that cancer patients experience is another important component in tipping the balance toward recovery. Psychologist Leonard Derogatis, in a study of 35 women with metastatic breast cancer, found that the long-term survivors had poor relationships with their physicians—as judged by the physicians. The survivors consistently questioned their doctors and expressed their emotions freely. Conversely, those who died within a year had relied heavily on repression, denial, and other psychological defenses.

National Cancer Institute psychologist Sandra Levy has further shown that seriously ill breast-cancer patients who expressed high levels of depression, anxiety, and hostility survived longer than those who showed little distress. As Levy reports in the September/October 1988 issue of *Psychosomatic Medicine,* she and other researchers also have found that aggressive "bad" patients tend to have more killer T-cells—white cells that seek and destroy cancer cells—than do docile "good" patients.

A group of London researchers under Keith Pettingale reported a 10-year survival rate of 75 percent among cancer patients who reacted to the diagnosis with a "fighting spirit," compared with a 22 percent survival rate among those who responded with "stoic acceptance" or feelings of helplessness or hopelessness.

Siegel agrees that "patients must be encouraged to express all their angers, resentments, hatreds and fears. These emotions are signs that we care to the utmost when our lives are threatened. Time after time, research has shown that people who give vent to their negative emotions survive adversity better than those who are emotionally constricted. Unexpressed feelings depress your immune system," he claims.

The social support provided by family members helps cancer patients strengthen their immune system while undergoing treatment. In a study of cancer patients between the ages of 25 and 70, reported by Levy in the January–February 1985 issue of *Psychosomatic Medicine,* patients who had a high quality of emotional support from a spouse or intimate other had higher levels of natural killer (NK) cell activity. Perceived support from the patient's physician, and actively seeking social support as a major coping strategy, also increased NK activity.

Traditional Chinese Medicine (TCM).

Chinese physicians regard cancer as an imbalance of chi, and treat the whole person rather than just the specific disorder. They claim that this approach avoids the phobia surrounding a diagnosis of cancer and focuses on returning the patient to optimal health once the cancer has been stabilized or reversed. Chinese physicians report having successfully treated cancer with acupuncture, herbs, nutritional therapies, meditation, and exercise therapies such as qi gong.

It is difficult for Western scientists to evaluate these therapies, because clinical trials in China are not randomized or controlled. Given these reservations, J. Han, writing in a 1988 issue of the *Journal of Ethnopharmacology,* states that TCM already has yielded a significant number of anticancer botanical therapies, including indirubin (from dang gui lu hui wan), irisquinone (from iris lactea pal-

lasii), and zhuling polysaccharide (from polyporous umbellata). A study by Eric J. Lien at the University of Southern California School of Pharmacy, published in 1985, concluded that Chinese herbs and plants from more than 120 species (belonging to 60 different families) have been used successfully to treat cancer.

Juzentaihoto (or JT-48, or JTT) appears to be one of the more promising Chinese herbs for treating cancer. It traditionally has been used to relieve anemia, anorexia, extreme exhaustion, and fatigue. In November 1988, G. Wang reported to the First Shanghai Symposium on Gastrointestinal Cancer that patients given this herbal remedy had three- to ten-year survival rates "significantly higher than commonly anticipated."

Herbal therapy using JTT in combination with chemotherapy and hormonal therapy has been shown to extend the life (and improve the quality of life) for metastatic breast cancer patients. A 1989 article by I. Adachi in the *Japanese Journal of Cancer and Chemotherapy* reported a controlled clinical trial at the National Cancer Center Hospital in Tokyo in which 119 advanced metastatic breast cancer patients were given either chemotherapy and endocrine therapy alone or in combination with JTT. After 38 months, the survival rate was significantly higher in the group receiving the herbal remedy. Quality of life was better for those receiving JTT, including physical condition, appetite, and temperature of hands and feet. In addition, herbally treated patients were protected from the bone marrow suppression associated with chemotherapy.

The *Journal of the American Medical Association (JAMA)* reported at a Special Hearing on Alternative Medicine convened by the U.S. Senate Subcommittee on Appropriations on June 24, 1993, that a Chinese herbal therapy called fu zheng significantly extends the life expectancy of patients with rapidly advancing cancers, when combined with Western treatment. The therapy, which consists of ginseng and astragalus, more than doubled the survival rate of patients with nasopharyngeal (nasal passage and pharynx) cancer, from 24 percent to 53 percent.

Visualization. Dr. Carl Simonton and Stephanie Matthews-Simonton were the first to develop imagery with the goal of physically reversing the development of cancer. They varied their image visualizations to accommodate the belief systems of their cancer patients, and also encouraged the use of meditation, biofeedback, and hypnosis. The most important factor, the Simontons state, was whether patients visualized themselves returning to a healthy life. If they had positive reasons to live, patients usually were able to visualize themselves as being free of cancer.

The Simonton's imagery may not work for everyone, and it remains controversial. Many clinicians, including Siegel, suggest that symbolic imagery may be more powerful than the anatomically accurate visualizations used by the Simontons. Siegel states that the key factor in recovery is ending the imagery session by focusing clearly and powerfully on a healing image that is relevant, understandable, and powerful.

Vitamin Therapies. Vitamin B6 is one of the most promising B vitamins for cancer treatment. Hans Ladner and Richard Salkeld, German and Swiss researchers, conducted a clinical trial treating cancer patients with vitamin B6 in addition to radiotherapy. As cited in L. Poirier's Essential Nutrients and Carcinogenesis, B6 was given over a seven-week period to 105 endometrial cancer patients, aged 45 to 65. These patients had a 15 percent improvement in five-year survival rates compared to 105 patients who did not receive the B6 supplements. No side effects from the B6 supplementation were observed.

Visualization Images

In their book *Getting Well Again* the Simontons describe common mental images that can help cancer patients in their visualizations:

- The cancer treatment (either radiation or chemotherapy) is strong and powerful.
- The cancer cells are weak and confused.
- The healthy cells can repair any slight damage the treatment might do.
- The army of white blood cells is vast and destroys the cancer cells.
- The white blood cells are aggressive and quick to find the cancer cells and destroy them.
- The dead cancer cells are flushed from the body naturally.
- I am healthy and free of cancer.
- I still have many goals in life and reasons to live.

Ladner and Salkeld also confirmed the beneficial effects of B6 on radiation-induced symptoms (nausea, vomiting, and diarrhea) in gynecological patients treated with high-energy radiation. They subsequently gave B6 to 6,300 patients with cervical, uterine, endometrial, ovarian, and breast cancers, and concluded that both quality of life and survival rates significantly improved with B6 supplementation.

Vitamin B6 also has proved effective in inhibiting melanoma cancer cells. One research team, as cited in *Essential Nutrients in Carcinogenesis,* developed a topical B6 pyridoxal that "produced a significant reduction in the size of subcutaneous cancer nodules and complete regression of cutaneous papules." While the results were considered preliminary, they may lead to a more successful topical B6 treatment for several forms of skin cancer.

Folic acid supplementation has been used to regress precancerous cells in patients with cervical dysplasia, an abnormal condition of the cells of the cervix, which usually is regarded as a precancerous lesion. When treated with folic acid, the regression-to-normal rate was observed to be 20 percent in one study and 100 percent in another, according to *Essential Nutrients and Carcinogenesis.*

Combined antioxidant treatments may extend survival times of cancer patients treated with chemotherapy or radiation. Twenty lung cancer patients in one study (five of which had advanced lung disease), reported in the May–June 1992 issue of *AntiCancer Research,* received antioxidant treatments of vitamins, trace elements, and fatty acids in combination with chemotherapy and/or irradiation at regular intervals. The average survival time for the entire group was 505 days. Fourteen (77 percent) survived for more than 12 months, and six patients (33 percent) for more than two years. One patient survived more than five years. Eight patients (44 percent) were still alive with a survival time of 32 months at the end of the study. Antioxidant treatments prolonged the survival time of patients with small cell lung cancer compared to combination treatment regimens alone. Patients receiving antioxidants also were able to tolerate chemotherapy and radiation treatment well.

Dr. Keith Block's Integrated Therapy

Block, creator of the Block diet, has developed a multifaceted cancer care program at Edgewater Medical Center in Chicago, an affiliate hospital of the Chicago Medical School. The therapy, described in a November 1988 monograph Block prepared for the Office of Technology Assessment (which was updated in 1990), is based on medical *caritas,* from the Latin meaning "compassionate caring for others." He says, "At the heart of the model is a carefully developed, very special doctor-patient relationship. The primary care physician seeks not only to understand and treat the patient's illness, but also to identify the patient's psychological, biomechanical, nutritional and physiological resources. In addition, the physician functions as a coordinator of medical care for patients."

Block's program is based on using the most effective, least invasive procedures first, before adopting more invasive procedures as, and if, they become necessary. He also uses innovative diagnostic and therapeutic tools that are noninvasive or low-invasive. One of Block's fundamental premises is that his model of compassionate caring focuses not only on the diagnosis of a physical disease, such as cancer, but also "on a deep understanding of that patient's total psychosocial-cultural gestalt. Without a clear recognition of what is deeply important to the patient—e.g., prestige, libido, safety needs, control issues—the physician may propose a treatment that the patient cannot psychologically, culturally or socially accept. As many physicians have found to their dismay, treatment urged on a frightened or unwilling patient often compounds the problem rather than alleviating it."

Biopsychosocial. Block has also developed a three-and-a-half-day training program that includes nutritional instruction, physical conditioning counseling, and stress-reduction exercises to give patients a sense of personal control and competence. Block believes that giving patients personal responsibility and a sense of personal power regarding their care is as important as prescribing the right medications. Minimizing negative physical or psychological factors and enhancing emotional vitality, he points out, "builds a foundation upon which invasive techniques, when needed, can work most effectively."

Botanicals. Block includes shiitake mushrooms (lentinus edodes) and laminaria sea vegetables (kombu, kelp) in his diet because of their potent anticancer properties, even at relatively low levels of dietary intake. He believes they boost the activity of interferon-like protein polysaccharides that attack and destroy cancer cells, and interfere with the initiation and promotion stages of carcinogenesis. He also recommends echinacea and garlic to strengthen the immune system and to counteract the side effects of cancer treatments.

Exercise. In determining what exercise regimen is best suited for a patient's condition, Block takes into account both what the patient is capable of doing and willing to do. His approach is cardiovascular, aerobic, isometric, structural, and neurokinesthetic to produce maximum possible efficiency in all life support systems: cardiovascular, pulmonary, skeleto-muscular, neurologic, metabolic, immunologic, and total organic functioning. These exercises are designed to help patients function at the level of peak performance; produce a heightened sense of well-being, vitality, and emotional resilience; and overcome the impact of psychological stress, whether caused by internal or external pressures. Block's basic physical conditioning program often starts with 30 minutes of vigorous walking five days a week for patients who are able to do so. Others may start with isometric, flexibility, or minimal aerobic exercises. All patients gradually work into a more comprehensive program.

Summary

Currently, one of every five Americans is likely to develop cancer during his or her lifetime, and of those persons, one in five is likely to die from it. Cancer is a group of diseases that involve abnormal cell growth and proliferation. The alternative approach focuses on prevention, early detection, and treatment with a variety of therapies that restrengthen the immune system to stabilize malignant tumor cells and eliminate them from the body.

Human healing systems are both complex and varied, and the most effective treatments combine nutritional, vitamin and mineral supplementation, botanical, and psychoimmunological therapies. The optimal therapeutic strategy will vary from patient to patient and from therapist to therapist.

Both alternative and conventional therapies, when given sufficient time to work, have helped people become healthier cancer patients—physically, emotionally, and mentally. These cancer patients often do better with conventional therapies because their outlook makes them more responsive to treatment and in some instances more resilient to the disease itself. Improved physical and mental health of patients who combine holistic and conventional cancer therapies may in some cases help shift the balance toward improved outcomes. Alternative approaches to cancer can make an enormous difference in extending life. The holistic psychoimmunological therapies developed by Siegel and others can help cancer patients achieve physical recovery. Conversely, long-term chronic depression, hopelessness, and cynicism tend to diminish resilience and increase physical vulnerability.

In summarizing the factors that lead to the onset of cancer and the most successful methods of treating it, Siegel concludes in *Peace, Love & Healing:* "Although there's no question that environment and genes play a significant role in our vulnerability to cancer and other diseases, the emotional environment that we create within our bodies can activate mechanisms of destruction or repair."

Resources

References

Adachi, I. "Role of Supporting Therapy of Juzenthaiho-to (JTT) in Advanced Breast Cancer Patients." *Gan To Kagaku Ryoho/Japanese Journal of Cancer and Chemotherapy* (1989, Volume 16): 1538–43.

Bishop, J. "Cancer Study Tries Lethal Warheads." *Wall Street Journal* (October 21, 1993): B6.

Block, Keith I. "Part I—Block Nutrition Program." *New Clinical Care Model: Applications to Cancer-Patient Care.* Prepared for Office of Technology Assessment (November 1989): 1–2.

Brown, Donald. "Phytotherapy Review & Commentary." *Townsend Letter for Doctors* (April 1994): 406–07.

The Burton Goldberg Group. *Alternative Medicine: The Definitive Guide.* Puyallup, WA: Future Medicine Publishing, Inc., 1993.

Burzynski, S. "Synthetic Antineoplastons and Analogs." *Drugs of the Future* (1986, Volume 11, No. 8): 679.

Chlebowski, R.T., et al. "Influence of Hydrazine Sulfate on Nutritional Status and Survival in Non-Small Cell Lung Cancer." *Journal of Clinical Oncology* (January 1990): 9–15.

Cichoke, Anthony. "Maitake—The King of Mushrooms." *Townsend Letter for Doctors* (May 1994): 432–34.

Filov, V., et al. "Results of Clinical Study of the Preparation Hydrazine Sulfate." *Voprosy Onkologii* (1990: Volume 36, No. 2): 721–26.

Gold, Joseph. "Hydrazine Sulfate: A Current Perspective." *Nutrition and Cancer* (1987, Volume 9): 59–66.

Han, J. "Traditional Chinese Medicine and the Search for New Antineoplastic Drugs." *Journal of Ethnopharmacology* (1988, Volume 24): 1–17.

Hooper, Judith. "Unconventional Cancer Treatments." *Your Health* (July 13, 1993): 34–38.

Howe, G. "A Collaborative Case-Control Study of Nutrient Intake and Pancreatic Cancer." *International Journal of Cancer* (May 1992): 365–72.

Kovacs, E. "Improvement of DNA Repair in Lymphocytes of Breast Cancer Patients Treated with Viscum Album Extract (Iscador)." *European Journal of Cancer* (1991, Volume 27): 1672–76.

Lane, William, and L. Cormac. *Sharks Don't Get Cancer.* Garden City Park, NY: Avery Publishing Group, 1992.

Levy, S.M. "Perceived Social Support and Tumor Estrogen/Progesterone Receptor Status." *Psychosomatic Medicine* (January–February 1985): 73–85.

Lien, Eric. *Structure Activity Relationship Analysis of Anti-Cancer Chinese Drugs and Related Plants.* Long Beach, CA: Oriental Healing Arts Institute, 1985.

Livingston-Wheeler, Virginia. *The Conquest of Cancer: Vaccines and Diet.* New York, NY: Franklin Watts, 1984.

———. *Physician's Handbook: The Livingston-Wheeler Medical Clinic.* San Diego, CA: Livingston-Wheeler Clinic, 1980.

Murray, Michael, and Joseph Pizzorno. *Encyclopedia of Natural Medicine.* Rocklin, CA: Prima Publishing, 1991.

Poirier, L. *Essential Nutrients in Carcinogenesis.* New York, NY: Plenum Press, 1986.

Samid, Dvorit. "Trials Underway at Several Research Centers and Antineoplastons: New Antitumor Agents Stir High Expectations." *Oncology News* (1990, Volume 16): 1, 6.

Siegel, Bernie, M.D. *Love, Medicine & Miracles.* New York, NY: Harper & Row Publishers, Inc., 1986.

————. *Peace, Love & Healing.* New York, NY: Harper & Row Publishers, Inc., 1989.

Simonton, Carl, and Stephanie Matthews-Simonton. *Getting Well Again.* Los Angeles, CA: Jeremy P. Tarcher, Inc., 1978.

"Special Hearing on Alternative Medicine." Subcommittee on Appropriations, United States Senate (June 24, 1993): 65, 69.

Spiegel, David. "Effect of Psychosocial Treatment on Survival in Patients with Metastatic Breast Cancer." *The Lancet* (October 14, 1989): 888–91.

"Supplements Improve Response to Chemotherapy for Lung Cancer." *AntiCancer Research* (May–June 1992): 599–606.

United States Congress Office of Technology Assessment. *Unconventional Cancer Treatments.* Washington, DC: U.S. Government Printing Office, September 1990.

Wang, G.T. "Treatment of Operated Late Gastric Carcinoma with Prescriptions of 'Strengthen the Patient's Resistance and Dispel the Invading Evil,' in Combination with Chemotherapy: Follow-up Study of 158 Patients and Experimental Study in Animals." *Meeting Abstract* (First Shanghai Symposium on Gastrointestinal Cancer, November 14–18, 1988): 244.

Williams, D.G. "The Final Results of the First Cuban Study." *Alternative Newsletter* (February 1993, Volume 4): 20.

Wolf, Michele. "Can Exercise Ward Off Cancer?" *American Health* (October 1993): 77.

Organizations

The Alliance for Alternative Medicine
PO Box 59, Liberty Lake, WA 99019.

American Cancer Society
1599 Clifton Rd. NE, Atlanta, GA 30329. Burzynski Clinic. 6221 Corporate Dr., Houston, TX 77036.

Cancer Control Society
2043 N. Berendo St., Los Angeles, CA 90027.

Foundation for Advancement in Cancer Therapy
PO Box 1242, Old Chelsea Station, New York, NY 10113.

International Association for Cancer Victors and Friends
7740 W. Manchester Ave., Ste. 110, Playa del Rey, CA 90293.

Livingston Foundation Medical Center
3232 Duke St., San Diego, CA 92110.

National Cancer Institute
Office of Cancer Communications, Bldg. 31, 9000 Rockville Pke., Bethesda MD 20892.

Society of American Gastrointestinal Endoscopic Surgeons
Thomas Jefferson University Hospital, 111 S. 11th St., Philadelphia, PA 19107.

Syracuse Cancer Research Institute
Presidential Plaza, 600 E. Genesee St., Syracuse, NY 13202.

Additional Reading

Butler, Kurt, and Lynn Rayner. *The Best Medicine: The Complete Health and Preventive Medicine Handbook.* New York, NY: Harper & Row Publishers Inc., 1985.

Clark, Larry. *Selenium in Biology and Medicine.* New York, NY: Van Nostrand Reinhold Co., 1991.

Gerson, Max. *A Cancer Therapy: Results of Fifty Cases.* 5th edition. Bonita, CA: Gerson Institute, 1990.

Lerner, Michael. *Choices in Healing: Integrating the Best of Conventional and Complementary Approaches to Cancer.* Cambridge, MA: The MIT Press, 1994.

Revici, Emanuel. *Research in Physiopathology as a Basis of Guided Chemotherapy with Special Application to Cancer.* New York, NY: American Foundation for Cancer Research, 1961.

Walters, Richard. *Options: The Alternative Cancer Therapy Book.* Garden City Park, NY: Avery Publishing Group, 1993.

Chapter 18

HEART DISORDERS

More than 1.5 million people in the U.S. suffer from heart attacks every year, and 500,000 die as a result, nearly half of them women. In fact, more Americans die each year from cardiovascular disease—44 percent—than from all other causes of death combined, including cancer, AIDS, infectious diseases, accidents, and homicides. Cardiovascular is a general name for more than 20 diseases of the heart and its blood vessels. Coronary artery disease (CAD), also referred to as coronary heart disease (CHD), is the most deadly of all heart disorders, accounting for approximately one out of every three deaths related to heart disease.

When people learn they have a heart disorder, they have two choices. They can consult a conventional heart specialist who will provide the heart treatments (including drugs and surgery) recommended by the American College of Cardiology, or they can choose a holistic cardiologist who will suggest noninvasive, low-risk therapies based on lifestyle changes in such critical areas as nutrition, stress reduction, and exercise that can lead to a better life, as well as a longer one.

In 1989, 48 patients with severe coronary heart disease enrolled in a very unusual one-year experimental study conducted by heart specialist Dr. Dean Ornish. In his study, reported in *Dr. Dean Ornish's Program for Reversing Heart Disease*, participants were randomly divided into two groups. Patients in the usual care comparison group were asked to follow their doctors' advice: to make moderate dietary changes (eat less red meat and more fish and chicken, use margarine instead of butter, and consume no more than three eggs per week), to exercise moderately, and to quit smoking. Patients in the other group were asked to

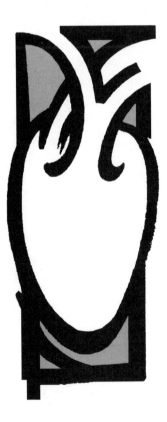

follow Ornish's holistic heart reversal program, which included cessation of smoking, a vegetarian diet that allowed no more than 10 percent of calories from fat, stress management (including meditation, relaxation exercises performed one hour a day, and group support), and moderate exercise (30 minutes daily).

Both groups were given angiograms at the beginning of the study and again a year later. After one year, 82 percent of the people who adopted Ornish's comprehensive lifestyle changes demonstrated "some measurable average reversal of their coronary artery blockages." Overall, the average blockage declined from 61.1 to 55.8 percent; more severely blocked arteries showed even greater improvement. Four arteries that had been completely blocked began to open, even those that had been occluded for years. This group also experienced a 91 percent decrease in the frequency and severity of chest pain. According to Ornish, most coronary blockages take decades to build up, but even a small amount of reversal after one year in a severely blocked artery causes a great improvement in blood flow to the heart. As a result, these participants began to feel better very quickly. In contrast, the majority of heart patients in the comparison (usual care) group who were following their doctors' advice became measurably worse during the same one-year interval.

Ornish's study provided the first solid evidence that major lifestyle changes can do what many scientists thought impossible— unclog arteries without the use of drugs or surgery. The findings were so conclusive that one major insurance company, Mutual of Omaha, announced it would cover the costs of this diet and stress-reduction program, making it the first nonsurgical, nonpharmaceutical therapy for heart disease to qualify for insurance reimbursement. This chapter analyzes the alternative therapies developed by Ornish

and others to prevent, treat, and even reverse major coronary heart disorders.

The Heart

The heart is one part of the cardiovascular system ("cardio" means heart and "vascular" refers to blood vessels). Its function is to pump blood (most adults have slightly more than a gallon of blood in their bodies) through more than 60,000 miles of blood vessels. Gordon Edlin and Eric Golanty estimate that the average adult's gallon of blood contains approximately 25 trillion red blood cells, which carry oxygen from the lungs to all of the body's tissues. More than 200 million new red blood cells are produced and released from bone marrow into circulation each day. Approximately the same number of old red blood cells are removed and recycled.

The heart, a strong and highly specialized muscle a little larger than a fist, pumps blood continuously through the circulatory system. It is divided into four chambers: the two upper chambers, called atria, receive blood returning from the body via the veins; the two lower chambers, called ventricles, pump blood out of the heart into the lungs and body through the heart's main artery, the aorta. The right atrium connects to the right ventricle and the left atrium connects to the left ventricle. A thin wall between the atria and ventricles divides the heart in half. Large blood vessels lead into the atria and leave the ventricles, passing through valves that separate these chambers and allow blood to flow in only one direction when the heart expands and contracts (beats). Each day the heart beats approximately 100,000 times, depending on the body's activity, and pumps about 2,000 gallons of blood.

The heart does not use oxygen and nutrients from the blood that passes through its chambers. Instead, it depends on a series of arteries found on the outside surface of the heart. These are called the coronary arteries, so named for their crown-like appearance as they branch out from the aorta girdling the outer surface of the heart.

Angina

When the heart muscle does not get sufficient blood (and oxygen) for a given level of work, even for just a few minutes, chest discomfort called angina pectoris can develop. The pain, which radiates outward from the heart, usually subsides in a short time if a person rests or uses nitroglycerine, a drug that dilates blood vessels. Angina typically occurs when extra demands are placed on the heart, such as during periods of physical exertion, exposure to extreme cold or wind, or emotional stress or excitement. Some people also develop angina after eating a large meal, when increased blood flow is required for digestion. Angina is not a heart attack, although it can be a warning sign that a person is at risk.

Heart Attack

A heart attack, or myocardial infarction, occurs when the blood supply to part of the heart muscle itself (the myocardium) is severely reduced or stopped because one of the coronary arteries (that supply blood and nutrients to the heart) is obstructed. A heart attack also can be caused by a blood clot lodged in a coronary artery, which is called coronary thrombosis or coronary occlusion. The underlying cause of most heart attacks suffered by Americans is arterial disease—atherosclerosis—which also accounts for 85 percent of all cardiovascular deaths (CVD) in the U.S. (see Chapter 9 for a more complete discussion of atherosclerosis).

If blood supply to the myocardium is cut off drastically or for a long time, muscle cells suffer irreversible injury and die. Depending

Heart Attack Facts

According to the American Heart Association:

- About 1.5 million Americans have heart attacks annually.
- About 500,000 of them will die as a result of a heart attack.
- Heart attacks are the leading killer of American men and women.
- 85 percent of heart disorders are caused by atherosclerosis.
- 33 percent of all heart attacks in the U.S. are caused by atherosclerosis.
- 60 percent of heart attack deaths occur before the person reaches a hospital.
- 55 percent of people who have heart attacks are 65 years old or older.
- 80 percent of people who die of heart attacks are over age 65.

on where the blockage occurs and the amount of heart muscle that is damaged, a heart attack can be extremely serious or relatively minor. Even after a heart attack, the heart can recover if the damaged area is not too extensive; over time, small blood vessels within the heart may gradually reroute blood around the blocked or clogged arteries, a process called collateral circulation.

Symptoms of Heart Attacks. According to the American Heart Association's *Fact Sheet on Heart Attack, Stroke and Risk Factors,* symptoms include feeling uncomfortable pressure, fullness, squeezing, or pain in the center of the chest (which may spread to the shoulders, neck, or arms) for more than a few minutes. Nausea, dizziness, sweating, faint-

Coronary Artery Disease:
Major Risk Factors that Can't Be Changed

- **Heredity:** People with a parent or sibling who had a premature heart attack (before age 55 in a man or 65 in a woman) are at increased risk of CAD.

- **Gender:** Before age 55, men have a much higher rate of CAD than women, but by the time they reach 60, women develop CAD at the samerate as do men at age 50. Women who have a heart attack, especially at older ages, are more likely to die from it than are men.

- **Increasing age:** Approximately 55 percent of all heart attacks, and more than 80 percent of fatal ones, occur after age 65.

- **Race:** African-Americans have an elevated risk of CAD, primarily because they have a higher risk of hypertension and diabetes than Caucasians.

ing, a feeling of severe indigestion, and shortness of breath may occur. Conversely, sharp, stabbing twinges generally are not signals of a heart attack. The importance of recognizing the symptoms and responding immediately cannot be overemphasized. More than 300,000 heart attack victims, the AHA warns, die before reaching the hospital each year, usually because they did not recognize the warning signals in time to receive emergency medical service.

Diagnosing Heart Disorders

Heart disorders are diagnosed on the basis of symptoms, medical history, and tests such as a treadmill exercise test or coronary angiograph, which allows the physician to examine the coronary arteries themselves to determine the nature and extent of the narrowing or blockage. Blood tests may be used to detect abnormal levels of certain enzymes in the bloodstream that indicate heart muscle damage. Additional tests may be needed in some cases to rule out other conditions such as muscle disorders, infection, structural abnormalities, anxiety, or indigestion. A doc-

tor also may test for signs of fluid accumulation in the lungs and tissues, or use an electrocardiogram (ECG or EKG) to discover any abnormalities of heart rhythm, insufficient blood flow to the heart muscle, or other problems. Ultrasound, another noninvasive procedure, defines heart size and pumping ability, and can be used to check for problems with the functioning of the heart valves. The key is to identify the symptoms of heart disease in time to implement alternative strategies to counteract their effects.

The importance of early detection and diagnosis is underscored by the fact that as many as 25 percent of Americans who die of sudden cardiac death (SCD) had no previous symptoms of a heart problem, according to the March 1994 issue of *Graboys Heart Letter.* SCD occurs when an already damaged heart muscle (caused by hardening of the arteries, viruses, drugs, or valve disorders) leaves a person susceptible to irregularities in the electrical signals that govern the heart's beating. When an incident occurs, the heart rhythm deteriorates into a fibrillation, or twitching, and blood flow stops. If blood flow is not restored quickly, death will result. SCD

Coronary Artery Disease: Major Risk Factors that Can Be Changed

Risk Factor	*Percent Attributable Risk*
• **High blood cholesterol** (> 240 mg/dl). For every 1 percent reduction in blood cholesterol,there is a 2 to 3 percent decline in the risk of heart attack.	42.7%
• **Inactivity.** Sedentary people who begin a regular program of exercise reduce their risk of a heart attack by 35 to 55 percent.	34.6%
• **Obesity.** About one in three American adults isseriously overweight or obese, which doubles the risk of CAD at a given age. People who put weight on around the waist (potbellied body) have a greater chance of CAD than those who accumulate weight on the hips (pear-shaped body).	32.1%
• **High blood pressure** (>140/90 mm Hg). For every one point drop in diastolic blood pressure, there is a 2 to 3 percent drop in the risk of heart attack.	28.9%
• **Cigarette Smoking.** Researchers believe 20 to 40 percent (100,000 to 200,000 people each year) of all CAD deaths are directly attributable to smoking. Smoking is also the leading cause of sudden cardiac death. Additionally, more than 35,000 nonsmoking Americans die annually from secondary smoking—exposure to other people's smoke.	25.1%

Contributing Factors

• **Diabetes.** Non-insulin-dependent diabetes, which afflicts about 12 million Americans, increases the risk of CAD in men 2- to 3-fold and in women 3- to 7-fold. Insulin-dependent diabetes is also a factor.

• **Stress.** Studies have found a link between anger and CAD risk, particularly in those people who suppress their emotions.

Fitness and Your Health. Copyright © 1993 Bull Publishing Company. All rights reserved. Reprinted by permission.

CORONARY ARTERY DISEASE RISK FACTORS

kills 300,000 Americans each year—or one victim every 90 seconds. The average age of victims is between 55 and 60.

Coronary Artery Disease Risk Factors

Unlike what happens in other organ systems of the body, most heart diseases are not caused by infection (although cardiac infections can occur), but by atherosclerosis of the coronary arteries. According to the American Heart Association, the major risk factors for coronary artery disease include heredity, increasing age, high blood cholesterol levels, high blood pressure, and cigarette smoking. Coronary artery disease also can result from contributing risk factors such as diabetes, obesity, physical inactivity, and emotional stress.

Conventional Treatments for Heart Disorders

Conventional heart specialists normally treat coronary artery disorders with drugs (which affect the supply of blood to the heart muscle or the heart's demand for oxygen) or surgery. Coronary vasodilators such as nitroglycerin, for example, cause blood vessels to relax which, in turn, causes the opening inside the vessels to enlarge. Blood flow then improves, allowing more oxygen and nutrients to reach the heart. Coronary vasodilators also reduce the amount of blood returning to the heart, thus lessening the heart's need to pump. Other drugs lower blood pressure and therefore reduce the heart's workload and need for oxygen. Drugs that slow the heart rate achieve a similar result. All of these drugs have side effects, however, and have not proven successful in reversing coronary artery disease by removing the plaque that blocks coronary arteries.

Coronary bypass surgery, one of the most frequently recommended surgical procedures

in the U.S., involves removing the diseased portions of the arteries and grafting a portion of a vein, usually taken from the patient's leg, onto the coronary arteries to replace the diseased segments, thus creating new pathways for blood flow to the heart. However, according to Ornish, heart attacks, strokes, infection, or death can occur as a result of bypass surgery, and up to one-third of patients who undergo this operation suffer some form of transient or permanent neurological damage. Fifty percent of bypassed arteries clog up again within five years, and eighty percent become blocked after seven years.

Edlin and Golanty report in *Health and Wellness: A Holistic Approach* that a study by the National Heart, Lung and Blood Institute showed the five-year survival rate for patients with mild coronary artery blockage was the same whether they had bypass surgery or used medication to treat symptoms. As a result of the study, the institute concluded that as many as 25,000 bypass operations a year are performed unnecessarily.

Heart specialist Dr. Thomas Graboys reports in *A Graboys Heart Letter Special Report* that he and his colleagues at the Lown Cardiovascular Center in Boston conducted a study in which they saw 168 patients who had been advised to undergo coronary bypass surgery and who were seeking second opinions. They advised 83 percent of these patients not to have the operation. After four years, the death rate for those patients who declined the procedure was actually lower than the death rate for those who chose bypass surgery. In other words, 83 people in the study would have needlessly undergone an expensive and invasive procedure if they had not sought a second opinion.

Balloon angioplasty, first employed by a Swiss cardiologist in 1977, is a relatively quick procedure that is less traumatic and expensive than bypass surgery, and is now used to treat hundreds of thousands of patients

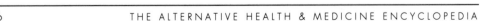

each year. In this procedure, a catheter with a deflated balloon on the end is threaded through an artery in the groin up into the patient's narrowed coronary artery. After the balloon is inflated to widen the artery, both the catheter and the balloon are removed. This compresses the plaque against the arterial walls (but does not remove it), and enlarges the inner diameter of the blood vessel so that blood can flow more easily to the heart. A newer form of angioplasty inserts a laser catheter and places it at the beginning of the blockage. The laser is activated and moved forward as it destroys fatty deposits; after the artery is cleared, the laser catheter is removed. According to Ornish, one-third of all patients who undergo balloon angioplasty find the same artery becoming narrowed or blocked within four to six months, to the point that another angioplasty is recommended. Despite this percentage, balloon angioplasty accounts for 90 to 95 percent of all angioplasty operations.

As serious as a heart attack can be, about 90 percent of patients who reach the hospital go home alive, and about 95 percent of those people live for at least a year. This survival rate is partly the result of new treatment strategies developed over the past three decades, including the use of aspirin and beta-blocking drugs (propranolol and atenolol, for example), to control the symptoms and reduce adverse outcomes of coronary artery disease. One of the most dramatic developments, according to the April 1994 issue of the *Harvard Health Letter,* has been the use of thrombolytic agents or clot-busting drugs that stop heart attacks in progress and thereby limit the amount of heart muscle that is damaged.

In a recent clinical trial called GUSTO (Global Utilization of Streptokinase and Tissue Plasminogen Activator [t-PA] for Occluded Coronary Arteries), reported in the April 1994 *Harvard Health Letter,* more than

40,000 patients in 15 countries were treated with either streptokinase or t-PA, the two most popular clot-busting drugs in the U.S. Both effectively dissolved the clots that had caused the heart attacks and kept the heart muscle alive. These medications are not always effective, however. In the GUSTO trial, 19 percent of patients who received t-PA still had blocked arteries 90 minutes after it was administered, as did 40 percent of patients who received streptokinase. Both drugs have been associated with some risks, particularly undesirable bleeding.

Alternative Treatments for Heart Disorders

Graboys asserts in the March 1994 *Graboys Heart Letter* that "everyone with a heart problem can benefit from an aggressive approach to the management of risk factors. Resetting life's priorities to include nutrition, exercise, and stress management is necessary to continued heart health. I've worked with hundreds of patients who have recovered from a life-threatening heart problem using a 'holistic' approach to heart health."

Botanical Medicines. According to *Alternative Medicine: The Definitive Guide,* garlic, ginger, and hawthorn berry extract may be valuable in preventing and treating heart disorders. Garlic contains sulfur compounds that work as antioxidants and help dissolve blood clots. Ginger has been shown to be effective in lowering cholesterol levels and making blood platelets less sticky.

A placebo-controlled, double-blind study reported by H. Kiesewetter in a 1993 issue of *Clinical Investigations* (Volume 71) found that garlic-coated tablets reduced platelet aggregation. In this 12-week study, patients who took garlic significantly increased their ability to walk longer distances by the fifth week of treatment. This increase was accompanied by a simultaneous decrease in platelet aggregation, blood pressure, plasma viscosity, and serum cholesterol levels.

Ginkgo biloba, according to nutritionist Donald J. Brown, writing in the May 1994 *Townsend Letter for Doctors,* is the premier botanical medicine used to treat intermittent claudication (clogging) caused by plaque or platelets. Brown suggests that using ginkgo biloba in conjunction with garlic should prove beneficial in treating coronary artery disease.

Michael Murray and Josephy Pizzorno report in the *Encyclopedia of Natural Medicine* that hawthorn berry extracts are widely used in Europe to treat cardiovascular problems, and they cite nine studies that have demonstrated the effectiveness of the extracts in preventing angina attacks as well as lowering blood pressure and serum cholesterol levels.

In their book *Prescription for Nutritional Healing,* James F. Balch and Phyllis Balch recommend barberry, black cohosh root, butcher's broom, cayenne pepper, dandelion, ginseng, hawthorn berries, red grapevine leaves, and valerian root. They suggest that some heart patients may benefit from suma herb tea, consumed three times a day with ginkgo biloba extract. All of these should be prescribed by a physician, herbalist, or health practitioner.

Estrogen Replacement Therapy (ERT). Declining estrogen levels in women after menopause are believed to contribute to an increased risk of osteoporosis and heart attacks. Estrogen therapy, according to the May 1994 issue of the *UC Berkeley Wellness Letter,* raises HDL ("good") cholesterol. Hormone replacement therapy usually includes progestin (a synthetic form of the hormone progesterone) along with estrogen. Recent studies cited by the *UC Berkeley Wellness Letter* suggest that the combined estrogen–progestin therapy also protects against heart disease. ERT is not appropriate for all women, however, and a physician

should be consulted before starting treatment. The link between estrogen deficiency and an increased risk of heart disease varies with the age, health status, and nutritional and lifestyle habits of each individual.

There is preliminary evidence that low levels of sex hormones in men may play an indirect role in heart disease. A study reported in the June 1994 issue of the *Harvard Health Letter* compared 49 heart attack victims, all of whom were under the age of 56, with an equal number of healthy volunteers. The two groups had similar levels of estrogen, the female hormone that also is present at low levels in normal men. Those who had suffered heart attacks, however, had levels of the male hormone dehydroepiandrosterone sulfate (DHEAS) approximately 20 percent lower than those of the healthy volunteers. How lower levels of male sex hormones might contribute to the development of heart disease is not known.

Exercise. In healthy people, Ornish claims exercise causes the arteries to secrete a substance called endothelium-derived relaxation factor (EDRF) that dilates the coronary arteries and allows more blood to flow to the heart. In people with coronary artery blockages, however, less EDRF is produced and the coronary arteries constrict during exercise. Smoking also decreases the production of EDRF. Therefore, people with a heart condition should consult with a physician before starting an exercise program. People over age 35 who have not exercised regularly for several years also should be examined by their physician before beginning regular exercise.

Vigorous exercise may actually increase the risk of heart attacks in people who have coronary artery blockages, eat a high fat diet, smoke, manage stress poorly, and use stimulants. Moderate exercise, however, if it is combined with lifestyle changes that include a low-fat diet, stress reduction, and the elimina-

What Does Exercise Do to Prevent Heart Disease?

- It exercises the heart, a muscle that must be exercised to stay fit.

- Exercise raises the maximal heart rate, but lowers the resting heart rate once exercise is completed. Thus, it lowers the resting heart rate for 23 hours of the day, causing the heart to beat less yet more efficiently.

- Exercise helps in weight loss, a key factor in avoiding heart disease.

- Exercise raises HDL cholesterol.

- Exercise lowers LDL cholesterol and triglycerides.

- Exercise lowers blood pressure levels. Following aerobic exercise, blood pressure falls for at least 90 minutes. Studies have shown that both physical fitness and aerobic activity (at least three times a week for 20 minutes each session) are associated with decreased risk of hypertension. Exercise training also is associated with lower blood pressure among hypertensive people.

tion of stimulants and smoking, is beneficial in the treatment of coronary disorders.

Graboys recommends for his heart patients any form of exercise that "breaks a sweat" for at least 20 to 30 minutes, three to four times a week, including brisk walking, jogging, rowing, swimming, low-impact aerobics, and outdoor (or stationary) bicycling. These aerobic exercises increase blood flow to the large muscle groups of the body, which keeps the heart and circulatory system healthier and more functional. Regular exercise also contributes to weight loss or weight control, helps moderate the effects of stress, decreases the tendency of blood to form clots, helps the body use insulin, lowers blood pressure, and may boost HDL cholesterol.

D. Nieman reports in *Fitness & Your Health* that the U.S. Centers for Disease Control reviewed 43 studies of North American and European working-age men. Controlling for age, blood pressure, smoking status, and total serum cholesterol levels, 68 percent of the studies reported a statistically significant relationship between physical activity and the risk of coronary heart disease (CHD). The studies confirmed that both

physical fitness and physical activity (whether on the job or during leisure times) are associated with reduced risk of CHD, and that regular physical activity should be promoted in CHD prevention programs as vigorously as blood pressure control, dietary modification to lower serum cholesterol, and smoking cessation. Next to high blood cholesterol levels, Nieman notes, lack of physical activity is the second most important risk factor for heart disease in the U.S.

Lowering Blood Pressure. High blood pressure levels can permanently damage the heart, and many Americans take antihypertensive drugs to lower their blood pressure. However, Ornish states that these drugs often have severe side effects, including impotence, fatigue, depression, and blood cell disorders. He believes that the safest and most effective way to lower blood pressure is to use natural stress reduction therapies such as yoga, meditation, and visualization. Most of the patients who followed Ornish's program were able to decrease or discontinue their blood pressure medications.

As discussed in Chapter 8, studies by Dr. Herbert Benson at the Harvard Medical

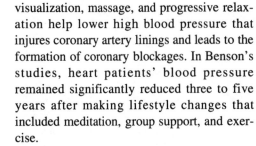

School clearly show that yoga, biofeedback, visualization, massage, and progressive relaxation help lower high blood pressure that injures coronary artery linings and leads to the formation of coronary blockages. In Benson's studies, heart patients' blood pressure remained significantly reduced three to five years after making lifestyle changes that included meditation, group support, and exercise.

Ornish believes that deep breathing and imaging techniques aimed at reducing stress should be conducted frequently throughout the day to reduce the output of adrenal hormones and lower the level of platelet aggregation. He encourages patients to do these techniques before meals and at bedtime, because they not only reduce stress but also improve digestion. Ornish's program is supported by Dr. William Lee Cowden, a cardiologist in Dallas, Texas, who notes in *Alternative Medicine: The Definitive Guide* that some nutrients which may help reverse coronary blockages (including magnesium and vitamins B, C, and E) must be absorbed out of the gastrointestinal tract. If the tract is in a stressed state, it cannot absorb these nutrients nearly as well as when it is relaxed.

Nutritional Therapies. Ornish claims that diet can almost immediately affect the heart. Even a single meal high in fat and cholesterol, he suggests, may cause the body to release a hormone, thromboxane, that causes the arteries to constrict and the blood to clot faster—one reason heart patients often get chest pain after eating a fatty meal. According to Ornish, the diet he developed "allowed participants' arteries to dilate and blood to flow more freely because the fat and cholesterol content was so low."

Ornish's nutritional therapy focuses on lowering high blood cholesterol levels that form plaque and injure (tear) the linings of the coronary arteries. His vegetarian diet eliminates cholesterol, which is found in animal products (including meats), poultry, fish, and dairy products. Not only are vegetarian foods cholesterol-free but, with rare exception, they are low in saturated fat, which has a direct relationship to blood cholesterol levels. Ornish's diet excludes all oils and animal fats except nonfat milk and yogurt, as well as coffee, colas, monosodium glutamate (MSG), tobacco, and other stimulants. All fried foods are prohibited. Dairy foods high in vitamin D also are eliminated, including homogenized milk, because these products contain the enzyme xanthine oxidase, which damages the arteries.

Ornish's diet allows only moderate use of salt and sugar. He advises that eating increased amounts of dietary fiber, especially flax seed, oat bran, and pectin; onions and garlic (both raw and cooked); vegetables; and fish, can help reduce the consumption of saturated fats, cholesterol, sugar, and animal proteins. The diet is not restricted in calories because Ornish believes that the type of food eaten is more important that the amounts consumed. An important adjunct is reducing fat consumption to 10 percent of total caloric intake. However, he suggests that omega-3 fatty acids (eicosopentanoic acid—EPA) may be beneficial for some patients, and these are provided by the fish included in his diet.

Balch and Balch recommend a well-balanced diet that contains adequate amount of fiber. They suggest raw foods, broiled fish, turkey, chicken, garlic, onions, lecithin, almonds and nuts (no peanuts), olive oil, pink salmon, trout, tuna, Atlantic herring, and mackerel. All of these foods contain essential fatty acids, are low in fat, and provide nutrients needed for normal heart functioning. Balch and Balch also counsel that no salt should be included in the diet.

Positive Thinking. Positive thinking and a healthy outlook help the heart to heal. One

ALTERNATIVE TREATMENTS FOR HEART DISORDERS

National Cholesterol Education Program/American Heart Association Dietary Guidelines for Prevention and Treatment of Coronary Heart Disease

- Total fat intake should be less than 30 percent of calories.

- Polyunsaturated fat intake should be less than 10 percent of calories.

- Saturated fat intake should be less than 10 percent of calories.

- Cholesterol intake should not exceed 300 milligrams per day.

- Carbohydrate intake should constitute 50 percent or more of calories, with emphasis on complex carbohydrates.

- Protein intake should provide the remainder of calories.

- Sodium intake should not exceed 3,000 milligrams per day.

- Alcohol consumption should not exceed one to two ounces per day.

- Total calories should be sufficient to maintain the individual's recommended body weight.

- A wide variety of foods should be consumed.

study conducted by Dr. Daniel Mark, a heart specialist at Duke University, and reported in April 15, 1994, edition of the *New York Times,* concluded that optimism was a powerful predictor of who will live and who will die after being diagnosed with heart disease. Mark conducted a follow-up study of 1,719 men and women who had undergone heart catheterization, a common procedure used to check the arteries for clogging. The patients typically underwent the test because of chest pain, and all were diagnosed with heart disease. When interviewed initially, 14 percent said they doubted that they would recover enough to resume their daily routines. After one year, 12 percent of these pessimists had died, compared with 5 percent of those who were optimistic about recovering. Even when the severity of people's conditions was taken into account, outlook was a crucial factor in survival. In fact, optimism often seemed to have little bearing on how sick people were. Some of those with very mild heart disease had the grimmest views of their prospects.

Mark concluded: "The mind is a tremendous tool or weapon, depending on your point of view." In his study, pessimism appeared to be even more damaging to recovery than depression, which also has been shown to lower a person's chance of recovery from heart disease.

Hostility, anger, and anxiety are thought to play a key role in heart disease. Psychologist Catherine Stoney of the American Psychosomatic Institute suggests that hostile, anxious people metabolize fats more slowly than positive, relaxed persons, which may be a key reason hostility and heart attacks are linked. Those who seethe with anger—and usually try to suppress it—are slowest at ridding their bodies of dietary fat. Experts have known that hostile adults have higher cholesterol levels, and Stoney's findings, which were summarized in the April 15, 1994, edition of the *Marin Independent Journal,* may provide a partial answer.

Deep Relaxation

1. Lie back with eyes closed.
2. Inhale deeply and progressively relax all the muscles.
3. Feel the gentle flow of air as it comes in and out of the nose.
4. Gradually allow the inhalations to become deeper with each breath.
5. Imagine breathing in light and healing energy, as well as oxygen, that are revitalizing and recharging both body and mind.

Alternate Nostril Breathing

1. Sit in a comfortable position and close the eyes.
2. Exhale fully.
3. Close off the right nostril with the thumb and inhale slowly through the left nostril.
4. Close off the left nostril and exhale through the right nostril.
5. Inhale through the right nostril.
6. Close off the right nostril and exhale through the left nostril.
7. Continue this pattern, changing the nostril after each inhalation.
8. Continue for 30 seconds to three minutes.
9. If there is a feeling of not getting enough air, simply resume breathing normally.

Progressive Deep Relaxation and Deep Breathing. In *Dr. Dean Ornish's Program for Reversing Heart Disease,* Ornish describes several progressive deep relaxation exercises that his patients have used to induce the relaxation response. Besides connecting the mind and body, this kind of breathing also decreases heart rate, blood pressure, muscular tension, and sympathetic nervous system stimulation.

Deep breathing, according to Ornish, is one of the most effective ways of preventing and relieving chronic stress. He has his patients practice alternate nostril breathing, as described on this page.

Quitting Smoking. According to Ornish, smoking causes "many more deaths" from heart disease than from lung cancer, in both men and women. The nicotine and other toxic substances in tobacco are absorbed into the blood and injure the lining of the coronary arteries. Nicotine also causes the coronary arteries to constrict, and can lead to the formation of blood clots.

Ornish cites recent studies that have demonstrated that quitting smoking reduces the risk of heart disease by 64 percent within the first three years after stopping. When people stop smoking, nicotine is eliminated from the body quickly, and the risk of blood clots or coronary artery spasms decreases rapidly.

Traditional Chinese Medicine (TCM). Traditional Chinese Medicine views heart disease as a problem stemming from poor digestion, which causes the buildup of plaque in the arteries. Chung San Yuan reports in a 1973 issue of the *Chinese Medical Journal* that the Chinese herb mao-tung-ching has been used successfully to treat coronary heart disease. Mao-tung-ching was administered daily (both orally and intravenously) to 103 patients. In 101 out of 103 cases, significant improvement resulted. The herb is believed to dilate the blood vessels, although its effectiveness in treating patients with coronary artery disease has not been confirmed in Western clinical trials. TCM practitioners often combine Chinese botanical therapies with acupuncture, which they believe is an effective multiple treatment for chronic coronary heart disease cases. Further clinical trials are necessary, however, to evaluate the effectiveness of acupuncture in the treatment of cardiovascular disorders.

Visualization. Visualization also directly produces the relaxation response, and lowers heart rate and blood pressure. According to Ornish, visualizing healing images can improve coronary blood flow by dilating the coronary arteries. Visualization also reduces the number and severity of irregular heartbeats. He suggests that people with coronary blockages ask their cardiologist for a diagram showing the exact location of each blocked artery.

Vitamin and Mineral Therapies. Atherosclerosis and heart disease take many

years to develop, and a daily regimen of vitamin and mineral supplements may be helpful in preventing or treating both. The best procedure is to consult a heart specialist who may recommend vitamin and mineral supplements based on a person's diet, body weight, medical status, and absorption levels.

Plaque formation in arteries usually follows prior damage to the inner lining of the arteries. A sudden increase in blood pressure due to chronic emotional stress, for example, can cause small tears in the arterial linings, as blood vessels do not always dilate rapidly enough to accommodate sudden increases in pressure. As noted in Chapter 3, deficiencies of vitamins B, C, and E, and magnesium can make this inner lining more susceptible to damage and subsequent plaque formation.

Vitamin B3 reduces cholesterol and triglycerides in the blood and helps dilate the coronary arteries. Vitamins B6 (pyridoxine) and B12 (necessary for the conversion of homocysteine to cystathionine) also help reduce cholesterol levels, especially oxidized cholesterols known as oxysterols. Homocysteine is derived from methionine (an amino acid found in red meat, milk, and milk products) and converted with the help of pyridoxine to a nontoxic derivative. A deficiency of pyridoxine leads to the accumulation of homocysteine, which is damaging to endothelial cells (which line the heart) and can contribute to atherosclerosis.

Vitamins C and E help prevent and dissolve coronary blood clots, prevent excessive scarring of the heart after a heart attack, and facilitate circulation by dilating capillaries and developing collateral blood vessels (see Chapter 3).

As cited in the May 20, 1993, editions of the *New York Times* and the *Wall Street Journal,* researchers at the Harvard School of Public Health and Brigham and Women's Hospital in Boston reported that people who take daily megadoses of vitamin E have a sig-

ALTERNATIVE TREATMENTS FOR HEART DISORDERS

Recovering from a Heart Disorder

Millions of people diagnosed with coronary artery disease recover fully and live long, happy, and productive lives. The following recommendations are an important part of this process.

- **Keep blood pressure low.** High blood pressure (hypertension) increases the risk of recurrence of cardiovascular problems, as well as kidney problems and strokes. Ways to help lower blood pressure include reducing salt intake, exercising regularly, and losing weight (if overweight). Medication also is effective.

- **Maintain low blood cholesterol.** Reduce fat in the diet by eating vegetables, grains (pasta, rice, breads), beans, and fruit. Avoid fatty animal products, dairy products, and snack foods. Cholesterol-lowering medications may help, but often a good diet will produce desired results.

- **Exercise.** The key is to gradually work up to a regimen of exercising three times a week that will raise the heart rate for 20 to 30 minutes. This can be as simple as brisk walking, bicycling, or swimming. Regular exercise helps to curb appetite, relieves stress, improves HDL cholesterol blood levels, conditions the heart and lungs, and teaches the body's large muscles to extract oxygen and nutrients more efficiently.

- **Return to work.** Following hospital discharge after a heart attack, rest fully, and then return to part-time work before resuming work full time. Patients should discuss the timing with their doctor and make sure the physician fully understands all the details about their level of stress and the physical and emotional demands of their job.

- **Lose weight.** The fastest way to lose weight is to eat less fat—ideally reducing fat to 10 percent of total caloric intake.

- **Reduce stress level.** Angry stress can create an excess release of adrenaline and various steroids in the body which, over time, cause hardening of the arteries. Exercise, biofeedback, yoga, meditation, and visualization all help reduce angry stress.

- **Join a heart rehabilitation support group.** Most community hospitals have programs that include exercise three to four times weekly and relaxation therapies. These programs are especially helpful for those who are having difficulty adjusting to the reality of their heart problem after discharge.

- **Resume sexual activity.** It is common for both men and women to experience reduced sexual desire for several months following a heart attack. Support groups are available to help people with these issues and others that arise during rehabilitation. If chest discomfort is experienced, nitroglycerin can be used preventively (before making love) to eliminate it.

Graboys Heart Letter, "The Road to Heart Health: Five Steps to Recovery" by Thomas B. Graboys. Copyright © 1993 GHL Publishing, Inc. All rights reserved. Reprinted by permission.

nificantly reduced risk of heart disease, although they cautioned that it is still too soon to recommend widespread use. Separate studies of more than 120,000 men and women who took daily vitamin E supplements of at least 100 International Units—more than three times the current U.S. RDA—showed that they had a 40 percent lower risk of heart disease than people who did not use the supplement.

The researchers found that the reduction in risk appeared after two years of taking the supplements, and that people who simply consumed a diet rich in vitamin E did not derive the same health benefits. They also found that the benefit was not enhanced when people took more than 100 units. The researchers concluded that vitamin E, as an antioxidant, might reduce heart disease by having an effect on low-density lipoprotein (LDL) cholesterol, the so-called "bad" cholesterol.

According to Murray and Pizzorno, carnitine, pantetheine, and coenzyme Q10 help prevent the accumulation of fatty acids within the heart muscle by improving the breakdown of fatty acids and other compounds. Pantetheine has been shown to reduce serum triglyceride and cholesterol levels significantly while increasing HDL cholesterol levels in clinical trials. It appears to accelerate fatty acid breakdown as well.

Coenzyme Q10, a vitamin that functions as a coenzyme, protects against atherosclerosis by helping to prevent the formation of oxysterols. Dr. Karl Folders, a biomedical scientist at the University of Texas in Austin, suggests in the March/April 1994 issue of *Natural Health* that many heart patients suffer from a coenzyme Q10 deficiency. One study found coenzyme Q10 deficiencies in 75 percent of 132 patients undergoing heart surgery. Dr. Peter Langsjoen, a cardiologist in Tyler, Texas, states in the same article: "In 80 percent of my (heart) patients, I see a clinical improvement within four weeks of adminis-

tering coenzyme Q10." According to Langsjoen, all forms of heart disease seem to respond to coenzyme Q10.

Other minerals linked with reductions in cholesterol and platelet levels include selenium, magnesium, calcium, chromium, and potassium. Dosages for these minerals should be prescribed by a heart specialist or physician.

Yoga. Both Ornish and Graboys recommend yoga as an adjunct to stress reduction therapies. The form of yoga used by Ornish's patients, hatha yoga, combines stretching and breathing techniques that produce a sense of equilibrium and rebalancing. It also includes visualization, progressive relaxation practices, self-analysis, and meditation.

Summary

Although heart disease causes nearly half of all deaths in the U.S., it is one of the most preventable chronic degenerative disorders. Eighty-five percent of all heart attacks are caused by atherosclerosis—hardening of the coronary arteries that blocks blood flow to the heart. Overwhelming evidence suggests that the risk of coronary artery disease, including angina and myocardial infarction, can be reduced through dietary changes, vitamin and mineral therapies, botanical therapies, exercise, and stress management, all of which help prevent excessive oxidation of cholesterol in the bloodstream.

In the past three decades, significant progress has been made in the war against heart disease. Although the U.S. population has increased in size and become more elderly, the total annual number of heart attacks has remained relatively constant. Thus, the rate of heart attacks per 100,000 people of any given age has declined by approximately 40 percent since the early 1960s. According to the April 1994 issue of the *Harvard Health*

Letter, prevention has played a major role in reducing the heart attack rate, and at least half of the credit for this improvement belongs to patients, who have modified their diets to reduce cholesterol levels, avoided cigarettes, controlled their blood pressure, and undertaken regular physical activity.

Resources

References

American Heart Association. *Fact Sheet on Heart Attacks, Stroke and Risk Factors.* Dallas, TX: American Heart Association, 1987.

———. *Heart and Stroke Facts.* Dallas, TX: American Heart Association, 1992.

Balch, James F., and Phyllis Balch. *Prescription for Nutritional Healing.* Garden City Park, NY: Avery Publishing Group, 1993.

Benson, Herbert. *The Relaxation Response.* New York, NY: William Morrow, 1975.

Brody, Jane. "Vitamin E Greatly Reduces Risk of Heart Disease, Studies Suggest." *New York Times* (May 20, 1993): B7.

Brown, Donald J. "Garlic for Intermittent Claudication." *Townsend Letter for Doctors* (May 1994): 546.

The Burton Goldberg Group. *Alternative Medicine: The Definitive Guide.* Puyallup, WA: Future Medicine Publishing, Inc., 1993.

Edlin, Gordon, and Eric Golanty. *Health and Wellness: A Holistic Approach.* Boston, MA: Jones and Bartlett Publishers, 1992.

Folders, Karl. "Heart Disease." *Natural Health* (March/April 1994): 3.

Graboys, Thomas B., M.D. "Avoiding Sudden Cardiac Death." *Graboys Heart Letter* (March 1994): 1–2.

———. "Choosing The Right Options for Heart Diagnosis and Treatment." *A Graboys Heart Letter Special Report* (1994): 1–4.

———. "Five Common Sense Ways to Stay Heart Healthy." *A Graboys Heart Letter Special Report* (1994): 1–4.

———. "Healing Your Own Heart: A Holistic Approach." *Graboys Heart Letter* (March 1994): 3.

———. "Nitroglycerine Can Eliminate Your Chest Pains." *Graboys Heart Letter* (May 1994): 3.

"Hostility and Heart Attacks." *Marin Independent Journal* (April 15, 1994): A1.

"How Risky is Physical Exercise?" *Harvard Health Letter* (May 1994): 13.

"Insurance to Cover Alternative Heart Treatment." *Natural Health* (November/December 1993): 18.

Kieswater, H. "Effects of Garlic Coated Tablets in Peripheral Arterial Occlusive Disease." *Clinical Investigations* (1991, Volume 71): 383–86.

McDonagh, E. "An Oculocerebrovascullometric Analysis of the Improvement in Arterial Stenosis Following EDTA Chelation Therapy," in *A Textbook on EDTA Chelation Therapy* by E.M. Cranston. New York, NY: Human Sciences Press, 1989: 155.

"Men, Hormones, and Heart Disease." *Harvard Health Letter* (June 1994): 8.

"Mind/Body: Stress and Anger." *UC Berkeley Wellness Letter* (May 1994): 5.

Murray, Michael, and Joseph Pizzorno. *Encyclopedia of Natural Medicine.* Rocklin, CA: Prima Publishing, 1991.

Nieman, D. *Fitness & Your Health.* Palo Alto, CA: Bull Publishing Company, 1993.

"Optimism Can Mean Life for Heart Patients and Pessimism Death, Study Says." *New York Times* (April 15, 1994): A11.

Ornish, Dean, M.D. *Dr. Dean Ornish's Program for Reversing Heart Disease.* New York, NY: Ballantine Books, 1990.

"Progress in the War Against Heart Attacks." *Harvard Health Letter* (April 1994): 1–5.

"Rating Your Risks for Heart Disease." *UC Berkeley Wellness Letter* (May 1994): 4–5.

Stipp, David. "Vitamin E Link Is Seen in Lowering Heart Disease Risk." *Wall Street Journal* (May 20, 1993): A10.

Yuan, Chung San. "Treatment of 103 cases of Coronary Diseases with Ilex pubescens." *Chinese Medical Journal* (1973, Volume 1): 64.

Organizations

American Heart Association
7320 Greenville Ave., Dallas, TX 75231.

American Physical Therapy Association (APTA)
PO Box 37257, Washington, DC 20013.

American Rehabilitation Foundation
Kenny Rehabilitation Institute, 2727 Chicago Ave., Minneapolis, MN 55407.

Additional Reading

Angell, Dwight. "Doctors Fight to Keep Blood Flowing: Cleared Arteries Too Often Clogged by Returning Clots." *San Jose Mercury News* (January 16, 1994): C1.

Butler, Kurt, and Lynn Rayner. *The Best Medicine: The Complete Health and Preventive Medicine Handbook.* New York, NY: Harper & Row Publishers, Inc., 1985.

Chesebro, J.H., et al. "New Approaches to Treatment of Myocardial Infarction." *The American Journal of Cardiology* (February 2, 1990): 12C–19C.

Freundlich, Naomi. "A Cardiac Crusader Heads for Main Street: Will Dr. Ornish's No-Surgery Heart Disease Plan Work on a Large Scale?" *Business Week* (November 29, 1993): 90–94.

Kemper, M. "Caloric Requirements and Supply in Critically Ill Surgical Patients." *Critical Care Medicine* (March 1992): 344–48.

Margolis, Simeon, and Hamilton Moses III. *The Johns Hopkins Medical Handbook.* New York, NY: Medletter Associates, Inc., 1992.

Chapter 19

AGING

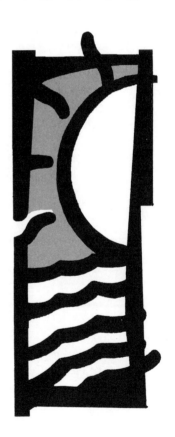

No matter how healthy their lifestyle, as people become older certain biological changes occur. They lose their hair or their hair turns grey, their skin wrinkles, they lose muscle tone and physical stamina, their lungs decrease in size, and their heart and immune systems become less efficient.

While scientists have not been able to stop the normal processes of aging, it is possible for people, as discussed in this chapter, to improve their strength, flexibility, and energy levels, thus helping to protect themselves against chronic illnesses associated with aging, including Alzheimer's disease, senile dementia, and osteoporosis.

Causes of Aging

One genetic theory suggests that the human body has a biological aging clock in which each cell is genetically programmed to live a proscribed life span. The longer the potential life span for a species, the greater the number of divisions a cell will undergo before its growth finally stops and the cell dies. Another theory, called the "error catastrophe" hypothesis, suggests that aging occurs as a result of accumulated genetic and cellular damage. The longer people live, for example, the more their bodies are exposed to radiation and cancer-causing chemicals. Eventually some essential cellular functions deteriorate because of mutations that inactivate the genes. Human cells possess a variety of enzymes that can repair damage to DNA and other vital cellular structures. If one or more of these enzymes becomes

Physiological Changes of Aging

- **Loss of vision and hearing:** Visual function starts to decline at around age 45. Gradual hearing loss generally begins at about age 20.

- **Loss of taste and smell:** With age, the taste buds diminish in number and size, which affects sweet and salty tastes in particular. Difficulty identifying common substances by smell increases.

- **Dental bone loss:** The majority of the elderly suffer bone loss and disease in the tissues around the teeth. This makes it more difficult to chew, leading to reduced consumption of fresh fruit and vegetables high in dietary fiber.

- **Loss of lean body weight:** As people age, their body fat tends to increase while their muscle and bone (lean body weight) decrease.

- **Loss of bone mass:** Women lose significant amounts of their bone mass by the age of 65, which can cause osteoporosis. If a bone is fractured, it often mends slowly.

- **Loss of mental clarity:** A large percent of the elderly show some signs of senile dementia and problems associated with it, including impairment of memory, judgment, personality, and the ability to speak.

- **Reduced ability to metabolize drugs:** The elderly less efficiently absorb, distribute, metabolize, and excrete nutrients as well as botanical and pharmaceutical drugs. The majority of the elderly regularly take more than one prescription drug, and these may interact with each other, causing severe side effects in some cases.

- **Urinary incontinence:** A large percent of the elderly cannot control their urination. This often leads to social isolation and embarrassment.

- **Reduction in heart and lung fitness:** With aging, there is a reduction every decade in the ability of the heart and lungs to supply oxygen to the muscles. Most of this is attributed to the reduced physical activity of the elderly.

Fitness and Your Health. Copyright © 1993 Bull Publishing Company. All rights reserved. Reprinted by permission.

defective, however, it is possible that essential cellular functions will begin to fail.

A third theory proposes that decline in immune system functioning is key to the aging process. As discussed in Chapter 7, weakening of the immune system often results in increased susceptibility to many diseases, including cancer and atherosclerosis. As the body ages, the immune system at some point cannot recognize and eliminate damaged or foreign cells efficiently—and the elderly become particularly susceptible to infections and chronic diseases that can be fatal.

Aging also has been attributed indirectly to the atrophy of the thymus gland. As people grow older, the thymus gland shrinks in size and produces less thymosin, an important hormone that may help regulate the biological aging clock. Another theory argues that aging is linked to cellular damage caused by free radicals—toxic molecules that can damage arterial walls and other healthy cells. Free radicals normally are neutralized or destroyed by protective enzymes in cells. However, cellular damage caused by free radicals may accumulate over time and contribute to the aging process.

A sixth theory suggests that aging may be related to dietary habits. Roy Walford, author of the book *Maximum Life Span,* has shown that the aging process in mammals is always in some degree related to caloric intake: the more calories they eat, the faster they age; the fewer calories they consume, the slower they age. Walford has successfully increased the life span of laboratory animals by reducing their caloric intake by 25 percent. The relationship between reducing caloric intake and extending normal life spans has not been conclusively proven in humans, however.

Finally, aging may be related to specific nutritional deficiencies, especially zinc. More than 100 enzymes in human cells require zinc to function properly. While a mild zinc deficiency may not produce any obvious clinical symptoms, a gradual depletion of zinc in the cells of older people could accelerate the aging process or increase their susceptibility to disease.

The most reasonable assumption about aging is that it is caused by both internal and external factors—including genetics—that interact in a complex way, and that those factors will affect each person differently. Because no scientific breakthroughs are anticipated to prevent normal human aging or death, everyone should strive to maintain good mental and physical health throughout all the stages of life.

Therapies for Coping with Aging

Ayurvedic Botanicals. As noted in Chapter 5, several Ayurvedic botanical supplements developed by the followers of the Maharishi Yogi, called Maharishi Amrit Kalash (MAK), have been effective in increasing cerebral functioning and may reverse some of the detrimental cognitive effects of aging.

Botanical Medicines. Dr. Ki C. Chen reports in the September 1993 issue of the *Journal of Traditional Chinese Medicine* that the Institute of Geriatrics at Xiyuan Hospital in Beijing is studying the anti-aging effects of 386 botanical medicines. Specifically, researchers are investigating the effects of each herb on cell generation, survival times, immunomodulation, improvement of visceral and metabolic functions, and inhibiting infections. Chen reports that preliminary results suggest that ginseng, radix astragali, radix angelicae sinensis, green tea, and ginkgo biloba compounds appear to delay some of the symptoms of aging and age-related diseases.

As noted in Chapter 5, green tea is believed to help prevent some cancers because its catechin and camellia sinensis act as powerful antioxidants that help control the activity of free radicals, the unstable compounds implicated in premature aging and a host of diseases. In addition, ginkgo biloba extract has been remarkably effective in treating insufficient blood and oxygen supply in the brain, which is associated with common symptoms of aging such as short-term memory loss, dizziness, headaches, ringing in the ears, hearing and energy loss, and depression. Research in China, summarized by Dr. C. Liu in the February 1992 issue of the *Journal of Ethnopharmacology,* indicates that panax ginseng "strengthens immune function and metabolism, possesses biomodulation action, and has effects on anti-aging and relieving stress."

As also discussed in Chapter 5, the Chinese regard the shiitake mushroom as a plant that gives eternal youth and longevity. The shiitake mushroom has been used in

Traditional Chinese Medicine (TCM) to increase immune resistance to disease.

Exercise. Can regular exercise lengthen life expectancy? Dr. Ralph Paffenbarger of Stanford University found that Harvard alumni whose weekly energy output in walking, stair climbing, and active sports totaled at least 2,000 calories had a 28 percent reduction in death rates from all causes. Paffenbarger suggests in a 1986 volume of the *New England Journal of Medicine* that this improvement in longevity—due to a reduced risk of major diseases—can be gained by walking or jogging eight to ten miles a week.

The 11 benefits of exercise described in Chapter 6 are especially important for the elderly. As people age, their hearts normally pump less blood. However, experiments conducted at the National Institute on Aging show that if the heart is free of disease, blood pumps just as efficiently in a 90-year-old as in a young adult. The aging heart apparently compensates for a slow rate of pumping in older people by enlarging, thereby increasing its capacity to pump more blood through the veins and arteries with each heartbeat.

The lungs, on the other hand, decrease in size with age, and, as a result, an elderly person has only half the maximum breathing capacity of a young person. Most elderly people, however, are able to engage in physical activities such as walking, shopping, and playing golf. Strength training makes the heart more efficient at delivering blood to the muscles, and it therefore does not have to work as hard. According to the winter 1993 issue of *Healthy Woman,* strength training also appears to relax the blood vessels so that blood flows through them more efficiently. Exercise increases cerebral blood flow, improves memory, and increases bone mass and bone density, which is especially important for postmenopausal women (see discussion of Alzheimer's disease and osteoporosis).

In addition, exercise increases immune resistance. Researchers at Purdue University and the University of Arizona examined the roles vitamin supplements and exercise play in immunity. They found that vitamins C and E help strengthen immune function, and that exercise strongly augments this effect. As reported in *Forever Young,* a group of volunteers was given a four-month regimen of vitamins C and E, a 1½-hour workout three times a week, both vitamins and workouts, or neither one. Participants who exercised and took vitamin supplements produced the most infection-fighting T-cells in their blood. Researchers concluded that both physical conditioning and a high intake of vitamins can stimulate cellular immune functions in adults.

Nutritional Therapies. "There is no doubt that life can be shortened by a variety of forms of malnutrition," writes Alfred E. Harper, Ph.D., of the departments of nutritional sciences and biochemistry at the University of Wisconsin. In Forever Young, published by Rodale Press, Harper goes on to say that "dietary modification can be used to reduce the severity of the signs and symptoms of a variety of genetic and pathological conditions that result in metabolic defects. Application of nutritional knowledge in these ways can prolong survival and increase longevity—within the biologically determined life span—just as can the application of other therapeutic measures or avoidance of environmental hazards."

To slow the general decline of bodily functions that occurs in aging, Dr. Sheldon Hendler, author of *The Complete Guide to Anti-Aging Nutrients,* suggests reducing fat intake to no more than 30 (preferably 20) percent of total calories. He also recommends limiting red meat and animal protein intake because they are harder for the kidneys of elderly people to absorb. On the other hand, evidence suggests that protein enhances calci-

Nutritional Recommendations to Increase Lifespan

- **Eat fruits and vegetables.** The National Cancer Institute recommends five daily servings of fruits and vegetables, which are the key sources of substances such as fiber, vitamins C and E, and beta-carotene—all of which reduce the risk of cancer. They also may help prevent heart disease, cataracts, and other age-related illnesses.

- **Eat less fat.** In a five-year Family Heart Study project conducted in Portland, Oregon, researchers found that people who adopted a low-fat diet suffered fewer day-to-day feelings of depression and anger. Reducing fat intake also will reduce the risk of heart disease and obesity.

- **Reduce the consumption of alcohol.** Excess alcohol consumption puts a strain on the liver.

- **Eat a healthy breakfast.** Research suggests that starting the day with a sensible meal is one of seven factors associated with longevity. A 10-year study of 7,000 men and women by UCLA's School of Public Health found that women who ate a healthy breakfast, along with never smoking, exercising regularly, drinking only moderate amounts of alcohol, sleeping seven to eight hours a night, maintaining proper weight, and not eating between meals, lived an average of eight years longer than women who followed only one to three of these practices.

- **Eat dinner at lunchtime.** The French (who suffer fewer heart attacks than Americans even though they ingest the same amount of fat) consume 57 percent of their calories before 2 p.m., while Americans eat only 38 percent of their calories by that time. Researchers speculate that when people eat the bulk of their calories earlier in the day, their bodies are better able to metabolize fat. As a result, blood cells called platelets are less likely to aggregate, reducing the incidence of clotting that can lead to strokes and heart attacks.

- **Eat foods rich in calcium.** The more calcium people store in their bones during their 20s and 30s, the less likely they are to suffer from osteoporosis in later years.

- **Eat foods containing chromium.** Fresh fruits and vegetables, dairy products, whole wheat, and meat all contain small amounts of chromium, a trace mineral. Research conducted at the Human Nutrition Research Center in Beltsville, Maryland, suggests that people who do not get enough chromium cannot use their insulin as efficiently to get sugar out of the bloodstream and into the body tissues, which could be an early warning sign of diabetes.

um absorption. Also, various illnesses in the elderly result in a decrease in the amount of nutrition absorbed from the food eaten, creating more loss of protein. For these reasons, older people should probably eat a little extra protein, preferably plant protein. Protein should comprise about 13 percent of total calorie intake, although some conditions such as surgery, chronic diseases, or skin ulcerations may increase this requirement.

Antioxidant Recommendations of the Alliance for Aging Research

- **Vitamin C:** 250 to 1,000 milligrams, or 4 to 16 times the U.S. RDA of 60 milligrams.
- **Vitamin E:** 100 to 400 International Units (IU), the equivalent of 3 to 13 times the U.S. RDA of 30 IU.
- **Beta-carotene** (a relative of vitamin A found only in plant foods): 17,000 to 50,000 IU, or 3 to 10 times the recommended vitamin A allowance of 5,000 IU.

James F. Balch and Phyllis Balch suggest in *Prescription for Nutritional Healing* that the elderly should restrict sugar and refined carbohydrates. Refined carbohydrates may increase glucose intolerance, which occurs to an extent in normal aging. They recommend increasing the amount of fruits, vegetables, and fiber as substitutes for sugary foods. High-fiber foods are protein-rich and help ease constipation, another common complaint of older people.

According to the American Heart Association, eating less fat and salt, and more fresh fruits, vegetables, and whole grains, can reduce the risks of heart disease, cancer, and obesity. Ongoing research at the USDA Human Nutrition Research Center on Aging at Tufts University has found that cutting back on fat and stocking up on key nutrients can help increase life span.

Relaxation Training. Psychosocial factors such as loneliness and stress also affect the immune system of people as they age. The hazards of loneliness can increase when they are combined with stress, according to an Ohio State University study reported in *Forever Young.* Researchers divided 30 residents of a retirement home into three groups: 10 people received relaxation training three times a week; 10 received individual "social contact" three times a week; and 10 had no contact with the researchers. Those who learned to relax experienced a 32 percent increase in white blood cell levels. Those who had social contact had an 18 percent rise. The people in the no-contact group suffered a 6 percent loss of white blood cells, and showed the least resistance to herpes virus infections.

Vitamin and Mineral Therapies. Although the role of vitamins and minerals in delaying the aging process is debated by scientists, one public health organization, the Alliance for Aging Research, recommends vitamin supplements to reduce the risk of life-threatening medical disorders such as heart disease and cancer. According to an article in the May 1994 issue of the *Tufts University Diet & Nutrition Letter,* the Washington, D.C.-based health advocacy group now officially advises people to take large doses of vitamins C, E, and beta-carotene—known as antioxidant nutrients—to supplement the amounts of these substances received from foods.

The alliance's recommendations were developed by a panel of scientific experts from research and academic institutions around the country. The panel reviewed more than 200 studies of antioxidants conducted over the last 20 years, which together suggest that much larger amounts than the U.S. RDAs are necessary to combat free radicals—the highly toxic molecules produced as a natural by-product during the chemical process of oxidation. Oxidation is triggered by environmental pollutants as well as by an individual's own metabolism. If free radicals are left unchecked, they can, according to the alliance, damage the cells inside various tissues, potentially leading to the development of clogged arteries, various cancers, and other debilitating conditions.

Alzheimer's Disease and Senile Dementia

Alzheimer's disease—the most common form of dementia among the elderly—is a neurodegenerative disorder in which people progressively lose their ability to memorize, perceive, speak, solve problems, or make judgments. It was first described in 1906 by Alois Alzheimer, a German neurologist who discovered abnormal microscopic structures in the brain tissue of women who died of senile dementia. These structures were found primarily in the hippocampus, the part of the brain related to memory and intellectual function.

According to the California Medical Association's April 1990 *Health Tips,* approximately 500,000 to 1.5 million older Americans are affected by Alzheimer's, although as many as 2.5 million may suffer from it. Alzheimer's is present in an estimated 25 percent of Americans who are 85 years or older, although it can occur in middle life as well. The Alzheimer's Association claims the disease is the fourth leading cause of death in the U.S.

Alzheimer's disease, previously classified as pre-senile dementia, is characterized by irreversible changes in nerve cells in certain vulnerable areas of the brain devoted to mental functions. This results in neurofibrillary tangles (tangles of thread-like nerve filaments in the outer layers) and many small plaques of a tough, fibrous protein called beta-amyloid, both of which indicate serious disruptions in the structural and functional connections between brain cells (neurons).

The disease usually has a gradual onset. People may begin to experience difficulty with memory, especially in terms of recent events. Other symptoms include language problems, such as inability to find the correct word when thinking abstractly. There may be poor or decreased judgment, disorientation, inability to learn new material or to concentrate, loss of initiative, changes in mood or behavior, changes in personality, paranoia, and motor activity problems. These symptoms typically cause difficulties in everyday activities. People may get lost in familiar surroundings, for example, or lose their way to a familiar destination. They may also find it hard to handle money, get dressed, read, write, use keys, or operate electrical appliances. The overall result is a noticeable decline in personal activity and work performance. How quickly these changes occur varies from person to person, but eventually the disease progresses to the stage where victims are unable to care for themselves.

Symptoms occurring before age 65 are designated presenile dementia of the Alzheimer's type (PDAT); after 65 they are called senile dementia of the Alzheimer's type (SDAT). Current diagnosis of Alzheimer's disease is extremely difficult as the only definitive diagnosis is a postmortem biopsy of the brain.

No cause has been identified for Alzheimer's disease, although it may be infectious (viral), degenerative, or auto-immune. The disease is thought to be associated with a loss of acetylcholine, which functions as a transmitting agent in the brain, although there is a general reduction in the concentration of all neurotransmitting substances. It is likely that a combination of genetic and environmental factors contributes to its development. For example, Alzheimer's disease has been linked to a genetic abnormality on chromosome 19, one of the 23 pairs of human chromosomes, and the disease tends to run in families.

The fact that older people exhibit the symptoms of Alzheimer's does not necessarily mean they have the disease. For example, many elderly persons develop "benign forgetting," in which they have trouble remembering a word or thought and need a brief period of time to recall it. This and other conditions that produce symptoms similar to Alzheimer's may be treatable if detected early enough. Regular medical checkups can help physicians determine the cause of the symptoms, which could include a previous stroke, depression, drug intoxication, thyroid disease, nutritional deficiencies, brain tumors, head trauma, or a condition such as hydrocephalus, a disorder in which an abnormal amount of spinal fluid in the skull causes widening of the brain ventricles.

Dementia refers to a general mental deterioration. In the elderly, it is referred to as senile dementia. It can be marked by progressive mental deterioration, loss of short-term memory, moodiness and irritability, self-centeredness, and childish behavior. This often is due to Alzheimer's disease, although there are many other causes of senile dementia.

Currently 1.3 million elderly people in the U.S. suffer severe dementia and approximately 3 million endure mild to moderate dementia, or a total of approximately 15 percent of all elderly Americans, report Simeon Margolis and Hamilton Moses III. Dementia in the elderly often is a result of insufficient blood and oxygen flow to the brain. Also associated with these insufficiencies are short-term memory loss, vertigo, headaches, ringing in the ears, and depression. Much of this is due to the presence of atherosclerotic cardiovascular disease.

Many cases of dementia are reversible. Michael Murray and Joseph Pizzorno, in the *Encyclopedia of Natural Medicine,* claim that more than 80 percent of the elderly are deficient in one or more vitamins or minerals

which may induce dementia. In addition, more than 30 percent of the elderly use a number of prescription drugs daily. Drugs and drug interactions probably play a greater role in creating symptoms of dementia and confused states than is currently realized.

Although senile dementia of the Alzheimer's type is not yet curable or reversible, there are ways to alleviate symptoms and to prevent or delay their onset.

Therapies for Coping with Alzheimer's Disease and Senile Dementia

Ayurvedic Medicine. Dr. Sodhi, director of the American School of Ayurvedic Sciences in Bellevue, Washington (as cited in *Alternative Medicine: The Definitive Guide),* has successfully treated both Alzheimer's and senile dementia using a combination of homeopathic and Ayurvedic therapies. Although each patient's condition is caused by a unique combination of factors, he claims that more than 80 percent have environmental toxicities that must be eliminated first. He prescribes herbs that cleanse the liver, along with triphala, a combination of three herbs, and gotu kola, which increases brain cell functioning. For cerebral functioning, he prescribes ginkgo biloba or macunabrure along with vitamin B1 and B3 supplements, as long as patients do not have liver disorders.

Botanical Medicines. Ginkgo biloba has been shown in several clinical trials to improve brain circulation and increase mental capacity, according to M. Allard, writing in the September 1986 issue of *Presse Medicale.* In one study involving 112 geriatric patients diagnosed with cerebral vascular insufficiency, the administration of 120 milligrams per day of ginkgo biloba extract (GBE) resulted in a statistically significant regression of the major symptoms. As reported by Dr. G. Rai in a 1991 issue of *Current Medical Research & Opinion,* volume 6, the regression of these symptoms suggests that a reduced blood and oxygen supply to the brain may be the major cause of the so-called age-related cerebral disorders (including senility), rather than a true degenerative process of nerve tissue. It appears that ginkgo biloba extract, by increasing blood flow to the brain, increases oxygen and glucose utilization and offers relief from these presumed side effects of aging. "The results show," Rai concluded, "that GBE may be of great benefit in many cases of senility, including Alzheimer's disease." Balch and Balch suggest that the herbs blue cohosh and anise also may be effective, in combination with ginkgo biloba, in improving brain functioning by increasing the flow of oxygen to the brain.

Estrogen Replacement Therapy (ERT). According to a University of Southern California study, reported in the March 8, 1994, edition of the *New York Times,* postmenopausal women who take ERT to prevent bone loss and heart disease are less likely to develop Alzheimer's disease. If they do develop the disease, their symptoms are less severe than those experienced by women who do not take ERT. Researchers examined 2,418 women over a period of 11 years and found that those taking estrogen were 40 percent less likely to develop Alzheimer's.

The research suggests that estrogen plays an important role in maintaining connections between neurons (brain cells). When estrogen levels drop sharply upon menopause, the complexity of connections may slowly diminish, perhaps making neurons more likely to degenerate and die. In contrast, because males do not go through menopause and therefore retain higher levels of their sex hormone (testosterone), much of which is converted into estrogen in the brain, far fewer suffer from Alzheimer's.

Preventing and Treating Alzheimer's Disease

- Avoid excessive exposure to aluminum and silicon.
- Consume supplemental antioxidants such as carotenes, flavonoids, vitamins C and E, zinc, and selenium.
- Correct any underlying thyroid abnormality.
- Maintain adequate blood and oxygen flow to the brain. The latter measure is particularly important if symptoms of cerebrovascular insufficiency exist, such as ringing in the ears, dizziness, depression, and headaches. An extract of ginkgo biloba has been shown to be especially effective in the treatment of these symptoms and capable of improving brain wave patterns in elderly individuals with senile dementia.

Lifestyle Changes. Toxins such as food and tap water chemicals, carbon monoxide, diesel fumes, solvents, aerosol spray, and industrial chemicals can cause symptoms of brain dysfunctions that may lead to an inaccurate diagnosis of Alzheimer's or senile dementia. Avoiding external toxins and eliminating internal toxins by using the detoxification programs outlined in Chapter 7 can be helpful in preventing the onset of these symptoms.

Tom Warren, in his book *Beating Alzheimer's,* describes his own poignant case in which he had his amalgam fillings removed; began an organic, whole foods diet (to eliminate allergic foods); took daily supplements of vitamin B3; began a regular exercise regimen; and avoided all household chemical pollutants. Four years after beginning this program, and 11 years after being diagnosed with Alzheimer's, Warren was able to return to work.

Nutritional Therapies.   Diet is extremely important for Alzheimer's patients. Many elderly people tend to be undernourished, have food sensitivities, eat non-nutritious foods, and experience digestion and elimination problems because of these or other factors. Dr. William Crook of Jackson, Tennessee, as reported in Alternative Medicine: The Definitive Guide, notes that many Alzheimer's patients have an overgrowth of the yeast candida albicans in their gastrointestinal tract, which often contributes to food allergies and poor nutrient absorption. The inability to absorb nutrients needed for normal cardiovascular and brain functioning can result in depression, anemia, and symptoms of dementia. Crook gives Alzheimer's patients a complete medical examination to isolate the cause or causes of symptoms, and urges them to follow a sugar-free diet, avoid antibiotic drugs, and consume adequate amounts of acidophilus (found in some yogurts) to restore their intestinal flora.

Balch and Balch also believe that nutritional factors can prevent or delay the onset of common symptoms such as memory loss associated with Alzheimer's disease and senile dementia. For example, patients with Alzheimer's disease tend to have lower body weight despite a high energy intake. Balch and Balch stress the importance of the B vitamins in maintaining memory, especially choline and B6, and recommend frequent consumption of whole grains, tofu, fresh eggs, legumes, wheat germ, soybeans, fish, brewer's yeast, nuts, millet, brown rice, and raw foods.

Traditional Chinese Medicine (TCM).   Dr. Maoshing Ni, vice president of Yo San University of Traditional Chinese Medicine in Santa Monica, California, reports in *Alternative Medicine: The Definitive Guide* that he has used a combination of acupuncture with Chinese herbs, nutrition, and exercise to halt the advance of Alzheimer's disease. He often urges patients to practice qi gong, a form of martial arts that restores deep breathing and improves cardiovascular functioning. Ni believes that because it combines concentration and visualization, qi gong balances the brain and body in very subtle ways that delay the development of hardening of the arteries in the brain.

Vitamin and Mineral Therapies. Nutritional deficiencies that have been tentatively linked to Alzheimer's disease include folic acid, niacin (vitamin B3), thiamine (vitamin B1), vitamins B6 and B12, vitamin C, vitamin D, vitamin E, magnesium, selenium, zinc, choline, L-glutamine, and lethicin.

Vitamins C and E, carotenes, flavonoids, zinc, and selenium are antioxidants that may neutralize the free radical-related processes thought by many to be involved in the development of Alzheimer's disease. Free radical damage is particularly detrimental to the immune system. Zinc supplements may help maintain the health of the immune system, and Murray and Pizzorno suggest that zinc picolinate is the best form of zinc supplementation for a majority of the elderly. Zinc also may play a role in normalizing cell replication, as zinc contains most of the enzymes involved in DNA replication and repair.

Balch and Balch claim that autopsies of victims of Alzheimer's disease show excessive amounts of silicon and aluminum in the brain. They cite a 1989 study by the British government that found the risk of contracting Alzheimer's disease had risen 50 percent in areas of Great Britain where drinking water contained elevated levels of aluminum. Environmental sources of aluminum and silicon include many antacids and nonprescription antidiarrheal drugs, processed foods, underarm deodorants, antidandruff shampoos, douches, buffered aspirin, bentonite clay, aluminum cookware, and drinking water.

Dr. Abraham Hoffer, former president of the Canadian Schizophrenia Foundation, suggests in *Alternative Medicine: The Definitive Guide* that serum vitamin B12 levels are significantly low, and vitamin B12 deficiency significantly common, in Alzheimer's patients. There often is mistaken reliance on the presence of anemia to diagnose vitamin B12 or folic acid deficiency. However, deficiencies of either vitamin are associated with mental symptoms, including dementia, long before changes occur in the blood. In addition, changes in the blood may never take place, despite the fact that severe deficiencies are affecting in other tissues. Supplementation of B12 and/or folic acid may significantly improve symptoms in some patients, but there is usually little improvement for the majority.

Some patients with Alzheimer's have cardiovascular disorders that prevent enough blood and oxygen from reaching the brain. Vitamin and mineral therapies such as those used by Hoffer may improve mental alertness and memory. He combines niacin, which improves circulation and lowers cholesterol levels, with large doses of vitamins C and E. He also recommends folic acid because 40 percent of all senile patients are deficient in this B vitamin. Recently he has begun adding low daily doses of aspirin, which he regards as safe and helpful in preventing the platelets from sticking to each other—thus improving circulation in the brain.

As reported by M. Imagawa in the September 1992 issue of *The Lancet,* studies in Japan have confirmed that daily supplements of vitamin B6, coenzyme Q10, and iron returned some Alzheimer's-diagnosed patients to "normal mental capacity." In another study cited in *Alternative Medicine: The Definitive Guide,* Alzheimer's patients who took a daily regimen of evening primrose oil, zinc, and selenium showed significant improvements in alertness, mood, and mental ability.

Osteoporosis

According to the June 1994 issue of the *Tufts University Diet & Nutrition Letter,* 24 million Americans, 80 percent of them women, suffer from osteoporosis, a progressive condition in which bones lose mass and become extremely brittle and prone to injury. Osteoporosis affects more women than heart disease, stroke, diabetes, breast cancer, or arthritis. It results in 1.5 million bone fractures annually, with yearly health care expenses exceeding $10 billion. If steps are not taken to reduce the incidence of the disease, its prevalence is expected to double in the U.S. in just 25 years due to the aging of the population, with annual health care costs related to osteoporosis reaching $30 billion.

Osteoporosis begins when the body cannot make new bone fast enough to replace bone that is lost. Both men and women lose some bone mass as they age, but the rate of loss is much slower in men (who have denser bones to begin with) than in women, and osteoporosis is less of a problem for them. Conversely, according to Kurt Butler and Lynn Rayner in *The Best Medicine: The Complete Health and Preventive Medicine Handbook,* women who live to the age of 80 usually lose a third to two-thirds of their entire skeletons and up to six inches of their height.

The process of bone loss typically begins in a woman's mid-30s, some 10 to 15 years before the onset of menopause, at a rate of 0.5 to 1 percent a year. This loss increases to 2 to 5 percent in the first 10 years following menopause, and then tapers off to about 1 percent per year. In the decade after menopause, women typically lose 5 to 10 percent of the

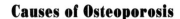

bone-sustaining minerals in their spines alone. As a result, according to the National Osteoporosis Foundation, one-third of American women over 65 suffer spinal fractures and 15 percent break their hips because of osteoporosis.

Causes of Osteoporosis

Estrogen deficiency, according to Balch and Balch, is the leading cause of osteoporosis in menopausal females. Other causes include the body's decreasing ability to absorb sufficient amounts of calcium through the intestines, a calcium–phosphorous imbalance, lack of exercise, jaundice, gastrectomy, and lactose intolerance. Smoking, excessive use of alcohol, exposure to the toxic chemical cadmium, and taking certain prescription drugs also have been linked to osteoporosis, as has excessive consumption of sugar (which depletes the body of phosphorous), soft drinks (which upset the calcium/phosphorous balance required by the body), and caffeine (which reduces blood-calcium levels).

Therapies for Coping with Osteoporosis

Botanical Medicines. One option for women who cannot take estrogen (those with congestive heart failure or migraines, for example) is to take plant estrogen (or "phytoestrogens"). Phytoestrogens such as soybeans, for example, may reduce osteoporosis without creating a risk of breast or uterine cancer. No clinical studies on the effectiveness of phytoestrogens have been reported, however.

According to Dr. John Lee, quoted in *Alternative Medicine: The Definitive Guide,* natural progesterone found in wild yams may be a safer and a more effective substitute for synthetic progesterone (progestin), currently used in combination with estrogen to treat osteoporosis. Progestin, he claims, does not keep sodium and water from moving into the cells as effectively, which can cause water retention and hypertension. Lee states that a treatment program combining diet, nutritional supplements, and natural transdermal (absorbed through the skin) progesterone is virtually 100 percent successful in building bone mass.

According to Lee, the average increase in bone mass is 15 percent in women with post-menopausal osteoporosis. He suggests that estrogen and natural progesterone supplements be taken together under the supervision of a physician or gynecologist. The Department of Obstetrics and Gynecology at Vanderbilt University now prescribes natural progesterone for both premenstrual syndrome (PMS) and menopausal hormone replacement therapy.

The July/August 1993 issue of *Natural Health* recommends obtaining calcium by using herbs that are rich in it, including nettles, oatstraw, horsetail, and raspberry leaves. Any of these can be made into a high-calcium tea by placing three tablespoons of the dried herb in a quart jar, filling the jar with boiling water, and immediately covering it. The tea should be steeped for at least 15 minutes before drinking. Maximum benefits are obtained by consuming three cups per day.

Estrogen Replacement Therapy (ERT). Butler and Rayner describe daily estrogen and calcium supplements as an effective and safe treatment that, while it cannot rebuild bone already lost, can greatly decrease the incidence of fractures and slow further bone loss. They claim that small doses of estrogen substantially lower the risk of breast cancer, and report that some studies suggest ERT also greatly decreases the incidence of heart attacks in postmenopausal women, perhaps by increasing HDL ("good") cholesterol levels. A *New England Journal of Medicine* study reported in the November 30, 1993, issue of *Your Health* indicates women should take estrogen for up to seven years after menopause to derive long-term protection from brittle bones.

Exercise. There is strong evidence that exercise helps prevent osteoporosis. Bone is a fluid tissue that is constantly being broken and reformed throughout a person's lifetime. Until the age of 35, more bone is deposited than removed, leading to a net gain in bulk and strength. After 35, and in some cases even earlier, the balance gradually begins to reverse, often leading to osteoporosis and subsequent fractures. This trend becomes particularly marked in menopausal women who lose the protective effect of estrogen against bone loss.

The best forms of exercise are those that increase calcium absorption and bone mass. Bones are living tissue that maintain their strength by having the muscles to which they are attached pull on them. As Jane Brody explains in the July 14, 1993, edition of the *New York Times,* this produces piezoelectricity, a force that results in bone deposition at the stress points. Exercise now appears to stimulate bone mineralization, particularly activities that involve high loads and high stresses, such as weightlifting. Brody maintains that such activities (including strength training or working out on resistance machines) build bone more-effectively than do activities that involve many repetitive cycles (running, walking, or swimming).

Women who exercise regularly tend to have lower estrogen levels and to be thinner (two states associated with higher risk for osteoporosis) then women who do not exercise regularly. However, the effect of exercise more than compensates for those factors, giving the more active women denser and stronger bones. A 1987 study at the Queen Elizabeth Hospital in Toronto, Ontario, cited by Brody compared bone densities of sedentary women between the ages of 50 and 62 with those of women who engaged in aerobic exercise and others who did both aerobic and strengthening exercises. The active women of both groups experienced similar significant gains in bone mass, while the sedentary women showed a loss.

Brody goes on to state that after puberty, the only way women can maintain their bone mass is to exercise regularly. Nancy Lane, a rheumatologist at the University of California in San Francisco, has extensively researched the bone density of older women runners. She suggests that exercise can slow the rate of bone loss during menopause and, by increasing a person's stability, strength, flexibility, and neuromuscular function, decrease the likelihood of bone-breaking falls.

Brody cites several studies that confirm that exercise can help maintain and even increase bone density. For example, a large study by researchers at Family Health International in Durham, North Carolina, found that women aged 40 to 54 who were physically active had significantly higher bone mineral density in their spines and arms than a comparable group of nonexercisers. At the University of Missouri, a one-year study among previously sedentary women who had recently gone through menopause found that both low-impact and high-impact exercise done for three 20-minute periods a week helped maintain their spinal bone. Another study of women in their 50s found that both brisk walking and aerobic dancing resulted in increased bone size and strength.

A study published in the *New England Journal of Medicine,* as reported in the June 23, 1994, edition of the *New York Times* confirmed that even among the very old, it is never too late to exercise. The study involved 100 male and female nursing home residents with an average age of 87—a third were in their 90s. Many had a variety of medical disorders, including dementia, arthritis, lung disease, and high blood pressure. Participants were randomly assigned either to take part in ordinary nursing home activities, or to work out vigorously for 45 minutes three times a week. Those assigned to work out used exercise machines to strengthen their thighs and knees. The exercising residents increased their walking speed by 12 percent and their ability to climb stairs by 28 percent. Four who had needed walkers to get around became able to walk with only a cane. The people who worked out were less depressed and more likely to take part in nursing home activities.

Together these studies indicate that older women clearly can maintain bone mass, and that, by adopting other good health habits as well, they can forestall or prevent the damaging effects of osteoporosis.

Nutritional Therapies. Many nutritionists and physicians believe that osteoporosis can be prevented by improved nutrition, calcium supplements, and lifestyles that include regular exercise and minimal use of alcohol and tobacco. Good sources of calcium are cheese, flounder, shrimp, clams, oysters, molasses, nuts and seeds, oats, seaweed, soybeans and soybean products such as tofu, wheat germ and whole wheat products, and yogurt. Kale, turnip and dandelion greens, leafy green vegetables, and broccoli are excellent vegetable sources. Sardines and salmon contain high amounts of calcium as well. Balch and Balch recommend avoiding cigarette smoking and alcohol consumption (which interfere with estrogen's bone-protecting effect), along with phosphate-containing drinks, high-protein animal foods (which deplete the body of calcium), and citrus fruits and tomatoes that may inhibit calcium absorption.

Butler and Rayner also counsel women to obtain adequate calcium and vitamin D well before their postmenopausal years, and to avoid too much phosphorous or protein. They recommend eating low-fat dairy products, soy products, sardines, salmon, beans, leafy greens, and a variety of vegetables.

Vitamin and Mineral Therapies. According to Balch and Balch, a diet that is adequate in protein, calcium, magnesium, phosphorus, and vitamins C and D can both prevent and treat osteoporosis. Since dietary calcium is so important, elderly people who have difficulty absorbing sufficient amounts may need calcium injections.

A July/August 1993 article in *Natural Health* entitled "Strong Bones" counsels women to consider supplemental calcium by their early 40s, before the onset of menopause. Particularly recommended are calcium citrate, calcium carbonate, or calcium lactate (forms that are easily absorbable by the body). Magnesium, another mineral essential for bone growth, can be found in nuts, seeds, fish, seafood, whole grains, legumes, and dark green leafy vegetables. In addition to calcium and magnesium, the body needs vitamin D to build bones. However, vitamin D is found in significant amounts in only a few foods—primarily egg yolks, fortified milk, butter, and fish liver oils. The article suggests that women consult a health practitioner to evaluate the advisability of taking calcium, magnesium, or vitamin B supplements.

Summary

As the ability to extend life through new technologies grows, so will the possibilities of improving the lifelong health of the elderly. New insights in molecular genetics and virology may allow most people to maintain full mental functions throughout their life span. Hormone replacement therapies also may prove effective in extending life span and reducing the incidence of chronic generative diseases. Natural substances within the body may be discovered that will preserve the strength of the immune system and slow the aging process. Once the loss of bone mass and bone density can be delayed, frailty, imbalance and walking disorders, now characteristic of many elderly, could be prevented. With more empirical studies of how nutritional, botanical, and psychoimmunological factors cause heart attacks and strokes, new gene-spliced drugs will help detect these disorders. The hope for an extended and healthy life is a wish of long standing. The difference today is that this generation could see that dream become a reality for the human family.

Resources

References

Allard, M. "Treatment of the Disorders of Aging with Ginkgo Biloba Extract: Pharmacology to Clinical Medicine." *Presse Medicale* (September 1986): 1540–45.

Allison, M. "Improving the Odds: Aging and Exercise." *Harvard Health Letter* (February 1991): 4.

Balch, James F., and Phyllis Balch. *Prescription for Nutritional Healing*. Garden City Park, NY: Avery Publishing Group, 1993.

"The Bare-Bones Facts for Avoiding Osteoporosis." *Tufts University Diet & Nutrition Letter* (June 1994): 3–6.

Brody, Jane. "Personal Health." *New York Times* (July 14, 1993): B6.

The Burton Goldberg Group. *Alternative Medicine: The Definitive Guide*. Puyallup, WA: Future Medicine Publishing, Inc., 1993.

Butler, Kurt, and Lynn Rayner. *The Best Medicine: The Complete Health and Preventive Medicine Handbook*. New York, NY: Harper & Row Publishers, Inc., 1985.

California Medical Association. "Alzheimer's Disease." *Health Tips* index 453 (April 1990): 1–2.

Casdorph, H. "EDTA Chelation Therapy: Efficacy in Brain Disorders," in E. Cranston's *A Textbook on EDTA Chelation Therapy*. New York, NY: Human Sciences Press, 1989: 131–53.

Chen, Li C. "Recent Advances in Studies on Traditional Chinese Anti-Aging Material Medica." *Journal of Traditional Chinese Medicine* (September 1993): 223–26.

Edlin, Gordon, and Eric Golanty. *Health and Wellness: A Holistic Approach*. Boston, MA: Jones and Bartlett Publishers, Inc., 1992.

"Estrogen Wards Off Alzheimer's." *Your Health* (January 11, 1994): 49.

"Exercise Found to Benefit Even the Very Old." *New York Times* (June 23, 1994): A12.

Forever Young: New Medical Evidence of Age Reversal. Emmaus, PA: Rodale Press, Inc., 1988.

Friend, Tom. "At 86, She's Running From Old Age." *San Jose Mercury News* (November 11, 1993): 7.

Gittleman, Ann Louise. "A Guide to Sturdy Bones." *Natural Health* (January/February 1994): 56–57.

Hendler, Sheldon, M.D. *The Complete Guide to Anti-Aging Nutrients*. New York, NY: Simon & Schuster, Inc., 1985.

Imagawa, M. "Coenzyme Q10, Iron and Vitamin B6 in Genetically Confirmed Alzheimer's Disease." *The Lancet* (September 1992): 671.

"Impotence Can Often Be Avoided, Study Finds." *San Jose Mercury News* (May 25, 1994): 7C.

Langreth, Robert. "Living to Be 150." *Your Health* (May 31, 1994): 33–38.

Lindner, Lawrence. "Smart Eaters Stay Healthier, Live Longer, Look Younger." *Fitness* (July/August 1993): 71.

Margolis, Simeon, and Hamilton Moses III. *The Johns Hopkins Medical Handbook.* New York, NY: Medletter Associates, Inc., 1992.

Murray, Michael, and Joseph Pizzorno. *Encyclopedia of Natural Medicine.* Rocklin, CA: Prima Publishing, 1991.

Nbiskane, L. "Resting Energy Expenditure in Relation to Energy Intake in Patients with Alzheimer's Disease." *Age & Ageing* (March 1993):132–37.

Nieman, D. *Fitness & Your Health.* Palo Alto, CA: Bull Publishing Company, 1993.

"Osteoporosis." *Your Health* (November 30, 1993): 45.

Paffenbarger, Ralph. "Physical Activity, All-Cause Mortality, and Longevity of College Alumni." *New England Journal of Medicine* (1986, Volume 314): 605–13.

Rai, G. "A Soluble-Blind, Placebo-Controlled Study of Ginkgo Biloba Extract ("Tanakan") in Elderly Outpatients with Mild to Moderate Memory Impairment." *Current Medical Research & Opinion* (1991, Volume 6): 350–55.

"Strong Bones." *Natural Health* (July/August 1993): 31–32.

"To Take Antioxidant Pills or Not? The Debate Heats Up." *Tufts University Diet & Nutrition Letter* (May 1994): 3–5.

Walford, Roy. *Maximum Life Span.* New York, NY: W.W. Norton and Co., Inc., 1983.

Warren, Tom. *Beating Alzheimer's.* Garden City Park, NY: Avery Publishing Group, 1991.

"You Can Prevent Many of the So-Called By-Products of Aging—Or Even Reverse Them—By Doing One Thing: Weight Lifting." *Healthy Woman* (winter 1993): 42–43.

Organizations

Alzheimer's Association
70 E. Lake St., Chicago, IL 60601.

Alzheimer's Disease Education and Referral Center
PO Box 8250, Silver Spring, MD 20807-8250.

National Council on Aging, Family Caregivers Program
600 Maryland Ave. SW, Washington, DC 20024.

National Institute on Aging Information Center
2209 Distribution Cir., Silver Spring, MD 20910.

National Osteoporosis Association
1625 Eye St. NW, Washington, DC 20006.

Additional Reading

Aronson, M.K., ed. *Understanding Alzheimer's Disease.* New York, NY: Scribners Educational Publishers, 1988.

Guthrie, Donna. *Grandpa Doesn't Know It's Me.* New York, NY: Human Sciences Press, 1986.

THE FUTURE OF ALTERNATIVE MEDICINE

To anticipate what advances might be made in the medical field and what role people will play in maintaining their own health in the future, Dr. Michael Murray, author of The Encyclopedia of Natural Medicine, *and the members of* The Alternative Health & Medicine Encyclopedia*'s Medical Advisory Board gathered to participate in a roundtable discussion.*

Q: In 2050, how will the way you conduct your practice be changed? What type of new equipment, if any, will you use? Will information that is inconceivable today be common knowledge?

ROGER KENNEDY: I think that certainly by the year 2050 we will begin to understand the limitations of our knowledge and be less arrogant about what technology can do. Instead we'll begin to judge therapy based on what it's going to do for the quality of life. For example, one vision of biotechnology is that we will be able to eliminate the gene for cystic fibrosis. While that may be a good thing, the gene is so widespread in single doses that it may actually be a very good gene. I think the assumption that all medical technology is positive is going to have to be seriously challenged, and I hope it takes less than 50 years to do that.

In the future, I think we'll have some highly specific ways of identifying people who are at high risk for certain diseases, malignant or metabolic, and be able to apply specific treatments. This will replace the shotgun approach we now have that may, in many instances, do more harm than good.

Hopefully what we will decide within the next couple of decades, as a lot of people have already figured out, is that as a nation our health is our own responsibility, not the responsibility

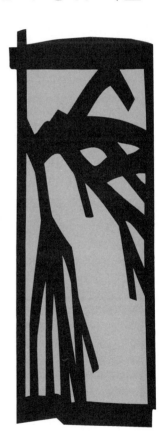

of technology or institutions. It is crucial that people begin to take full responsibility for their own health and well-being. My expectation is that by the year 2050 we will have developed effective ways to educate patients so that I won't be treating 90 percent of the ailments that currently show up in my office. People will be able to care for themselves, or they will avoid those things that lead to the ailments in the first place.

DANA ULLMAN: There will be several schools of thought and practice in homeopathy in 2050. There will still be the conventional or classical model of homeopathy which will be highly individualized and highly computerized. The expert systems for IBM and Macintosh users already in existence will be much more widely known and used. Another difference is that these expert systems are presently based on outdated documentation. In the future, new information on cured cases will be added into the system to expand the knowledge base and improve the practice.

Also, a greater number of medicines will be used by homeopaths, including many drugs that conventional medicine will have long ago discarded. Both low potency and high potency medicines will also continue to be an integral part of homeopathy, as each of them have a place.

Another advancement in homeopathy will be the use of electronic diagnostic equipment to measure subtle reactions to homeopathic medicines by having the patient hold the medicine in their hands to test for hypersensitivity. With these machines, an electrode is applied to an acupuncture point to measure both physiological and energetic responses. Recurrent testing will replace the classical tradition of interviewing the patient.

Although both these homeopathic schools of thought sound somewhat futuristic, what I'm describing has been happening over the past several years, so it's not all that new.

JONATHAN SHORE: Personally, I don't feel the way I conduct my practice will differ 50 years from now. One of the things that first attracted me to Chinese medicine and then to homeopathy was that the truth never changes. In a sense, what was true 2,000 years ago is still true today. That's what bothered me so much about conventional medicine—the half-life of medical knowledge. What was absolute when I was in medical school is regarded today as nonsense.

I suspect that if anything changes, it will be the subtlety of understanding of the practitioners. Homeopathy has to do with deeper and deeper penetration of the patterns of nature—and the patterns of people's behavior—and how the two interact. The deeper understanding of homeopathic materia medica won't change. And the remedies won't change. I understand more about the remedies I use now than I did 10 years ago, but the remedies themselves haven't changed.

LARRY ROSE: Although I'm not in practice and actually seeing patients, I'm still involved in alternative medicine in the sense that my work with California's Division of Occupational Safety and Health focuses on alerting the public to dangerous chemicals in the environment and the workplace that can affect their health. Much of my answer therefore depends on whether we have an informed, democratically functioning government and a citizenry that is really participating. There are some very promising developments along those lines, such as the growing environmental movement and an increased awareness among numbers of young people. As my work entails looking at worker health and safety, and toxins in the workplace and the environment, our functioning depends on the state of information possessed by the general population.

For example, hundreds of untested new chemicals are put on the market every year, and a lot of current corporate behavior is going to change as people understand that they lose far more than they gain from these toxic chemicals. Although there was a 50-year lag between the time when a link between cigarette smoking and cancer was first known, and a change in public policy occurred, let's hope public policy changes much more quickly in terms of environmental toxins.

JONATHAN COLLIN: I have to admit that I have an innate aversion to predicting the future because of the medical profession's propensity to say to patients, for example, that they will be dead in six months or three months. This type of prediction is frequently wrong, and other things can occur that greatly change the outcome of what is expected based simply on biology text books. I've come to have a great deal of respect for the point of view that a person's health is not determined by a medical recipe because there are so many variables involved.

JUDITH ASTON: By 2050, many alternative therapy systems will have proven invaluable in prevention, treatment, rehabilitation, and improving the overall quality of people's lives. New strides in biomechanics and product design will offer consumers far greater comfort, efficiency, and health enhancement.

ED WEISS: I don't believe the field of acupuncture will change very much in terms of particular treatments, styles of treatments or combinations of herbs, although there will be some access to new information. What I would hope for is that there will be more alternative practitioners and that this kind of medicine will be more widespread. I think it's a much better way of treating people.

GARY LINDSEY: The wave of the future in dentistry is high technology advances in cosmetics and augmentation, even on the cellular level. You'll probably be seeing vaccinations that will protect against caries, and perhaps even technologies that will be topically applied between the gums

and the teeth to eliminate gum disease. For example, with adhesion as it is today, we no longer have to cut teeth or dig holes to fill them. We can adhere such things as porcelain inlays to the teeth. A tooth is not a piece of rock in which you have to put a filling. It's a viable living dental tissue you can use as a substrate which you bond. Dental implants for the mouth and jaws will also become more common.

Dentists will continue to play an important role in the diagnosis of whole body diseases. At last count, some 200 to 250 pathologies are recognizable first in the head and neck, and I always make it a practice to give my patients a thorough examination in these areas.

YUAN-CHI LIN: In 2050, people's views of maintaining good health and preventing disease will differ from today's. They will be more interested in health and alternative medicine. Genetic research will allow us to diagnose and alter genetic abnormalities in utero.

STEPHEN VAN PELT: As a sports medicine physician, I hope that in the next 50 years we will understand something called overtraining, or what happens to people when they work out or train too hard. We know they start to get injuries not because they train unsafely, but because they push their bodies too hard, and do too much too soon for what their bodies can stand at that time. We currently have very general indicators of overtraining, but we still do not have clinical tests.

THOMAS WEISMAN: My practice has changed tremendously in just the last five years. People are just barely coming out of a dark age emotionally and haven't been too aware of what they feel. They have tended to deny feelings that are unpleasant, hostile or angry, or if they do express them, do so in a violent manner. A lot of what I do is enable people to come to grips with what they feel. Whatever pain is in their body, their back, their neck, or any type of health problem invariably involves denial of what they're feeling. So I see in the next 50 years a real positive trend toward people getting much more in tune with what they feel, accepting feelings that are now totally unacceptable, and expressing opinions and hostilities in a way that doesn't offend. It's going to be much healthier world.

In the future, instead of taking medication to mask the discomfort of tension in their back or neck people will try to find out what causes that tension. My practice, network chiropractic, is really powerful in doing that. Through light touching in the right spot at the right time with the right amount of intent, people automatically start breathing deeper and begin releasing the tension.

I think that as people get more into their feelings, they will be able to use more than just the left side of their brain (which is logical, analytical, and sequential) in approaching life. They will also be able to use the right side (which is emotional, creative, and visual) simultaneously. If people go one way or the other, they're not in touch with their true energy. But if they integrate the two sides of the perceptual mechanism that is our brain, then they think with their feelings and feel with their thoughts. Evidence of that integration is already apparent in a big shift away from technology (a kind of left brain product), which has reached the point of costing outrageous amounts of money.

MICHAEL MURRAY: I think what you're going to see is a continual evolution in medicine. That means what is true and founded on good scientific principles will continue to evolve. Naturopathy is certainly founded on strong scientific principles. I think people's attitudes on health and preventing illness will be much more enlightened by the year 2050. It is ironic that people who care about their health and what they put into their

bodies are still considered health nuts. In the future, this attitude of really valuing a person's health will become the dominant attitude.

I also think we will see continued improvements in genetic engineering and in helping people with genetic defects. A good example is the research currently underway on cystic fibrosis. I think we will see the same sort of engineering in treating those forms of cancer which have a strong genetic link. Eventually, we may be able to use genetics to change a person's disposition to such illnesses as heart disease and Alzheimer's.

Q: Dr. Deepak Chopra, Dr. Bernie Siegel, and others argue that positive thinking plays an important role in healing. Do you support that contention?

LARRY ROSE: Absolutely. The effect of state of mind on the various systems—the endocrine system, the nervous system, the immune system, even the reproductive system—is profound. Various studies prove that time and time again.

JONATHAN COLLIN: Some of the medical journals in the last year and a half have taken a backlash on this thinking and report that in experimental situations there was no major benefit in doing mind/brain interaction on a particular group of patients. Of course this is just the opposite of what was printed up in the years before when mind/body interaction was shown to have an extremely positive effect on basic physiology with cellular mechanisms right on up to the way individuals face their basic disease process.

STEPHEN VAN PELT: In my experience, people who exercise regularly tend to handle stress better and have a better outlook on life. Because of that outlook, they monitor their nutrition better, cut down on smoking, and limit their fat and salt intake. Exercise also helps speed up metabolism and cycles toxins through the body without as much damage.

JEFFREY FLATGAARD: I see two limitations to this concept. One, wishful thinking can deter a person from seeking competent medical help when it is really needed. Second, it's hard to gauge the effectiveness when you see only the survivors. You never talk to the people who had a positive attitude and didn't live.

The most practical benefit of a positive attitude is that it enables people to carry out all the other things they should be doing to keep themselves in good health.

JONATHAN SHORE: Of course positive thinking plays a role in healing. We see this in the placebo effect. Classic experiments have been conducted in which medical school students are given amphetamines and told that they are tranquilizers—they go to sleep. For another example, in a single blind trial with arthritis patients, the expectation of the physician proved to be the most powerful factor.

THOMAS WEISMAN: Sure, it's true. The model of man when I was growing up was a chemical machine. If something goes wrong with it, you put in a new part if you possibly can or at least give it a chemical to help correct the malfunction. Personally, I think that model is outdated. Now in medicine we have an electrical model of man. The emphasis is on the central nervous system and its effect on organizing and controlling all the body's chemical reactions. That model is actually ancient, corresponding very closely to the acupuncture model that is getting more popular all the time.

According to this electrical model, as you think, you can create a positive electric field. But it requires more than just saying you're going to think positive thoughts. You also have to work on the emotional, feeling aspect of yourself. You can't just say I like potatoes when you can't stand potatoes. Everything has to be truthful and integrated on all levels. If you have a deep aversion and keep pretending you like potatoes, it's not going to work.

GARY LINDSEY: If you tell people that certain things are going to work and they have a positive attitude, generally it's just going to work better. If the patient has a positive enough motivation and the power of positive thinking, I'm not so sure that's not a more critical factor in the healing process than we give it credit for.

DANA ULLMAN: Positive thinking is a helpful, but not necessary, component. I mean, there are a lot of very hopeful people who have died. However, those who encourage a hopeful attitude do more than meets the eye. They're also encouraging other alternative treatment modalities—natural therapies can be very effective.

Gravity isn't just a good idea, it's the law. Likewise, homeopathy is not just a good idea. And it doesn't matter if you believe in it or not. While hope is nice and often effective, unless you also provide some other immune augmentative therapies, hope can easily be neutralized by day-to-day life.

I think consciousness and matter are intertwined and as much as consciousness affects matter, matter affects consciousness. However, even yogis die and they don't seem to live longer than the average person. I'm reminded of the story of Joe E. Smith, an American who lived to be 106 years old. He smoked, he drank, he chased women, and he said that if he knew he was going to live this long, he would have taken better care of himself.

So yes, positive thinking is a good idea, and some mental states do seem to speed up recovery faster. But as much as the mind has a consciousness, the body has a consciousness too. And there are stronger psychological forces that can overcome the physical, and sometimes stronger physical forces that can overcome the psychological. I'm a proponent of more energetic therapies such as homeopathy—the most sophisticated Western energy medicine—and acupuncture, representing the most sophisticated Eastern form of energy medicine.

ED WEISS: What people usually call positive thinking is often a euphemism for denial. I think true positive thinking—such as saying "I sure would like to get better" or "I could envision myself being well in the future"—can play a useful role, although it's only a limited one. As soon as people say, "I know this is going to help," the odds are about 99 to one that it won't. People convince themselves that something good is going to happen when inside they are afraid, and really expect a negative outcome. It is much better to start with the truth.

ROGER KENNEDY: I think that our mind, our beliefs, and our thinking have an enormous impact on our body. I think that by 2050, we will have learned more and more, although not so much exactly how that interaction works. Buddhists don't understand exactly why certain behavior creates a certain state, but I think we will have a large amount of data that shows how certain states of mind create disease.

I think perhaps in 50 years we'll discover we've gone down this blind alley—the technological imperative—and that isn't where it's at. The human mind and the energy we all share in the universe have so much more power than all of the things we create that we will begin to turn away from technology.

Q: Much is being written about how people can delay—or even in some cases reverse—the aging process. Which if any of the holistic specialty areas offers the most promise in this regard?

STEPHEN VAN PELT: I am not sure we can reverse the aging process. By 2050, we will know much more about what aging is

at the sub-molecular level. We will be able to diagnose each person in a much deeper way. We'll be able to say: "Here is your diet. This is how much you should be exercising. Here are the exercises that will help you delay aging most effectively. This is how much stress you can take."

This approach will be a little like the Russian model of sports figures that produced world champions. We'll test patients and tell them the optimal way to maximize the cards they've been dealt. We'll try to help them be the best they can be, and maximize their health and performance.

DANA ULLMAN: I have no doubt that using healing methods will extend the average life span—not just in quantity but in quality. That said, it depends on how much we are able to deal with some of the environmental factors that surround us.

There is no homeopathic medicine that singularly extends life, because all of them do. Each provides a healing benefit that tends to relieve pain and improve the overall healing process. I foresee a new way of looking at pharmacological actions and homeopathic medicines, leading to immunomodulating drugs or smart medicines that fit the unique body/mind characteristics of the patient and are like designer drugs because of that individualization.

JONATHAN COLLIN: Particularly during the last five years the so-called yuppie population, and even a lot of older folks, continue the hunt for the fountain of youth using an unusual biological program of drugs, nutritional supplements, herbs, and amino acids in varying doses for extended periods of time. It's created something that is quite different for medicine and society: an experiment involving perhaps thousands if not millions of individuals, using unapproved agents without medical oversight. In the short run, it appears that many are experiencing benefits of so-called life extension.

Unfortunately, the data on this type of long-term experimentation is not really in, but it's obvious that these intriguing life-extenders are showing a variety of benefits. Enzyme systems are known to function poorly during the aging process, with calcification of the enzyme systems essentially minimizing the enzyme's activity. Many of these life-extending agents appear to reverse the enzyme calcification process, restoring normal enzyme functioning. In addition, cross-linking of enzyme systems, through the inappropriate cross-linking of sulfide groups between amino acid chains, leads to destructive polymerization reactions, somewhat akin to the change in rubber as tires age and crack. Evidence is accumulating that such cross-linking degradation is being reversed through these life extension programs.

Cellular biochemistry is particularly important when the cellular wall fails to convey waste products out of the cell and oxygen and nutrients within the cell. The free radical pathology model is predicted on cell wall destruction coming about by peroxidation of lipid components of the cell wall. Antioxidant supplementation has been hypothesized to stop the peroxidation mechanisms that destroy normal cell wall physiology. Life extension biological agents will probably be critical in health examination recommendations in the future.

I think the functional medicine concept that Jeffrey Bland and others have been talking about involves trying to move the chronological window of aging toward the higher age categories. Basic pathologies and sub-diseases will begin at age 60 instead of 40; typical aging mechanisms will begin at age 80 instead of 60; diseases will start at age 100 instead of 80.

JEFFREY FLATGAARD: I don't think aging is actually going to be reversed. I think aging is a more profound phenomenon than something that is merely the result of bad habits or random chance. Aging is a general process developed in a large number of species; virtually all animals age. If you look around, aging is not an accident.

In terms of what offers the most hope for extending life span, I would say two things. One would be minimizing genetic damage, both environmental and inherited. The second would be more holistic—having people live a healthier life from birth. That would probably extend the life span dramatically. People live longer and have healthier lives than they did a couple of generations ago. One only has to go back and look at history to realize that people maintain an active role in public life at ages that would be thought suitable only if they were in a retirement home 100 years ago. Considerable evidence supports the contention that factors such as exercise, diet, and a healthy lifestyle have already significantly prolonged people's effective life span.

LARRY ROSE: From a public health standpoint, if you observe people's behavior, knowing all we know now, it's a society in denial. People are doing things that are absolutely destructive to their health. Vitamin and mineral intake, diet and exercise, lifestyle, the air you breathe, the water you drink, all of those things make an enormous difference in the quality of life for people as they grow older. And that's what we're really talking about, not immortality but quality of life.

ED WEISS: I think the whole list—vitamins and minerals, botanicals, exercise, nutrition, and lifestyle—is good for living a long life, but not extending life. So you can live to be 90 and be healthier, but I don't think any of those things will extend it. The only thing that might possibly change is that some Western biochemical products may actually extend life by extending the number of life cycles in cells before they die. However, I am not sure this would be good for us as individuals, or as a species.

GARY LINDSEY: In the dental area, I think once Mother Nature has aged something, it's pretty hard to make it young again. Slowing the progress of dental deterioration down to a snail's pace is the most likely thing I see. Right now, using fluoride gels on root structures is minimizing the amount of root decay. As a result, we're getting a lot of older people living a lot longer having more roots exposed in the mouth. If a way can be found to keep teeth hydrated at the same level when you're 80 as when you're a teen, then we'll be on to something.

THOMAS WEISMAN: I think something like tai chi is the most cost-effective way to slow the onset of aging, or something of that order where people are taught to move energy through their body, relax their body, relax their mind, and breathe. The less we rely on physical substances, and the more we use our natural physical resources built into our own body chemistry—with the mind helping to control them—I think that's the way to go.

Q: Do you see any of the disciplines currently under the holistic or alternative banner—such as homeopathy, naturopathy, Chinese medicine, or acupuncture—assuming greater prominence by 2050? Do you feel alternative medicine as a whole will have more adherents?

THOMAS WEISMAN: I think in the next 15 years there's a good probability that chiropractors will have a mainstream impact for two reasons. First, we finally got our act together and will continue to get better to the point that we are real in a universal way and can stand up under scrutiny. The second thing is that heavy reliance on technology is becoming too inefficient from a cost point of view. It will take another five years before those in the medical profession give up, try to find simple ways to deal with problems, and only use technology when they have to use it. Spending more money with no end in sight

cannot continue indefinitely, especially with the insurance crisis and lack of funding being chronic problems.

If people have a health problem, they need not run to their doctor or their chiropractor. The first thing they should do is use their own intelligence. More and more people are educating themselves, taking care of themselves, and becoming increasingly self-reliant.

JEFFREY FLATGAARD: In terms of a particular field being most useful, I would imagine it to be a field that enables us to look for chemicals and natural products already in existence to see whether they have a role in our own bodies or mimic other chemicals that do have a role. This is a continuation of how scientists and doctors have investigated the potential for human health over the last several thousand years, and will probably be a fruitful way of finding new tools, products, or insights.

LARRY ROSE: I see possibly naturopathy—if it's developed in a certain way—as having the greatest positive effect. This is because naturopathy involves what I consider to be key elements, as we discussed earlier, including nutrition, exercise, and lifestyle. I think there also needs to be an element of spiritual connection to the mysteries of life.

YUAN-CHI LIN: Alternative medicine as a whole will play a much greater role in health maintenance and care in the future, and acupuncture will be on the cutting edge for treating most disorders.

JONATHAN SHORE: Of course, this may sound prejudiced, but I think homeopathy will be most important. While it is unlikely that homeopathy as I define it will become a broad operation, it is the closest to a real holistic medicine. It is the only discipline to use a single substance incorporating the mind, feelings and body. When we practice this way, we do not separate illness into physical illness and psychological illness. For us, it is all one organism—just one unit. And a disturbance in that unit produces different manifestations, some of which are deeper and some more superficial.

GARY LINDSEY: It's about time we got back to looking at herbal medicines since all of our pain relievers and high blood pressure medications came from herbs in the beginning. There's high efficacy in some of these herbal remedies.

ED WEISS: I think alternative fields, and maybe some fields nobody has heard of yet, will become more prominent. People are looking for alternatives because there is so little humanity left in Western medicine. There will probably be some kind of revolution in Western medicine making it more human again, because people hate being treated mechanically.

A combination of two things will lead more people to turn to acupuncture: its success, and dissatisfaction with the conventional way of doing things. Acupuncture will prove itself in this culture. For example, I see and help a lot of people, and the ones who are helped send their friends.

DANA ULLMAN: In 2050, I don't think the words "holistic" or "alternative" will be used. These are simply relative terms that only have a temporal value right now. The methods presently thought to be alternative that will probably be most commonly used will be homeopathy, acupuncture, and botanical remedies, with conventional medicines and surgery as backups if other safer therapies do not work rapidly or adequately enough.

There will also be the use of super foods, or certain food items in concentrated doses, either alone or mixed with herbs. These include spirulina and bee pollen products, ginseng, and garlic. I don't want to call them a regular part of the diet, however, because these super foods are so strong that they are really medicinal agents. And you shouldn't need to take medicinal agents every day.

JONATHAN COLLIN: I think you're going to see two different areas of medicine in the future. One of these areas is going to be terribly high tech medicine that's going to get involved in some incredible breakthroughs. For example, I think we're going to come up with an entirely different mechanism for handling infectious diseases besides antibiotics. In diseases like diabetes, we might overcome the barrier that prevents insulin production so you will get insulin repair in the body.

We'll make some headway in relationship to heart attacks so that this whole bypass area is going to become a terribly bad joke. Rather than severing the arteries, we'll use laser technology or insert devices into the arteries that will clean them out. Another possibility is seeking out viruses and reprogramming their DNA, that kind of thing.

In terms of depression, I think we're going to be making major jumps beyond Prozac. While the whole neurotransmitter area is still a big mystery at this point, I think advances will change how these neurochemicals are internally produced so as to eliminate the need for using antidepressants or other substances to prevent depression.

On the other side, I don't think most alternative or holistic doctors will want to be involved with high technology. I think that they're going to want to create a more basic form of medicine that falls back on some older traditions and belief systems. Because they'll be angered at having to be constantly involved with technology in dealing with problems, they'll want to deal from non-technological solutions such as holistic mind/body interaction or something similar to the old Indian sweat lodges. I think a certain percentage of the population will be constantly wanting that approach rather than getting involved with all this technology.

ROGER KENNEDY: I don't think that any one discipline will particularly provide the answer because homeopathy, for example, is no more than a way of utilizing the body's own resources. Some of the Eastern philosophies, as exemplified by someone like Deepak Chopra and his very holistic approach to medicine, make a lot of sense to people.

We'll still have a need for the Western concept of medicine, but I don't think that is really going to be the answer. Hopefully, the way people will be viewed both in sickness and in health will be a reflection of taking what is applicable from various disciplines, not rigidly consigning treatment to any single one of them.

MICHAEL MURRAY: I don't think that what today is labeled alternative medicine will be labeled such in 2050 because it will have become the dominant form of medicine. What we'll see in 2050 is a greater appreciation of mind/body medicine. We will have documented how people's attitudes, thoughts, and emotions affect their individual health.

I think medical practice in the year 2050 will incorporate many of the practices and principles currently comprising naturopathy. For example, naturopaths use some genetic information today. If we do a detailed medical history, and see that the person's parents and grandparents all died of heart disease and the person has a cholesterol level over 300, we will know to immediately lower the person's cholesterol. In the future, we will be able to be even more specific and insightful.

Q: Do you have any final thoughts you would like to share?

ED WEISS: I think that being a human being, acting like a human being, being perceptive like a human being, and expressing love for your patient leads to health. That's the most important thing holistic medicine should offer.

GARY LINDSEY: As I stress to my patients, if you take good care of your body and are healthy in all other respects, over the years your mouth will follow right along.

DANA ULLMAN: Plato once said that a sure sign of a bad city is one with lots of doctors and lots of hospitals. So if things go well, there will be as few hospitals and doctors in the future as possible. There will be very few doctors because present doctors are going to have to retool themselves—or go the way of the typewriter or the rotary telephone—and many doctors are not going to want to go back to school. That's fine because once doctors are practicing the real healing sciences, there will not be as much of a need for them. The vast majority of conditions such as headaches and respiratory and digestive problems will be treated at home with software systems that will teach people alternatives that are available right now.

ROGER KENNEDY: My fervent hope is that it will finally dawn on us that technological solutions aren't getting us anywhere, which implies a greater ability of the human species to be self-correcting. Another very important thing we will certainly have by 2050 are very accurate computer models that predict, given a set of well-defined variables for an acutely ill patient, the patient's chances of survival. This will allow us to make a societal decision on whether or not to allocate resources in the final few days of life. I'm hoping we come around more to the Eastern views instead of clinging to that last little thread of life as we do now in our society.

There are certain basic things people can do that contribute to a better state of health, the most obvious being to stop smoking and exercise on a regular basis. But I also think we need to become aware of what our health is, understand what is actually going on in our bodies, and become active participants. We also need a much bigger understanding of, and appreciation for, the incredible power of our mind and emotions.

MICHAEL MURRAY: One area that will especially benefit from genetic research is the development of new botanical medicines. I think by 2050 that most plant-based drugs will not be grown in the soil, but rather in cell cultures. Some of those cell cultures will be producing more concentrated, standardized botanical medicines.

A number of the current chemotherapeutic drugs are derived from plants—for example, vincristine and vinblastine extracted from the periwinkle plant and taxol from the Pacific yew, which recently has received a lot of press attention. We are already using botanical substances in cancer treatment. In the future, drugs will become more sophisticated. For example, we will use monoclonal antibodies to deliver the plant substance directly to the cell, or we will develop other targeted cell delivery systems which will essentially transport these botanical substances to the targeted cell.

I also think we all will become more informed about nutrition. Most people would be better off decreasing animal foods and eating more plant foods. Most of the chronic degenerative diseases such as cancer, heart disease, stroke, and diabetes can be viewed as almost deficiencies of nutritional factors that are contained in plant foods. If we shift from animal-based diets to natural plant-based diets, most of these chronic diseases will fall by the wayside.

After the roundtable discussion, the author summarized his thoughts on the future of alternative medicine.

JAMES MARTI: Alternative, or "holistic," medicine, as several of the Medical Advisory Board panelists have stated, puts the human touch back into medicine. Alternative medicine combines safe and proven therapies of many different medical traditions, including ancient systems such as Chinese and Ayurvedic medicine, as well as allopathic (conventional) medicine. Alternative medicine is based on a philosophy that a patient's body must be maintained whenever possible and acknowledges that patients recover most effectively when they are informed, relaxed, and feel empowered to control their own healing process.

Over the next 50 years, I believe that alternative medicine will change in astonishing ways. By 2050, for example, the most revolutionary technology in medicine will be the most familiar—the computer and the telephone—and will rank with antibiotics, X-rays, and transplant surgery as milestones in the history of medicine. The life-saving potential of these new technologies will be most obvious in medical emergencies where dying patients—for example, at the scene of an automobile accident—will be treated by paramedics with video cameras and microphones that are patched directly through to a hospital physician who can treat patients remotely.

Perhaps more importantly, advances in computer technology will give physicians a more precise method of predicting any person's genetic predisposition to disease. Collaborative Research, a Massachusetts company, and the Human Genome Project at Stanford University are currently developing maps of the 23 pairs of human chromosomes which they hope will help them isolate the genes linked to more than 25 chronic illnesses, including heart disease and cancer. As Dr. Yuan-Chi Lin commented, genetic research may allow scientists in the near future to diagnose and alter genetic abnormalities in utero.

Because alternative medicine is whole body medicine, precise genetic information about each individual will give physicians an unprecedented ability to tailor safe, holistic, noninvasive therapies. For example, people will be able to customize their personal intake of foods, vitamins, minerals, and botanical supplements to correct possible genetic defects. The current system of RDAs will probably be replaced by more sophisticated computer-based programs that allow people to design a specific diet given their genetic makeup, physical fitness, body weight, and body composition. One such program, the Saturation Kinetics Model (SKM), describes the functional relationship between physiological responses and nutrients fed in graded amounts. Also, as Dana Ullman observes, superfoods will be scientifically produced in concentrated doses, either alone or mixed with botanicals such as spirulina, bee pollen products, ginseng, and garlic.

The increasing reliance on genetic information and computer technology to predict, prevent, and reverse serious diseases and increase life span might seem "anti-alternative," but they will most likely constitute an essential element of alternative medicine by 2050. Genes are, after all, not only part of the body, they are perhaps the that most heavily influence how the body functions and how long it will live.

Computers will play a critical role in diagnosing and treating serious diseases which now needlessly claim millions of lives each year and cause untold human suffering for both patients and their families. By 2050, computerized scans of regional heart wall motion, for instance, will yield new methods of treating coronary heart disease. Cardiologists will routinely use lasers or nanotechnology to insert devices into the arteries that will dissolve atherosclerotic blockages. Human life ends when the heart stops beating and the ability to prolong life by delaying the degeneration of the cardiopulmonary system will become a milestone.

The average human brain contains billions of cells and only recently, with the development of enormously powerful computers, have neuroscientists begun to understand how these tiny switches interconnect in astonishingly complex ways to produce our thoughts and emotions. Scientists now hope that precise neurological models of the human brain will enable them to more effectively treat many troubling mental health disorders such as depression, schizophrenia, phobias, Alzheimer's disease, and dementia. Dr. Roger Trabu, working with scientists at Columbia University has developed a computerized model that simulates the workings of 10,000 cells in the hippocampus, the area of the brain that is essential in forming new memories and is involved in epileptic seizures. By 2050, these computer models may also explain how neurochemicals are internally produced so as to eliminate the need for using antidepressants or other substances to prevent and treat depression.

The digital highway may make possible by 2050 what I would call "holistic telemedicine." Video therapy and surgery will become standard, and, in fact, this procedure is already being used on an experimental basis at the Erie County Medical Center in Buffalo, New York, where physicians employ two-way video systems to help rehabilitate paraplegics confined to their homes. The system allows video images and radiological films to be transmitted from the patients home to a computer monitor in the physician's office at the hospital, where doctors can view them. This futuristic form of fax is also in use at the clinic at Yellowstone National Park, where X-rays of injured hikers can be read by radiologists at West Park Hospital in Cody, Wyoming. Heart specialists at Baylor University Hospital in Dallas, Texas, to use another example, now perform remote surgery via video on heart patients in Russia, Turkey, and Saudi Arabia.

Recuperation and post-operative treatment will be more home-based in 2050 because studies have shown that most patients heal faster in familiar environments, and that keeping them in the hospital is not always cost-effective. As Judith Aston notes, new biochemical products will be available in 2050 which will help patients with neuromuscular disorders rehabilitate safely in their own homes. Their therapy will be monitored daily by a physician via interactive video services that combine X-rays and full motion video, voice, and text into packages, or "multimedia sessions." The exchange of images will take place simultaneously or be stored as electronic mail.

The administration of medicine will also change by 2050. Patients admitted to hospitals will have miniaturized medical cards that can be inserted into a computer. The patient's predisposition to diseases, medical history, nutritional status, physical fitness status, record of past botanical and antibiotic treatments (along with patient's reaction to them), and insurance information will be immediately available to physicians. The New Haven hospital has already implemented such an automated patient care information system, as have 10 to 15 percent of U.S. hospitals overall, according to the American Hospital Association.

Certainly hospital environments will change by 2050. Current market forces will motivate hospitals, health management organizations (HMOs), and insurance companies to make hospitals more effective healing environments where treatment, food, room settings, and rehabilitation combine holistically to optimize healing outcomes. Hospitals in Florida and Arizona now offer nutritious vegetarian food, soothing music, hydrotherapy, mineral spas, massage, and classes on yoga, visualization, meditation, exercise, and rehabilitation.

Dana Ullman projects that by 2050 the vast majority of nonchronic conditions such as headaches and respiratory and digestive problems will be treated by people themselves, with the help of software programs.

Patients will use computer databases and CD-ROMs at home to diagnose their own symptoms and conduct simple physiological tests. Using a computer, home patients will have access to hundreds of databases of traditional and alternative medicine. Home-based patients can already access the World Research Foundation's database in Sherman Oaks, California, which offers access to more than 5,000 medical journals from 100 countries.

Three major advances in botanical and pharmaceutical medicines will be underway by 2050. First, scientists will use computers to design new and safer pharmaceutical drugs to treat life-threatening diseases. Researchers at Affymans Research Institute in Palo Alto, California, have already created a variety of peptides, amino acids, nucleic acids, and other complex compounds on computer chips, and screened them for their reactions to other molecules such as monoclonal antibodies and the receptors on the membranes of immune system cells. Second, as Dana Ullman suggests, scientists may well trace the pharmacological actions of homeopathic medicines and create new immunomodulating drugs, or "smart medicines," that fit the unique body/mind characteristics of the patient. And third, as Michael Murray points out, botanical medicines will be grown in standardized cell cultures, and physicians will know how to safely deliver these botanical substances to specific tissues and organs of the body. These three research areas will also lead to a more detailed understanding of the human immune system. In many ways, the human body is its own best apothecary and often the most successful prescriptions are those filled by the body itself.

It is, however, the human touch of alternative practitioners combined with cutting-edge technology that will distinguish holistic telemedicine in 2050. Technology will do us little good if it does not help all patients become better informed, more relaxed, and empowered to heal themselves. Holistic medicine in the future will not only heal you, it will *transform* you. Thus, when you walk into a holistic practitioner's office, it will be likely that you might first receive a head massage, listen to relaxing music, or take a mud bath to eliminate toxins. Your physician may suggest that you meditate, or ask you to recite a mantra to heighten your consciousness. If you should require surgery, you might be asked, as part of a preoperative education program, to watch a videotape of the procedure beforehand, or talk with former patients who went through the same procedure. Preoperative care might involve acupressure, naturopathy, massage, and vitamin, mineral, amino acid, and botanical supplements.

During the procedure, the surgeon might choose a local anesthetic that would allow you to watch the surgery and talk with the surgical team throughout the operation. Your family might be asked to watch the procedure via videocamera in an adjacent room. This holistic approach to surgery gives patients more confidence, comfort, and support, and increases their chances of recovery, because patients tend to take better care of themselves when they feel they are controlling their own healing. It doesn't matter what you call your medical treatment—surgery, therapy, cure, or healing—the result will be that you heal faster and feel better,

This healing/transformation approach is at the center of alternative medicine and, in fact, the leading proponents use words like "transformation" or "transcendence" to describe their therapies. Dr. Dean Ornish states in *Dr. Dean Ornish's Program for Reversing Heart Disease,* that, while a cardiologist, he is "even more interested in the power of the program to transform our lives in deeper ways." In *Peace, Love & Healing,* leading cancer surgeon Dr. Bernie Siegel calls disease "an agent of transformation.... We all

have the ability to train our bodies to heal and eliminate illness," he states. "I think we can use meditative and lifestyle-altering techniques...to gain access to the superintelligence I'm convinced resides within each of us." Dr. Deepak Chopra, the leading proponent of Ayurvedic medicine and author of *Perfect Health: The Complete Mind/Body Guide,* observes, "If you live in tune with your quantum mechanical body, all of your daily activities will proceed smoothly...breathing, eating, digestion, assimilation and elimination. The most important routine to follow is transcending, the act of getting in touch with the quantum level of yourself." The accounts of patients who have been treated by Dr. Chopra, Dr. Ornish, Dr. Siegel, or other holistic physicians suggest that they were not just healed of a disorder— their lives were transformed.

Interestingly, the holistic treatment programs of these leading practitioners are remarkably similar. They each stress vegetarian diets, yoga, meditation, group support, stress reduction, and visualization. They document in their books that when their patients do yoga postures, their bodies become more limber, and when patients meditate, their bodies activate the "relaxation response" which escalates healing. When Dr. Ornish's patients adopt a vegetarian diet, they often find the foods so delicious that they choose not to revert back to animal foods. Dr. Chopra's patients report that his Ayurvedic diet increases their sense of smell and helps them to sleep more soundly. Clearly, once they are "touched" by the holistic practitioner, patients "get in touch" with deeper healing energies inside themselves, and they do not only feel better, they feel more beautiful. Perhaps this is why physicians such as Dr. Ed Weiss regard medicine as more art than science. This is the evolutionary future of alternative medicine—to merge science and technology with human aesthetics. The promise of alternative medicine for 2050 lies in its ability to give people more beautiful bodies, thoughts, and feelings. And feeling beautiful all the time, I believe, is why we are here.

GLOSSARY

absorption   the process by which nutrients are taken up by the intestines and passed into the bloodstream.

acetylcholine   one of the chemicals that transmits impulses between nerves.

acquired immune deficiency syndrome (AIDS)   a disease involving a defect in cell-mediated immunity that has a long incubation period, follows a protracted and debilitating course, is manifested by various opportunistic infections, and has a poor prognosis.

acupressure   a form of acupuncture where certain points of the body are pressed with the fingers and hands to release energy blocks.

acupuncture   Chinese practice of insertion of needles into specific body locations to relieve pain, to induce anesthesia, and for therapeutic purposes.

acute   having a rapid onset, severe symptoms, and a short course; not chronic.

adenosine triphosphate (ATP)   the energy source for muscular contraction.

adrenal gland   the organ that sits on top of each kidney and makes epinephrine (adrenaline) and norepinephrine—which regulate blood pressure and heart rate.

adrenaline   *See* epinephrine

aerobic exercise   any exercise that requires additional effort by the heart and lungs to meet the increased demand by the skeletal muscles for oxygen.

AIDS   *See* acquired immune deficiency syndrome (AIDS)

alkaloids   a group of organic compounds produced by plants (including caffeine, morphine, and nicotine) which can also be made synthetically.

allergen   a foreign substance (such as pollen, house dust, and various foods) that can produce a hypersensitive reaction in the body but is not necessarily intrinsically harmful.

allopathy   the conventional method of medicine that combats disease by using active techniques specifically against the disease.

Alzheimer's disease   a form of senile dementia associated with atrophy of parts of the brain.

amenorrhea   the absence of menstruation.

amino acid   a group of nitrogen-containing chemical compounds that form the basic structural units of proteins.

amniocentesis   the obstetric procedure used to aid in diagnosing fetal abnormalities in which a small amount of amniotic fluid is removed for analysis.

anabolic steroids   a group of synthetic, testosterone-like hormones that promote muscle growth and masculinizing effects.

analgesic   a substance that reduces the sensation of pain.

androgen   a steroid that stimulates male characteristics.

anemia   a condition in which hemoglobin, the oxygen-carrying pigment in the blood, is below normal limits.

aneurysm   a localized abnormal dilation of a blood vessel due to weakness in the vessel wall.

angina   a choking or suffocating pain in the chest (angina pectoris) usually caused by insufficient flow of oxygen to the heart muscle during exercise or excitement.

anodyne   a pain reliever.

anorexia nervosa   a psychoneurotic disorder that involves a long-term refusal to eat, resulting in emaciation, lack of menstrual cycles, emotional disturbance regarding body image, and an abnormal fear of becoming fat.

anovulation   failure of the ovaries to produce, mature, or release ovum (eggs).

antibody   a molecule made by lymph tissue that defends the body against bacteria, viruses, and other foreign bodies (antigens).

antidote   a substance that neutralizes or counteracts the effects of a poison.

antigen   any substance or microorganism that, when it enters the body, causes the formation of antibodies against it.

antihypertensive   of or pertaining to a substance or procedure that has a blood-pressure lowering effect.

antioxidant   a substance capable of protecting other substances from oxidation; some are made by the body to inhibit the destructive actions of chemicals called free radicals; some, such as vitamins C and E, are nutrients.

antispasmodic   any agent that relieves spasms.

aorta   the major trunk of the system of arteries that carries blood away from the heart to the tissues.

apnea   a cessation of breathing, usually temporary.

arrythmia   an irregular heartbeat.

arteriosclerosis   a variety of conditions that cause the artery walls to thicken, lose elasticity, and calcify, resulting in a decreased blood supply, especially to the cerebrum and lower extremeties.

arteries   vessels that carry blood away from the heart to the tissues of the body.

asthma   a respiratory disease characterized by wheezing or coughing which is caused by a spasm of the bronchial tubes or by swelling of their mucous membranes.

astringent a substance that causes a contraction of the tissues upon application.

atheroma abnormal mass of fat, or lipids; as in deposits in an arterial wall.

atherosclerosis the most common form of arteriosclerosis in which the inner walls of the arteries are narrowed by deposits of cholesterol and other material.

atrophy the wasting or shrinking of muscles or glands due to disease, malnutrition, or lack of use.

Ayurvedic medicine in Sanskrit "Ayurveda" means "science of life and longevity"; based on the premise that health is a state of balance among physical, emotional, and spiritual systems.

basal metabolic rate the minimum energy required to maintain the body's life functions at rest.

benign not recurrent; favorable for recovery.

beta-carotene a previtamin A compound found in plants that the body converts to vitamin A.

binge eating the consumption of large quantities of foods within short periods of time.

biofeedback the use of electronic devices that amplify body electricity in order to help people monitor otherwise unconscious physiological processes such as heart rate and body temperature.

bioflavonoid a term for any of a group of substances found in many fruits and essential for the absorption and processing of vitamin C.

blood pressure the pressure exerted by the blood on the walls of the arteries. It is measured in millimeters of mercury (as 120/80 mm Hg).

blood purifier a term used by herbalists to refer to an antibiotic action of certain botanical medicines.

body composition the proportion of fat, muscle, and bone making up the body. Body composition is usually expressed as percent of body fat and percent of lean body mass.

body mass index (BMI) body weight and height indices for determining a person's degree of obesity.

bone density the specific gravity of the body, which can be measured by underwater weighing.

botanical medicine therapies of or derived from plants.

bulimia an eating disorder characterized by episodes of continuous eating, often followed by self-induced vomiting.

cachexia malnutrition and wasting usually linked with diseases such as tuberculosis and cancer.

calisthenics systematic rhythmic bodily exercises performed usually without apparatus.

calorie a measure of the chemical energy provided by food. One calorie equals the amount of heat needed to raise the temperature of one gram of water one degree Celsius at 1 air pressure. One gram of carbohydrate or protein provides about four calories, while one gram of fat provides about nine calories.

canker an ulceration, usually of the mouth and lips.

---

capillaries   tiny blood vessels that link the arteries and the veins.

carbohydrate   a large group of sugars, starches, celluloses, and gums that all contain carbon, hydrogen, and oxygen in similar proportions.

carbon dioxide   a colorless, odorless gas that is formed in the tissues by the oxidation of carbon and is eliminated by the lungs.

carbon monoxide   an odorless, colorless, poisonous gas, produced mainly during combustion of fossil fuels, such as coal and gasoline.

carcinogens   substances that can cause cancer.

cardiac output   the volume of blood pumped out by the heart in a given space of time. A normal heart in a resting adult ejects from 2.5 to 4 liters of blood per minute.

cardiovascular   refers to the heart and blood vessel systems.

cataract   a partial or complete opacity of one or both eyes, especially an opacity impairing vision or causing blindness.

cesarean section   incision through the abdominal and uterine walls for the delivery of a baby.

chemotherapy   the treatment of disease by chemical agents; as in radiation chemotherapy used to treat cancer patients.

chiropractic   literally "done by hand," a science based on the theory that health and disease are life processes related to the function of the nervous system; a method of restoring wellness through adjustments of the spine.

cholesterol   a fat-like substance found in all animal fats, bile, blood, and brain tissue.

chromosomes   thread-like structures in the nucleus of a cell that carry genetic information.

chronic   a disease or disorder that develops slowly and persists for a long period of time.

cocarcinogens   substances that promote the action of a carcinogen.

coenzymes   substances necessary for the action of any enzyme; many vitamins are coenzymes.

collagen   a protein consisting of bundles of tiny fibers that forms connective tissue including the white inelastic fibers of the tendons, ligaments, bones, and cartilage.

colon   the part of the large intestine that extends to the rectum.

congenital   an inherited physical characteristic that is present at birth, such as congenital heart disease.

conjuctiva   the mucous membrane that lines eyeballs and inner eyelids.

constipation   infrequent or difficult evacuation of the feces.

coronary arteries   the arteries that feed oxygenated blood to the heart muscle.

corticosteroid   any one of the hormones made in the outer layer of the adrenal gland that influence or control key functions of the body, such as making carbohydrates and proteins.

cortisone   a steroid hormone made in the liver, or produced artificially, which is used to treat inflammation.

Crohn's disease a chronic inflammatory bowel disease of unknown origin affecting any part of the gastrointestinal tract from the mouth to the anus, but most commonly the ileum, the colon, or both structures.

cystitis a inflammation of the urinary bladder and ureters that may be caused by a bacterial infection, stone, or tumor.

cytoplasm the protoplasm of a cell exclusive of that of the nucleus; the site of most of the chemical activities of the cell.

degenerative diseases diseases that cause permanent deterioration of the structure or function of tissues, such as osteoarthritis and arteriosclerosis.

dementia a disorder in which mental functions break down, characterized by personality change, confusion, and lack of energy.

demulcent oily substance used to soothe and reduce irritation of the skin.

detoxification the body's natural process of neutralizing or eliminating toxic substances, primarily through the skin, liver, kidneys, feces, and urine.

diaphoretic a substance that promotes perspiration and helps control body temperature.

diastolic the second number in a blood pressure reading that measures the pressure in the arteries during the relaxation phase of the heartbeat.

dilution making a solution less potent.

disaccharides sugars composed of two simple (monosaccharide) sugars, such as lactose and sucrose.

disc cartilage between the backbones.

diuretic a drug or other substance such as a botanical that promotes the formation and release of urine.

DNA (deoxyribonucleic acid) a large nucleic acid molecule found in the chromosomes of the nucleus of a cell; carries genetic information.

double-blind study a way of controlling against experimental bias by ensuring that neither the researchers nor the subjects know which treatment any subject is receiving.

douche a method in which a medicated solution or a cleansing agent in warm water is flushed into a body cavity under low pressure.

duodenum the upper part of the small intestine into which the stomach empties.

dysmenorrhea pain linked with menstruation that typically occurs in the lower stomach or back.

edema the abnormal pooling of fluid in tissues that can be caused by conditions such as congestive heart failure, cirrhosis, draining wounds, excessive bleeding, and malnutrition.

electrocardiography (ECG) a device that records the electric activity of the heart to detect abnormal electric impulses through the muscle.

electroconvulsive therapy (ECT) inducing convulsions by means of electric shock; also known as "electric shock therapy."

elimination diet a way to test for food to which a person is allergic. Certain foods are eliminated from the diet one at a time until the allergy is identified.

embolism the sudden obstruction of an artery, usually in the heart, lungs, or brain, by a clot or foreign substance.

emetic substance that promotes vomiting.

endocrine system the network of ductless glands and other structures that secrete hormones into the bloodstream.

endometrium the membrane lining the uterus.

endorphins substances composed of amino acids and produced by the pituitary gland that act on the nervous system to reduce pain.

enzymes substances, usually proteins formed in living cells, that cause or speed up chemical reactions such as the breakdown of protein to amino acids in the gastrointestinal tract.

epidemiology the study of disease as it affects a particular part of the population.

epilepsy any of various disorders marked by disturbed electrical rhythms of the central nervous system and usually demonstrated by convulsive attacks.

epinephrine the hormone secreted by the adrenal gland that produces the "fight or flight" response.

epithelium the cells that cover the entire surface of the body and line most of the internal organs.

essential amino acids the nine amino acids that the body needs for protein synthesis and cannot produce itself.

essential fatty acids fatty acids that the human body cannot manufacture, such as linoleic and linolenic acids.

estrogen one of a group of hormonal steroid components that aid the development of female secondary sex traits such as breast development. Males also have estrogen in lesser amounts.

expectorants substances that help to expel mucus or other fluids from the lungs.

fallopian tubes the two tubes that carry the eggs from the ovaries to the uterus and through which sperm move toward the ovaries.

fibrin a white insoluble protein formed by blood clotting which serves as the starting point for wound repair and scar formation.

fibrocystic breast disease (FBD) the presence of single or multiple cysts in the breasts, usually benign and fairly common.

flavonoids plant pigments that contain several compounds which have beneficial physiological effects in the human body.

free radicals highly reactive molecules that bind to and destroy cellular compounds.

fu zheng Chinese herbal therapy, mostly ginseng and astragalus, that extends life expectancy of patients with rapidly advancing cancers.

gene a segment of the DNA molecule that carries physical characteristics from parent to child.

gingivitis inflammation of the gums.

glaucoma a disease of the eye marked by increased pressure within the eyeball that can result in damage to the optic disk and vision loss.

glucose a simple sugar found in foods, especially fruits, which is a major source of energy in body fluids.

glutamine an amino acid found in many of the body's proteins that helps remove ammonia.

glycogen the major carbohydrate stored in animal cells, which is changed to glucose and released into circulation as needed for energy.

helper T-cells white blood cells that help in immune system response.

hemorrhoid a mass of dilated veins in swollen tissue near the anus or within the rectum.

homeopathy system of therapeutics founded by Samuel Hahnemann in which diseases are treated by drugs which are capable of producing in healthy persons symptoms like those of the disease to be treated.

hormones chemical substances produced in one part or organ of the body that trigger or regulate the activity of an organ or group of cells in another part of the body.

hydrotherapy the application of water in any form, usually externally, in the treatment of disease.

hyperglycemia a condition characterized by too much sugar (glucose) in the blood.

hypertension a common disorder, often without symptoms, marked by high blood pressure persistently exceeding 140/90.

hypertropy the enlargement or overgrowth of an organ or part due to an increase in the size of its constituent cells; as in benign prostatic hypertropy.

hypoglycemia a less than normal level of sugar in the blood, usually caused by being given too much insulin, excessive release of insulin by the pancreas, or low food intake.

hypotension an abnormal condition in which the blood pressure is too low for normal functioning.

hysterectomy removal of the uterus by surgery.

immunoglobulins any of five distinct antibodies in the serum and external secretions of the body.

immunotoxic poisonous to the human immune system.

impotence inability of the adult male to achieve penile erection, or less commonly, to ejaculate having achieved an erection; weakness.

in vitro biological reactions produced in laboratory apparatus.

infarction the development of an area of decay in a tissue, vessel, organ, or part resulting from an interruption of the blood supply to the area or, less often, by the blockage of a vein that carries blood away from the area.

inflammation heat, redness, swelling, and pain caused by trauma, infection, allergic reactions, or other stress or injury to the tissue.

insomnia the inability to sleep; abnormal wakefulness.

insulin a hormone secreted by the pancreas that lowers blood sugar levels and promotes the entry of glucose into muscle, fat, and certain other cells.

interferon a substance produced by living tissues following infection by a bacteria or virus.

international unit (IU) a standard measurement of an antibiotic, vitamin, enzyme, or hormone, the amount of which produces a specific biological result.

intrauterine device (IUD) birth control device implanted within the uterus.

irritable bowel syndrome (IBS) chronic disorder of the small and large intestine causing abnormally increased motility of the bowels.

ischemia poor blood supply to an organ or part, often marked by pain and organ disorder.

jaundice a condition caused by elevation of bile pigment (bilirubin) in the body and characterized by yellow discoloring of the skin, mucous membranes, and eyes.

keratin a fibrous, sulfur-containing protein found in human skin, hair, nails, and tooth enamel.

ketones substances produced in the body through a normal change fats undergo in the liver.

lactase an enzyme that increases the rate of the change of milk sugar (lactose) to glucose and galactose.

lesions wounds, injuries, or other damage of body tissue.

lethargy abnormal tiredness, drowsiness, or lack of energy.

leukocytes white blood cells.

leukotrines a group of chemical compounds that occur naturally in white blood cells; they are able to produce allergic and inflammatory reactions, and may play a part in the development of asthma and rheumatoid arthritis.

libido the instinctual energy or drive associated with sexual desire.

ligaments white, shiny, flexible bands of fibrous tissue binding joints together and connecting various bones and cartilages.

lipid any of the various fats or fat-like substances in plant or animal tissues that serve as an energy reserve in the body.

lipoprotein a complex of protein and fat in one molecule.

lipotropic promoting the flow of lipids to and from the liver.

lymph a thin, clear, slightly yellow fluid originating in many organs and tissues of the body which circulates through the lymphatic vessels and is filtered by the lymph nodes.

lymphocytes white blood cells found primarily in lymph nodes.

macrophages large cells that can surround and digest foreign substances such as bacteria in the body. They are found in the liver, spleen, and loose connective tissue.

malabsorption a failure of the intestines to absorb nutrients, which may result from a birth defect, malnutrition, or an abnormal condition of the digestive system.

malignant a term used to describe a condition that tends to worsen and result in death.

malnutrition the condition of not receiving a proper balance of essential nutrients.

malocclusion abnormality in the coming together of teeth.

mandala a Hindu or Buddhist graphic symbol of the universe, specifically a circle enclosing a square with a deity on each side.

mastectomy surgical removal of one or both breasts.

materia medica the branch of medical study that deals with drugs, their sources, preparations, and uses; pharmacology.

megadose a large dose, often 100 to 1,000 times as much as that recommended, to prevent or treat diseases believed to be caused by nutrient deficiencies.

megavitamins   massive quantities of a specific vitamin usually given for therapeutic purposes.

Meniere's disease   a chronic disease of the inner ear characterized by recurrent episodes of vertigo, progressive nerve deafness, and tinnitus.

menopause   cessation of menstruation in the human female, usually occurring around the age of 50.

menorrhagia   abnormally heavy or prolonged blood loss during menstruation.

menstruation   the monthly (approximately) discharge through the vagina of blood, secretions, and tissue debris from the shedding of the endometrium from the nonpregnant uterus.

metabolism   a collective term for all the chemical processes that take place in the body by which energy is produced and new material is assimilated for the repair and replacement of tissues.

metastasis   the spread of cancerous cells via the blood or lymph from one part of the body to another.

microbial   of or pertaining to or caused by microbes.

microflora   microorganisms present in or characteristic of a special location, e.g., the colon.

molecules   the smallest complete unit of a substance that can exist independently and still retain the properties of an element or compound.

monoclonal antibodies   genetically engineered antibodies specific for one particular antigen.

monosaccharide   a carbohydrate made up of one basic sugar unit such as fructose and glucose.

morning sickness   nausea and vomiting that occur on rising in the morning, especially during the early months of pregnancy.

mucous membrane   the soft, pink tissue that lines most of the cavities and tubes in the body, including the respiratory system, gastrointestinal tract and genitourinary tracts, and the eyelids.

mucus   the slimy substance that acts as a lubricant and mechanical protector of the mucous membranes. It is composed of mucin, white blood cells, water and castoff tissue cells.

music therapy   a form of psychotherapy in which music is used as a means of recreation and communication and as a way to elevate the mood of depressed or psychotic patients.

myocardial infarction   death of an area of the heart muscle from the cessation of blood flow to the area due to arterial blockage.

myocardium   the middle and thickest layer of the heart wall.

naturopathy   a system of therapeutics based on natural foods, light, warmth, exercise, fresh air, massage, and the avoidance of medications. Advocates the belief that illness can be healed by the natural processes of the body.

neoplasm   a new and abnormal tissue growth which may be benign or malignant.

neurofibrillary tangles   a cluster of degenerated nerves.

neuron   the basic nerve cell of the nervous system.

neurotransmitters chemicals such as nor-epinephrine, serotonin, and acetylcholine that travel across the synapse and communicate impulses.

norepinephrine a neurotransmitter that functions mostly in the sympathetic nervous system and increases blood pressure by narrowing the blood vessels.

obesity body weight beyond the limitation of skeletal and physical requirement, so much that the body cannot function normally.

occlusion a blockage in a canal, artery or vein, or passage of the body. It can refer to any contact between the biting or chewing surfaces of the upper and lower teeth.

osteopathy a system of medical practice based on the theory that diseases and illness are due to the loss of structural integrity, which can be restored by manipulation of the joints and the spine supplemented by therapeutic measures.

osteoporosis the common condition, found usually in aging women, of weak, demineralized bones.

otitis inflammation or infection of the ear.

otosclerosis growth of a spongy bone in the inner ear that results in gradual tinnitus, then deafness.

ovulation the release of an egg from an ovary. This cycle usually occurs once a month in most women.

oxidize to cause a substance to chemically combine with oxygen.

palpitation a rapid or excessively forceful heartbeat.

panic disorder a neurotic disorder characterized by persistent, uncontrollable anxiety.

Pap test (or Pap smear) short for Papanicolaou's test, an examination of the cells of the cervix and vagina for precancerous or cancerous abnormalities.

parasympathetic nervous system the branch of the autonomic nervous system that tends to slow the heart, constrict the pupils, and promote digestive and sexual functions.

Parkinson's disease a chronic progressive nervous disorder marked by tremor and weakness of resting muscles and by a peculiar gait.

pathogens microorganisms that are able to cause a disease.

phobia an anxiety disorder characterized by an obsessive, irrational, and intense fear of a specific object, activity, or physical situation.

phytoestrogens plant compounds that exert estrogen-like effects.

placebo an inactive therapeutic substance, agent, or procedure that works (or appears to work) by suggestion, not by consistent physical effects on the body.

platelets tiny disc-shaped cells in the blood that have no hemoglobin but are needed for blood clot formation.

polyp a small tumor-like growth that projects from a mucous membrane surface.

polysaccharides carbohydrates such as starch that contain three or more simple carbohydrate molecules.

polyunsaturated fats fats, mostly from plants, with double bonds that can bind to hydrogen; these tend to be liquid at room temperature and are called oils.

premenstrual syndrome (PMS) syndrome of nervous tension, irritability, weight gain, headache, and edema occurring just before the onset of menstruation.

progesterone a natural hormone produced by the corpus luteum—the part of the ovary that the egg vacated—that prepares the uterus for the reception and development of the fertilized egg.

progestin any of a group of natural hormones released by the corpus luteum, placenta, or adrenal cortex; also made synthetically.

prostaglandins hormone-like compounds manufactured from essential fatty acids.

prostate the male gland that wraps around the neck of the bladder and produces a thin fluid that makes semen into a liquid.

prostatitis inflammation of the prostate gland.

pulmonary alveoli the tiny air sacs in the lungs from which oxygen enters the blood.

pyruvate an intermediate product in the breakdown of glucose to carbon dioxide and water.

qi gong a Chinese meditative exercise that relieves stress and improves cardiovascular functioning.

recommended dietary allowance (RDA) the proper amount of nutrients needed for optimum health.

retinopathy a noninflammatory eye disorder resulting from changes in the retinal blood vessels.

rheumatoid arthritis a chronic disease characterized by pain, stiffness, inflammation, swelling, and destruction of joints.

RNA (ribonucleic acid) similar to DNA; there are several types that carry gene data from the nucleus to the cytoplasm.

saccharide any of a large group of carbohydrates, including all sugars and starches.

saturated fats fats that have no double bonds and cannot accept more hydrogen atoms; such fats tend to be solid at room temperature and are mostly from animal sources such as meat, whole milk, butter, and eggs.

SIDS *See* sudden infant death syndrome (SIDS)

sinusitis inflammation of the sinuses.

sorbitol a sugar-alcohol made from glucose which, in diabetics, accumulates in peripheral nerves, the lens, and certain other tissues.

steroids the broad term includes a large number of chemicals including vitamin D, cortisone, testosterone, estrogen, and bile acids.

subluxation a partial dislocation.

sudden infant death syndrome (SIDS) the sudden, unexpected, and unexplained death of an apparently healthy infant, typically occurring between the ages of three weeks and five months.

suppressor T-cells lymphocytes that are controlled by the thymus gland and suppress the immune response.

sympathetic nervous system the branch of the autonomic nervous system that tends to promote motor and mental excitation and is responsible for the "fight or flight" response, symptoms of which include a faster heartbeat, dilated pupils, and digestive and sexual inhibition.

synapse the junction between two nerve cells.

syndrome a group of signs and symptoms that occur together in a pattern characteristic of a particular disease or abnormal condition.

systolic the pressure in the arteries during the contraction phase of the heartbeat. This is the first number in a blood pressure reading.

T-cells lymphocytes that are under the control of the thymus gland.

tinnitus tinkling or ringing in one or both ears.

toxicity a poisonous effect produced when people ingest an amount of a substance that is above their level of tolerance.

triglyceride a compound found in most animal and vegetable fats that is made up of a fatty acid and glycerol.

urinalysis a physical, microscopic, or chemical examination of urine for color density, acidity, and other conditions.

vaginitis inflammation of the vaginal tissues, as in a yeast infection.

varicose veins unnaturally and permanently distended veins, usually in the legs.

vasoconstriction the narrowing of any blood vessel, especially the arterioles and veins in the skin, stomach, and intestines.

vertigo a disordered state in which the individual or his/her surroundings seem to whirl dizzily.

visualization a variety of visual techniques used to treat disease based on inducing relaxation in the patient and having them actually will their disease away.

XJL Chinese herb that interacts with neurotransmitters in the brain to curb the desire for alcohol.

GENERAL BIBLIOGRAPHY

A

Altman, Nathaniel. *Everybody's Guide to Chiropractic Health Care*. Los Angeles, CA: Jeremy P. Tarcher, Inc., 1989.

Anderson, Robert A., M.D. *Wellness Medicine*. New Canaan, CT: Keats Publishing, Inc., 1990.

B

Balch, James F., and Phyllis Balch. *Prescription for Nutritional Healing*. Garden City Park, NY: Avery Publishing Group, 1993.

Benson, Herbert, and William Proctor. *Beyond the Relaxation Response*. New York, NY: Berkeley Publishing Group, 1987.

Benson, Herbert. *The Relaxation Response*. New York, NY: William Morrow, 1975.

Beverly, Cal, ed. *Natural Health Secrets Encyclopedia*. Peachtree City, GA: FC&A Publishing, 1991.

Bricklin, Mark. *The Practical Encyclopedia of Natural Healing*. New York, NY: Penguin Books, 1990.

Brody, Jane. *The Good Food Book*. New York, NY: Bantam Books, 1990.

———. *Jane Brody's The New York Times Guide to Personal Health*. New York, NY: Avon Books, 1982.

Bunyard, Peter. *Health Guide for the Nuclear Age*. London, England: Macmillan, 1988.

The Burton Goldberg Group. *Alternative Medicine: The Definitive Guide*. Puyallup, WA: Future Medicine Publishing, Inc., 1993.

Butler, Kurt, and Lynn Rayner. *The Best Medicine: The Complete Health and Preventive Medicine Handbook*. New York, NY: Harper & Row Publishers, Inc., 1985.

C

Carper, Jean. *The Food Pharmacy Guide to Good Eating*. New York, NY: Bantam Books, 1988.

———. *Food—Your Miracle Medicine: How Food Can Prevent & Cure over 100 Symptoms & Problems*. HarperSanFrancisco: HarperCollins, 1993.

———. *Creating Health: How to Make Up The Body's Intelligence.* Boston, MA: Houghton Mifflin, 1987.

Chaitow, Leon, M.D. *The Body/Mind Purification Program.* New York, NY: Simon & Schuster, Inc., 1990.

———. *The Stress Protection Plan.* HarperSanFrancisco: HarperCollins, 1992.

Chopra, Deepak, M.D. *Ageless Body, Timeless Mind.* New York, NY: Harmony Books, 1993.

———. *Perfect Health: The Complete Mind/Body Guide.* New York, NY: Harmony Books, 1991.

———. *Quantum Healing: Exploring the Frontiers of Body, Mind, Medicine.* New York, NY: Bantam Books, 1993.

Culbreth, D. *A Manual of Materia Medica and Pharmacology.* Portland, OR: Eclectic Medical Publications, 1983.

Cummings, Stephen, M.D., and Dana Ullman. *Everybody's Guide to Homeopathic Medicine.* New York, NY: St. Martin's Press, 1991.

D

Dharmananda, S. *Your Nature, Your Health— Chinese Herbs in Constitutional Therapy.* Portland, OR: Institute for Traditional Medicine and Preservation of Health Care, 1986.

Duke, J. *Handbook of Medicinal Herbs.* Boca Raton, FL: CRC Press, 1985.

E

Edlin, Gordon, and Eric Golanty. *Health and Wellness: A Holistic Approach.* Boston, MA: Jones and Bartlett Publishers, Inc., 1992.

Eisenberg, D.M., et al. "Unconventional Medicine in the United States: Prevalence, Costs, and Patterns of Use." *New England Journal of Medicine* 328 (March 1993): 246–52.

Ellingwood, F. *American Materia Medica, Therapeutics and Pharmacognosy.* Portland, OR: Eclectic Medical Publications, 1983.

Epstein, Gerald. *Healing Visualizations.* New York, NY: Bantam Books, 1989.

F

Felter, H. *The Eclectic Materia Medica.* Portland, OR: Eclectic Medical Publications, 1983.

G

Girdano, Daniel, and George Everly. *Controlling Stress and Tension: A Holistic Approach.* Englewood Cliffs, NJ: Prentice-Hall, 1986.

Goldstar, Rosemary. *Herbal Healing for Women.* New York, NY: Simon & Schuster, Inc., 1993.

Goleman, Daniel. *The Meditative Mind.* Los Angeles, CA: Jeremy P. Tarcher, Inc., 1988.

Goodhart, R., and V. Young. *Modern Nutrition in Health and Disease.* Philadelphia, PA: Lea & Febiger, 1988.

Griffith, H. Winter. *Vitamins.* Tucson, AZ: Fisher Books, 1988.

Guiton, Arthur, M.D. *Textbook of Medical Physiology.* Philadelphia, PA: Harcourt Brace Jovanovich, 1991.

H

Hahnemann, Samuel. *Organon of Medicine.* Translated by W. Boericke, M.D. New Delhi: B. Jain Publishers, 1992.

Hausman, Patricia, and Judith Been Hurley. *The Healing Foods.* Emmaus, PA: Rodale Press, Inc., 1989.

Hendler, Sheldon, M.D. *The Complete Guide to Anti-Aging Nutrients.* New York, NY: Simon & Schuster, Inc., 1985.

Hoffer, A. *Orthomolecular Nutrition.* New Canaan, CT: Keats Publishing, Inc., 1978.

Hoffman, David. *The New Holistic Herbal.* Rockport, MA: Element Books, 1992.

K

Kabat-Sinn, J. *Full Catastrophic Living: Using the Wisdom of Your Body and Mind to Face Stress, Pain, and Illness.* New York, NY: Delacorte Press, 1990.

Kahan, Barbara. *Healthier Children.* New Canaan, CT: Keats Publishing, Inc., 1990.

Kirchheimer, Sid. *The Doctor's Book of Home Remedies.* Emmaus, PA: Rodale Press, Inc., 1993.

Kutsky, Roman J., Ph.D. *Handbook of Vitamins, Minerals and Hormones.* New York, NY: Van Nostrand Reinhold Co., 1973.

L

Lane, William, and L. Cormac. *Sharks Don't Get Cancer.* Garden City Park, NY: Avery Publishing Group, 1992.

Leung, A. *Encyclopedia of Common Natural Ingredients Used in Food, Drugs, and Cosmetics.* New York, NY: John Wiley & Sons, 1980.

M

Margolis, Simeon, and Hamilton Moses III. *The Johns Hopkins Medical Handbook.* New York, NY: Medletter Associates, Inc., 1992.

May, L. *Drug Information.* St. Louis, MO: Mosby Year Book, Inc., 1993.

Mills, Simon. *Out of the Earth: The Essential Book of Herbal Medicine.* New York, NY: Penguin Books, 1991.

Monte, Tom, and the editors of *EastWest Natural Health. World Medicine: The EastWest Guide to Healing Your Body.* New York, NY: Putnam Berkley Group, Inc., 1993.

Murphy, Michael. *The Future of the Body.* Los Angeles, CA: Jeremy P. Tarcher, Inc., 1992.

Murray, Michael. *The Healing Powers of Herbs.* Rocklin, CA: Prima Publishing, 1992.

Murray, Michael, and Joseph Pizzorno. *Encyclopedia of Natural Medicine.* Rocklin, CA: Prima Publishing, 1991.

N

Newberry, Benjamin H., Janet Madden, and Thomas Gertsenberger. *A Holistic Conceptualization of Stress & Disease.* New York, NY: AMS Press, Inc., 1991.

Nieman, D. *Fitness & Your Health.* Palo Alto, CA: Bull Publishing Company, 1993.

O

Ody, Penelope. *The Complete Medicinal Herbal.* London, England: Dorling Kindersley, 1993.

Ornish, Dean, M.D. *Dr. Dean Ornish's Program for Reversing Heart Disease.* New York, NY: Ballantine Books, 1990.

———. *Eat More, Weigh Less.* HarperSanFrancisco: HarperCollins, 1993.

Ornstein, R. *The Human Ecology Program.* San Francisco, CA: San Francisco Medical Research Foundation, 1987.

P

Panos, Maesimund B., and Jane Heimlich. *Homeopathic Medicine at Home.* Los Angeles, CA: Jeremy P. Tarcher, Inc., 1980.

Pauling, Linus. *How to Live Longer and Feel Better.* New York, NY: W.H. Freeman and Co., 1986.

———. *Vitamin C and the Common Cold.* New York, NY: W.H. Freeman and Co., 1971.

Porkett, Manfred, M.D. *Chinese Medicine.* New York, NY: Henry Holt & Co., 1992.

R

Reid, Daniel. *Chinese Herbal Medicine.* Boston, MA: Shambhala Publications Inc., 1993.

Riggs, Maribeth. *Natural Child Care: A Complete Guide to Safe & Effective Herbal Remedies & Holistic Health Strategies for Infants & Children.* New York, NY: Crown Publishing Group, 1992.

S

Santillo, Humbart. *Natural Healing with Herbs.* Prescott, AZ: Hohm Press, 1991.

Schroeder, Steven. *Current Medical Diagnosis & Treatment.* Norwalk, CT: Appleton & Lange, 1992.

Selye, Hans. *Stress Without Distress.* New York, NY: New American Library, 1975.

Shangold, Mona. *The Complete Sports Medicine Book for Women.* New York, NY: Simon & Schuster, Inc., 1992.

Siegel, Bernie, M.D. *How to Live Between Office Visits.* New York, NY: Harper & Row Publishers, Inc., 1993.

———. *Love, Medicine & Miracles.* New York, NY: Harper & Row Publishers, Inc., 1986.

———. *Peace, Love & Healing.* New York, NY: Harper & Row Publishers, Inc., 1989.

Simon, Harvey B., and Steven R. Levisohn. *The Athlete Within: A Personal Guide to Total Fitness.* Boston, MA: Little, Brown, 1987.

Stanway, Andrew, M.D. *The Natural Family Doctor.* New York, NY: Simon & Schuster, Inc., 1987.

Stein, Diane. *The Natural Remedy Book for Women.* Freedom, CA: The Crossing Press, 1992.

Stewart, Felicia. *Understanding Your Body: Every Woman's Guide to a Lifetime of Health.* New York, NY: Bantam Books, 1987.

T

Tierra, Lesley. *The Herbs of Life.* Freedom, CA: Crossing Press, 1992.

U

Ullman, Dana. *Discovering Homeopathy.* Berkeley, CA: North Atlantic Books, 1989.

W

Walford, Roy. *Maximum Life Span.* New York, NY: W.W. Norton and Co., Inc., 1983.

Walters, Richard. *Options: The Alternative Cancer Therapy Book.* Garden City Park, NY: Avery Publishing Group, 1993.

Weil, Andrew, M.D. *Health and Healing.* Boston, MA: Houghton Mifflin Company, 1983.

————. *Natural Health, Natural Medicine.* Boston, MA: Houghton Mifflin, 1990.

Weiner, Michael. *Weiner's Herbal.* Mill Valley, CA: Quantum Books, 1990.

Y

Yoder, Barbara. *The Recovery Resource Book.* New York, NY: Simon & Schuster, Inc., 1990.

Z

Zimmerman, David. *Zimmerman's Complete Guide to Nonprescription Drugs.* Detroit, MI: Gale Research Inc. and Visible Ink Press, 1993.

INDEX

to, 156; calcium and, 63, 312; depression and, 175; limiting consumption of, 28, 31; panic attacks and, 181; physiological consequences of abuse of, *157*; ulcers and, 150

alcohol headaches, 141

alcoholic cirrhosis, and ulcers, 150

alcoholics, 42, 46, 64, 156

Alcoholics Anonymous (AA), 159, 170

alcoholism, 3, 156; alternative treatments for, 158–59, 162

aletris farinosa, 191

Alexander technique, 17, 141, 144

alfalfa, 122

alfalfa leaf, 138

algae, 81

algin, 115

alkoxyglycerols, 270

Allard, M., 306

allergic antibodies (IgE), 84

allergies, 68, 117

Alliance for Aging Research, *304*

The Alliance for Alternative Medicine, 279

allopaths, 90

aloe vera, 82, 121

aloe vera emodin, 82

alpha brain waves, 11

alpha-fetaprotein, 214

AlphaFetaprotein Screening, 214

alternate nostril breathing, 292

alternative care, 19

alternative medicine; specialties comprising, 1; future of, 315–29; life extension and, 320, 321; nutrition and, 13; philosophy of, 19; quality of life and, 321. *See also* individual specialties (i.e. biofeedback, hypnosis, meditation, osteopathic medicine, relaxation, visualization, yoga)

Alternative Medicine: The Definitive Guide (The Burton Goldberg Group), 85, 86, 89, 138, 146, 306, 308, 309, 310; on benign prostatic hypertrophy, 194–95; on bodywork thera-

pies, 144; on cancer, 269, 271, 272; on cataracts, 245, 247; on depression, 176, 177; on dysmenorrhea, 204, 205; on ear wax, 251, 253; on fibrocystic breast disease, 200; on glaucoma, 247; on heart disorders, 287, 290; on impotence, 192; on irritable bowel syndrome, 147; on Meniere's disease, 253; on otitis media, 254–55; on premenstrual syndrome, 207–8; on prostate gland, 195–96, 197; on refractive eye disorders, 249; on schizophrenia, 184; on sinusitis, 257, 258; on tinnitus, 256; on ulcers, 149; on yeast infections, 210

Alternatives Newsletter, 270

Altman, Lawrence, 189

aluminum, 308

Alzheimer, Alois, 305

Alzheimer's Association, 305, 314

Alzheimer's disease, 56, 175, 203, 299, 305–6; botanical medicines for, 306–7; coping therapies for, 306–9; estrogen replacement therapy and, 307; ginkgo biloba, 86; lifestyle changes and, 307–8; nutritional therapies and, 308; preventing and treating, 307; Traditional Chinese Medicine, 308; vitamin and mineral therapies for, 308–9; vitamin E and, 53

Alzheimer's Disease Education and Referral Center, 314

AMA. *See* American Medical Association (AMA)

amalgam fillings, 234, 307; mercury in, 234

amblyopia, 249

American Academy of Implant Dentistry, 241

American Academy of Ophthalmology, 248

American Academy of Pediatrics, 224

American Academy of Periodontics, 236

American Academy of

Periodontology, 241

American Academy of Sciences, 272

American Anorexia/Bulimia Association, Inc., 36

American Association of Acupuncture and Oriental Medicine, 21, 94, 149, 257

American Association of Homeopathic Pharmacists, 21

American Association of Naturopathic Physicians, 94

American Association of Orthodontics, 237

American Botanical Council, 85, 95, 141

American Cancer, 98

American Cancer Society, 8, 98, 170, 197, 265, 266, 272, 279

American Chiropractic Association, 21

American College of Cardiology, 281

American College of Nurse-Midwives (ACNM), 221

American College of Obstetricians and Gynecologists, 204, 228, 266

American College of Sports Medicine, 98, 110

American Council on Alcoholism, 170

American Council for Drug Education, 170

American Council on Science and Health, 31, 163

American Dental Association (ADA), 230, 231, 232, 236, 241

American Dietetic Association, 36

American Family Physician, 33, 35, 178

American ginseng, 86

American Health, 142, 203, 217, 234, 250, 251, 265

American Heart Association, 112, 135, 152, 168, 272, 283, 286, 297, 304

American Herbalists Guild, 95, 200

American Holistic Medical Association (AHMA), *16, 273*

Psychophysiology and
Biofeedback, 5, 21
Association for Voluntary
Sterilization, Inc., 198, 228
asthma, 117, 166; bronchial, 64;
exercise-induced, 102, 110;
office pollution and, 117
astigmatism, 248, 249
Aston, Judith, 18, 317
Aston patterning, 18
Aston Training Center, 18
astragalus, 275
astrocytoma, 269
atenolol, 287
atherosclerosis, 134, 137–39, 293,
295, 300, 306; alternative
treatments for, 138; botanical medicine for, 138; of
coronary arteries, 286; exercise for reducing, 138; heart
disorders and, 283; nutritional therapy for, 138–39;
underlying heart attacks,
283, 295; vitamin and mineral therapies for, 293–94
Atkins, Robert, 147
Atkins Center (New York,
NY), 147
atria, 282
Aubuchon, Paul A., 2
Auerback, Sanford, 179
*Australian/New Zealand Journal
of Medicine,* 142
*Australian-New Zealand Journal
of Psychiatry,* 42
Austria, banning of amalgam fillings in, 234
autogenic training, 129
autoimmune diseases, and microbial toxins, 117. *See also*
AIDS; immune system(s)
autoimmune thyroiditis, 117
Awang, D., 141
Awareness Through Move-
ment, 18
Aylsworth, J., 222
Ayurvedic medicine, 1, 4;
Alzheimer's disease and,
306; for atherosclerosis,
138; for enlarged prostates,
194; exercise and, 8; for
hypertension, 144; for
Meniere's disease (vertigo),
253; for otitis media, 254;
physicians practicing, 6; for

prostatitis, 196; senile
dementia and, 306

B

B vitamins, 42, 47, 290; alcoholism treatment and, 158;
for Alzheimer's symptoms,
308; disease prevention and,
47; for fibrocystic breast disease, 201; folic acid in, 214;
for osteoporosis, 312; phosphorus and, 65
B-complex vitamins, 73
Bacillus Calmette-Guerin (BCG)
vaccine, 271
back disorders, 3
back pain, exercise for, 100
back thigh, stretch exercise, 110
bacteria, 29
Balch, James F., and Phyllis
Balch, 304, 307, 308, 312;
on aloe vera, 82; on benign
prostatic hypertrophy, 193,
194, 195; on blood pressure,
145; on depression, 178; on
fibrocystic breast disease,
200, 201; on glaucoma, 247;
on headaches, 142; on heart
disorders, 288, 290; on
impotence, 191, 192; on irritable bowel syndrome, 147;
on Meniere's disease (vertigo), 254; on menopause,
202, 203; on pokeweed
extracts, 91; on premenstrual
syndrome, 206, 208; on prostatitis, 196–97; on sinusitis,
258; on throat cankers, 260;
on ulcers, 149, 150
balloon angioplasty, 286, 287
balsam pear, 82
barberry, 122
barbiturates, 156, 175
Bartisch, Ernst, 203
basal ganglia, 56
basketball, 106
Bastyr College (Seattle, WA), 12
Bayer Pharmaceutical Com-
pany, 164
Baylor College of Medicine, 75
BDS. *See* biochemical defense
system (BDS)
Beating Alzheimer's (Warren),

307–8
bee pollen products, 195, 323
behavior modification (BMOD),
33, 34
Belch, J., 82
bench aerobics, 104
benign prostatic hypertrophy
(BPH), 189, 193, 194, 195
benign tumors, 264
Benninga, M. A., 5
Benotti, Peter N., 33
Benson, Herbert, 11, 129, 131,
133, 260, 289
benzedrine, 161
benzene, 119
Ber, Abram, 89, 239
Berard, Yamil, 224
berberine, 86
Bergner, Paul, 149
beriberi, 42
Berkman, Lisa, 132
Berson, Eliot, 250
*The Best Medicine: The Complete
Health and Preventive
Handbook* (Butler and
Rayner), 99, 143, 219, 256,
309, 312; on atherosclerosis,
137, 139; on headaches,
142; on hypertension, 146;
on migraines, 140; on morning sickness, 220; on peptic
ulcers, 148, 150; on prostate
problems, 195
beta-amyloid, 305
beta-blocking drugs, 287
beta-carotene, 121; Alzheimer's
disease and, 53; for cancer
protection, 266, 304;
cataracts and, 6, 48, 246;
cholesterol and, 49; converted to vitamin A, 40, 41; disease prevention and, 304; for
ear infections, 255; for fibrocystic breast disease, 201;
longevity and, 56; for sinusitis, 258; for smokers, 168; in
spirulina, 81; for yeast infections, 210
*Better Health Through Natural
Healing* (Trattler), 12, 54, 56
Beyond Biofeedback (Green and
Green), 9
bicycling, 103, 104
bilberry, 248
bile acids, 28

binge eating, 35

Binnie, N. R., 5

biochemical defense system (BDS), 268, 269

biofeedback, 19; descriptions and treatment with, 5; for glaucoma, 247; hypertension and, 146, 150; for macular degeneration, 248; for panic disorder and phobias, 181; for stress management, 66, 126, 134, 143; for ulcers, 150

Biofeedback and Psychophysiology Center, 14

biological aging clock, 300

biomechanics, 317

biotechnology, 315

biotin, 42

bipolar disorder, 174, 176, 182

birth control pills, 6, 200, 215

birth defects (fetal), 219; from alcohol, 114, 157; drugs and, 219; folic acid and, 46; testing for, 214, 215

bisabolol, 83

bites, 236

bitter melon (momordica charantia), 82–83

Blackburn, George, 33

bladder, 83, 189, 196

bladder cancer, 45, 119

blade implants, 238

Blakeslee, Sandra, 226

Bland, Jeffrey, 321

bleeding ulcers, 150

blindness, 41, 225, 244

Block, Gladys, 49

Block, Keith, 272

Block diet, 272, 276

Bloksma, N., 89

blood cholesterol, 27

blood lipids, 28

blood pressure, 160, 289. *See also* hypertension

Bloom, Pamella, 17

blueberry extract, 248

blue-green algae, 80

Blumberg, Jeffrey, 56

BMOD. *See* behavior modification (BMOD)

The Body/Mind Detoxification Program (Chaitow), 168

bodywork therapies, 17–18; for headaches, 141; for hypertension, 144

Boesler, D., 205

bonding, between mother and child, 222, 224, 227

bone marrow suppression, 274

bone(s), 52, 62, 68, 311

"Bones of Contention," 8

The Boomer Report, 6

Boston University School of Medicine, 255

botanical extracts, 80

botanical medicines, 1, 5, 19, 79, 91, 184, 325; aging and, 301; for alcoholism, 158; aloe and, 82; Alzheimer's disease and, 306; for atherosclerosis, 138; choosing, 80; encapsulated, 80; for enlarged prostate, 194, 195; for irritable bowel syndrome, 147; for menopause, 202; osteoporosis and, 310–11; for otitis media, 254; schizophrenia and, 183; side effects of, 80; for sinusitis, 258; stress reduction with, 130, 134; for vaginitis, 210

Boyle, Wade, 16

BPH. *See* benign prostatic hypertrophy (BPH)

braces, orthodontic, 237

bradyarrhythmia, 88

brain abscesses, 254

brain tumors, 14, 15

bran, 28

Brandeis University, 169

Branewmark, Per-Ingvar, 238

breast cancer, 200, 264; botanical treatments for, 6; exercise and, 98; fat consumption and, 29; female obesity and, 33; iodine deficiency and, 69; vitamin D and, 51, 52

Breast Center (Los Angeles, CA), 200

breast milk, 222, 223; infant formulas vs., 222–23; infant teeth and, 230

breast removal, 199

breastfeeding, 216, 222; baby's immune system and, 223; benefits for baby of, *223,* 227; maternal mineral loss

and, 224

Bricklin, Mark, 64, 66, 74

Brigham and Women's Hospital, 293

British Institute of Homeopathy and College of Homeopathy, 21

British Journal of Cancer, 85

British Journal of Psychiatry, 47, 184

British Medical Journal, 68, 71, 106

Brodey, Denise, 217

Brody, Jane, 191, 230, 237, 245, 311

bromelain, and platelet aggregation, 139

bromocriptine, 200

bronchitis, 166

Brown, Donald J., 91, 288

Brunner, E., 64

bruxism headaches, 141

buckthorn, 122

Buddhism, 133, 320

bulimia, 34–35, 229

buprenorphine, 162

bursitis, ginger and, 85

Burzynski, Stanislaw, 268, 269

Burzynski Research Institute, 268

Butler, Kurt, 137, 256, 309, 312; on exercise, 99, 104; on headaches, 142; on hypertension, 146; on morning sickness, 220; on peptic ulcers, 148, 150; on prostate problems, 195, 196

butyl methacrylate, 119

C

CAD. *See* coronary artery disease (CAD)

Cade, J., 42

cadmium, 68

caffeine; consumption of, 159; effect on pregnancy, 217; effects on body, 160; fibrocystic breast disease and, 201; panic attacks and, 181; sleep quality and, 179; treatment for caffeinism, 160; ulcers and, 150

Calan, 190

calciportiol, 52

calcitrol, 51, 52

calcium; in algae, 81; deficiency, 62–63; fluoride and, 68; food sources of, 312; for healthy teeth, 229; in herbs, 310; magnesium and, 64; for menopause symptoms, 203; for osteoporosis, 312; phosphorus and, 65; for pregnant women, 218; sources of, 62; vitamin D and, 52, 62

calcium carbonate, 63, 312

calcium channel blockers, 190

calcium citrate, 63, 312

calcium lactate, 312

calcium supplements, 70, 224

calf muscle stretch exercise, 109

California Division of Occupational Safety and Health, 316

California Medical Association, 34, 226, 305

calisthenics, 106–7

calories, 26

Camp, Joe, 236

Canada Health and Welfare Department, 141

Canadian Schizophrenia Foundation, 184

canadine, 86

cancer, 263, 264; aging and, 39, 115, 300; alternative treatments for, 268, 277; antineoplaston therapy, 268–69; Ayurvedic medicine for, 4; bladder, 269; bone, 269; botanical treatments for, 79, 264, 269–70, 277; breast, 269, 271; causes of, 264; colorectal, 269; conventional treatments for, 266–68, 277; diagnosing, 266; Dr. Block's therapy for, 276; early detection of, 267, 277; endometrial, 203; exercise and, 98, 265; fat consumption and, 28; fiber and, 28; garlic and, 85; germanium and, 69; hormone-related, 265; hydrazine sulfate for, 270–71; hypnosis and, 9; lentinus edodes and, 91; Livingston therapy for, 271; lung, 118, 269, 271; meat protein and, 29, 30; mistle-

toe and, 89; nutritional therapies for, 266, 272, 277; obesity and, 33; positive mental states and, 272–74; preventing, 265, 277; prostate, 269, 271; selenium and, 72; skin, 98, 118; smoking and, 317; social supports and, 272–74; spirulina and, 81; stomach, 269; symptoms, 265; toxins and, 7, 114, 122; Traditional Chinese Medicine for, 274; vaginal infections and, 209; visualization and, 275; vitamin A and, 41; vitamin and mineral therapies for, 275, 276, 277; vitamin B6 and, 45–46; vitamin C and, 48, 49, 50, 51; vitamin E and, 54, 56; water toxins and, 119; zinc and, 74

Cancer Control Society, 279

Cancer, Immunology, Immunotherapy, 89

Cancer Treatment Centers of America, 89, 269

Cancer Weekly, 49, 51, 54

candida albicans; in Alzheimer's disease patients, 308; chamomile oil and, 83; effect of diet on, 210; licorice and, 88; selenium and, 73

Cannabis sativa plant, 163

canola oil, 28

Capoten, 190

caprylicacid, 122

captopril, 190

Carbamazapine, 162

carbohydrates, 26, 35, 40, 291; children and, 31; complex, 27, 31; dietary balancing of, 30

carbon dioxide, 63

carbon monoxide, 166

carbon tetrachloride, 119

carcinomas, 264

cardamom, 233

Cardene, 190

cardiac surgery, 10. *See also* heart disease

cardiologist, holistic, 281

cardiovascular disease, 281; risk factors, 31; death and, 283;

exercise and, 98, 109; manganese and, 71

cardiovascular disorders, 69

Cardizem, 190

Careiello, A., 65

Cargile, William, 149, 257

Carl Pfeiffer Treatment Center, 184

carnitine, 295

carnivora, 270

carotenoids, 53, 84

carrots, 84

cassia, 121

cassia senna, 122

Castelman, Michael, 239

cataracts, 247; blindness and, 244; botanical medicines and, 245; factors contributing to, 244; germanium and, 69; nutritional therapies for, 245; prevention and treatment of, 245; selenium and, 73; stress management and, 245; surgery for, 245; Traditional Chinese Medicine for, 245; vitamin C and, 48, 56; vitamins and minerals for, 245–46

cavities. *See* dental cavities

CCD. *See* charged-couple device

CD-4 cell levels, 89

CD4+ lymphocyte levels, 74

CDA Journal, 234

CDC. *See* Centers for Disease Control and Prevention

Cesarean sections, 221

Cellular & Molecular Biology Research, 83

Center for Applied Psychophysiology–Menninger Clinic, 247

Center for Balance and Fitness, 131

Center for the Improvement of Human Functioning International, 176

Center for the Study of Anorexia and Bulimia, 36

Centers for Disease Control and Prevention (CDC) (U.S.), 98, 106, 115, 166, 213, 289

Central Middlesex Hospital, 53

central nervous system depressants, 165

cerebral palsy, 5, 225

certified nurse-midwives, 221
cervical dysplasia, 73
Cesarean deliveries, 10, 222
chair aerobic programs, 110
Chaitow, Leon, 63, 116, 168, 178, 181
chamomile (matricaria rucutita), 83, 130
charantin, 82
charged-couple device (CCD), 239
CHD. *See* coronary heart disease (CHD)
Chemical & Pharmaceutical Bulletin, 83, 84
Chemical Pharmacology Bulletin, 83
chemotherapy, 267–68, 271–73, 274, 276
Chen, Ki C., 301
chi, 2, 129, 133; botanical medicine and, 6; detoxification and, 123; qi gong channels, 132; rebalancing, 3, 274
chi stagnation, and menstrual cramps, 205
Chicago Medical School, 276
childbirth, 213, 220, 226; attended by nurse-midwives, 221
children; air pollution and, 114; exercises for, 98; immunotoxins and, 116; iron deficiency in, 61, 71; lead toxicity and, 115; learning and behavior disorders in, 68; nutrient requirements for, 30, 31, 32; protein and, 29; second hand smoke and, 166; simple phobias in, 181; zinc levels in, 75
China, 274; acupuncture in, 3; botanical medicine in, 5; cataract treatment in, 245; esophageal cancer study in, 50; exercise in, 107; kudzu in, 159; martial arts in, 8; massage education in, 17; selenium deficiency in, 72; spirulina growing project, 81; traditional medicine in, 13
Chinese Journal of Integrated Traditional & Western Medicine, 183

Chinese Medical Journal, 138, 292
Chinese medicine. *See* Traditional Chinese Medicine (TCM)
Chinese skullcap (scutellaria baicalensis), 83
chiropractic medicine, 1; benefits of, 7; for headaches, 142; history, 6; osteopathic medicine and, 14
chiropractors, 7, 9, 15, 322; kinesiology used by, 18
Chlebowski, Rowan T., 271
chlorhexidine, 236
chloride, 63
cholecalciferol. *See* vitamin D (cholecalciferol)
cholesterol, 27–28, 291; beta-carotene and, 6; chromium and, 67; coronary artery disease and, *285;* drugs to lower, 28; exercise lowers, 99, 138; fiber and, 139; hawthorn berry and, 87; heart attack risk and, 285; impotence and, 191; lipids and, 28; meditation and, 11; spirulina and, 81; testing for, 28; vitamin B3 and, 43; vitamin C and, 48, 51
Chopra, Deepak, 4, 10, 318, 324
"The Chopra Prescriptions," 4
chorionic-villus sample testing (CVS), 214
chromium, 67, 72
chromium chloride supplementation, 67
chromosome 19; Alzheimer's disease and, 305
Chronic Fatigue and Immune Dysfunction Syndrome Association, 152
chronic illness; massage benefits for, 17; preventing, 2, 40
Chung-Kuo Chung Hsi i Chieh Ho Tas Chih, 88
Chuong, C. James, 75
Cichoke, Anthony, 89, 269
cigarettes, 169; cancer and, 115, 166, 263; stopping use of, 324; ulcers and, 150
circumcision, 224
Clark, Gregory, 178
Clark, Larry, 72

Classical Medicine Center, 255
claustrophobia, 181
Clinical Investigations, 287
Clinton, Bill, 179
clot-busting drugs, 287
Clozapine, 183
cluster headaches, 140, 141
CNMs. *See* certified nurse-midwives
cobalamin, 42
cobalt, 67; in cancer treatment, 267
coca plant, 162
cocaine, 155, 161, 162; alternative treatments for addiction to, 162–63; dangers of addiction to, 162; effect on body, *161;* withdrawal from, 162, 168
cochlear implants, 251
codeine, 164
coeliac disease, 46
coenzyme Q10, 201, 254, 295, 309
coenzymes; vitamin B2, 42; vitamin B9, 46
coffee; calcium and, 63; decaffeinated, 150; limiting consumption of, 28; substitutes for, 160; ulcers and, 150
coitus interruptus, 193
colds, 48
collateral circulation, 283
Collin, Jonathan, 318, 320–21, 323
colon cancer, 265; fat consumption and, 29; male obesity and, 33; meat consumption and, 29; prevention of, 28; toxins and, 122; vitamin D and, 52
colonic therapy, 147
colorectal cancer (Stage IV), 89, 269
Columbia School of Public Health, 217
The Complete Guide to Anti-Aging Nutrients (Hendler), 302
The Complete Sports Medicine Book for Women (Shangold), 208
complex carbohydrates, 26; cellulose and, 28; in fruits and vegetables, 27; stress reduc-

tion and, 131
composite fillings, 233
Comprehensive Headache Center
    at Germantown Hospital and
    Medical Center, 142
condoms, 193
conductive hearing loss, 251
congenital glaucoma, 246, 247
Connecticut, 12
*Conquest of Cancer: Vaccines
    and Diet* (Livingston), 271
constipation; during pregnancy,
    220; preventing, 28
Consumer Product Safety
    Commission, 118, 124
*Consumer Reports Health Answer
    Book,* 194
contact lenses, 244
Contributions to Nephrology, 16
copper, 67; in algae, 81; deficien-
    cy, 61, 68; excess of, 68;
    schizophrenia and levels of,
    184; sources of, 68
cornea, 243, 245; radial keratoto-
    my and, 249; reshaping, 249
coronary angiograph, 284
coronary arteries, 283
coronary artery disease (CAD),
    281, *284*; botanical medicine
    for, 287, 288; bypass
    surgery, and 286; exercise
    and, 288, *289*; plaque
    deposits and, 1; risk factors,
    284, 285, 286; Traditional
    Chinese Medicine for,
    292–93; vitamin and mineral
    therapy for, 293
coronary blockages, 282, 290
coronary bypass surgery, 286
coronary heart disease (CHD),
    281; prevention and treat-
    ment of, *291*
coronary occlusion, 283
coronary thrombosis, 283
Corsello, Serafina, 131
Corsello Centers for Nutritional
    Medicine, 131
Corti's arch, 256
corticosteroids, 62
cortisol, 17, 126, 177
cosmic consciousness, 11
Council on Chiropractic
    Education, 21
Cowden, William Lee, 290
crack cocaine, 162

cranberries, 83; treatment for
    bladder infections, 121
crash diets, 32
crataegus monogyna, 87–88
cretinism, 69
Crohn's disease, 68; folic acid
    deficiency and, 46; intestinal
    toxins and, 117
Crook, William, 308
cross-country skiing, 103, 104
Cummings, Stephen, 142, 180,
    258, 259
*Current Medical Diagnosis and
    Treatment* (Schroeder), 158
*Current Medical Research &
    Opinion,* 85, 307
CVS. *See* chorionic-villus sample
    testing (CVS)
cycling, 99
cylindrical implants, dental, 238
cystic fibrosis, 315; testing
    for, 215
cystic mastitis, 199. *See also*
    fibrocystic breast disease
cytomegalovirus, 219

D

daidzin, 159
dairy products, 30
danazol, 200
dance aerobics, 105
dandelion (taraxacum officinale),
    84, 121
danocrine, 200
Das, Arabinda, 253
Data, Katie, 251
Dausch, J., 85
D.C. *See* Doctor of Chiropractic
DDT, 114
de Keyser, J., 55
deafness, 250–51, 255
death; leading causes of, 13, 281;
    obesity and, 32
deep relaxation, *292*
deep-tissue muscle therapy, 18
degenerative bone condition, 17
degenerative diseases, 27
dehydration, 102
dehydroepiandrosterone sul-
    fate, 288
Delicious, 131
dementia, 306
DeNardo, Gerald, 268

dental amalgams, 253
dental care, 229–31, 240
dental cavities, 240; chromium
    and, 67; fluoride and, 232;
    kinetic cavity preparation
    and, 234; plaque and, 229;
    sweets and, 231; types of
    fillings for, 233–34. *See also*
    oral hygiene
dental chewing gum, 232
dental hygienists, 235
dental implants, 238–39; guide-
    lines for, *238*; risks associat-
    ed with, 239
dental infections, 229
dental insurance plans, 232
dental plaque, 68
dental sealants, 232
dental surgery, 3
dental X-rays, 239
Dental Products Report, 240
dentine, 230
dentistry, 317
dentists; diagnosing disease, 229;
    guidelines for choosing,
    240; holistic, 233, 236, 239;
    tartar removal and, 235
dentures, 237–38
depression, 173, 184, 323;
    biofeedback and, 5; botani-
    cal therapies for, 176; caf-
    feine and, 160; causes of,
    175; in children, 178–79;
    deep breathing exercises for,
    176; in the elderly, 175–76;
    exercise for, 8, 177; heart
    disease and, 291; homeo-
    pathic therapies for, 177;
    lithium for, 177; major, 174;
    massage therapy for, 17,
    177; nutritional therapies
    for, 177–78; post-delivery,
    222; psychotherapy and,
    178–79; symptoms of, *174*;
    treatments for, 175; types of,
    174; vitamin and mineral
    therapies for, 179; vitamin
    B1 and, 42
"Depression: Lifting the Cloud,"
    175, 177
*Depression Is a Treatable Illness:
    A Patient's Guide,* 175
Derogatis, Leonard, 273
desipramine, 162
DET, 164

Medicine (Murray and Pizzorno), 28, 32, 42, 43, 63, 82, 288; on alcoholism treatments, 159; on bitter melon, 82; on botanical medicines, 130; on carnitine, 139; on chamomile, 83; on dementia, 306; on depression treatments, 176; on detoxifying kidneys, 121; on dong quai, 84; on ear inflammations, 254; on echinacea, 90; on goldenseal, 87; on hawthorn berry extracts, 144; on heart disease, 288; on high blood pressure, 146; on irritable bowel syndrome, 147, 148; on lymph system, 121; on ma huang, 88; on migraines, 143; on milk thistle, 89; on mistletoe, 89; on morning sickness, 220; on prostate health, 195; on sinusitis, 258; on sore throats, 259; on spleen, 121; on throat cankers, 260; on toxic heavy metals, 115; on ulcer treatment, 150; on yeast infections, 210

endometrial cancer, 45, 203
endometritis, 209
endorphins, 3, 17
endothelium-derived relaxation factor (EDRF), 288
endotoxins, 117
English chamomile, 83
enlarged prostate, 189, 194, 197. *See also* benign prostatic hypertrophy
Environmental Nutrition, 48, 50, 51, 246
Environmental Protection Agency (EPA), 118, 124, 166
EPA. *See* Environmental Protection Agency (EPA)
ephedrine, 88
epididymitis, 196
epidural anesthesia, 221
epigallocatechin gallate (EGCG), 87
Epilepsia, 55
epilepsy, 72
epileptic seizures, 55
episiotomies, 221
Epstein-Barr virus, 87

Ergonomics, 5
"error catastrophe" hypothesis, 299
esophageal cancer, 50, 67
esophagus, 259
essential fatty acids (EFA), 81, 206, 208
essential hypertension, 143, 146
Essential Nutrients in Carcinogenesis (Poirier), 45, 275, 276
estrogen, 200, 222; Alzheimer's disease and, 307; cancer risks and, 265; fibrocystic breast disease and, 201; menopause and, 201, 288, 307; osteoporosis and deficiency of, 310
estrogen replacement therapy, 202–3, 288; slowing of bone loss and, 310–11
ethyl alcohol, 156
ethylene dibromide (EDB), 238
European Archives of Psychiatry and Clinical Neuroscience, 10
European Cytokine Network, 90
European Journal of Cancer, 270
eustachian tube, 250, 254
evening primrose oil, 143; for ear infections, 255; for premenstrual syndrome, 206; prostate gland and, 196
Everybody's Guide to Homeopathic Medicine (Cummings and Ullman), 142, 180, 258, 259
Exceptional Cancer Patients, 273
exercise, 1, 8, 11, 26, 288, 318, 322; aerobic, 32, 102, 103; aging and, 302; benefits of, 8, 19, 97, 99–100, 131, 302, 321, 324; bulimia treatments and, 35; caffeinism and, 160; cancer and, 265; for children, 108–10; choosing program of, 99; depression and, 176; detoxification and, 123; disabled and, 108; elderly and, 109–11; goals, 101; for headache relief, 142; heart disease reversal and, 1, 97; for hypertension, 145–46; isometric, 101; lowering cholesterol and, 28,

138; maximum pulse rate and, 101; menopause and, 203, 311–12; precautions for, 101–2; pregnancy and, 180, 217; to prevent osteoporosis, 311–12; "Reversal Program" and, 13; starting program of, 98; for stress management, 66, 130, 133, 134; to treat alcoholism, 159; treating mental disorders with, 184; water-based, 109; for women, 199; at work, 107
exercise-induced asthma (EIA), 102, 110
exercise-talk test, 217
exhaustion, 126
exotoxins, 117
expectorant, 88
expert systems, 316
Exsosurf, 225
eyedrops, 247
eyeglasses, 249
eyes, 260; common problems with, *250*; drops for, 244; preventing damage to, *244*; vitamin A deficiency, 243

F

FA. *See* ferulic acid (FA)
Fackelmann, Kathy A., 54, 75
Fact Sheet on Heart Attack, Stroke and Risk Factors, 283
Fahrion, Steve, 247
fallopian tubes, 216
Family Health International, 311
Family Heart Study, 303
Farley, Dixie, 34
Farnsworth, N., 190
Farris, R. P., 31
farsightedness, 248
fats, 28–29, 35; in diets, 40; lowering, 31; polyunsaturated, 291; saturated, 27, 28, 291
fatty acids, 26
FDA. *See* Food and Drug Administration (FDA)
FDA Center for Devices and Radiological Health, 238
FDA Consumer Reports, 34, 232, 234, 237, 238
FEBS Letter, 82

146–47; vitamin C and, 50; vitamin, mineral, and botanical therapies for, 147. *See also* high blood pressure

hyperventilation, 181

hypervitaminosis A, 41

hypnosis, 9, 10, 150

hypnotherapists, 10

hypoglycemia, 177; vitamin D and, 52; zinc and, 74

hypothalamus, 17

hypothyroidism, 60, 176

hysterectomies, 3, 199

I

ibuprofen, 149

Idaho State University Senior Enhancing Lifelong Fitness program, 109

IDL. *See* intermediate-density lipoproteins (IDL)

IHD. *See* ischemic heart disease (IHD)

Imagawa, M., 309

immune augmentive therapies, 319

immune system; aging and decline in, 300; caffeine suppresses, 160; cancer and, 263, 264, 272, 277; dysfunction, 70; exercise and, 8, 110, 130; fighting and, 122; healthy teeth and, 229; meditation and, 11; protein and, 29; selenium and, 72, 73; social support and, 132; spirulina and, 82; toxins and, 2, 113, 114, 123; vitamin A and, 40; vitamin B12 and, 47; zinc and, 75

Immunobiology, 89

immunocompetence, 7

immunomodulating drugs, 320

immunostimulants, 69

immunotoxins, 116

impotence, 15

in vitro fertilization (IVF), 216

inactivity, *285*

inappropriate affect, 182

India; Ayurvedic medicine in, 4; exercise in, 107; spirulina growing project in, 81; traditional medicine in, 13;

xerophthalmia cases in, 41; yogic exercise from, 8

Indian Journal of Medical Research, 88

Indian sweat lodges, 333

indoor toxins and pollution, 119

indrubin, 274

industrial gases, 116

INED, 14

infant care, 213, 216, 222; feeding crying baby, *225;* formulas for, 222–23; nutrients for, 31; starting solid foods for, 225; Sudden Infant Death Syndrome, 226; teething and tooth care, 226, 230

infant massage, 224

infant mortality, 224

infertility, 215–16

influenza virus, 82

infusion, 80

injection therapy, 192

injuries; during exercise, 104–5

inner ear, 250

insecticides, 115

Insight, 249

insoluble salts, 61

insomnia, 173; botanical therapies for, 179; exercise and, 179; guidelines for good sleep, *180;* homeopathic therapies for, 180; hormone therapy for, 180; sleep therapy and, 180

Institute for Aerobics Research, 98, 265

Institute of Geriatrics, Xiyuan Hospital, Beijing, 301

insulin, 82; zinc and, 74

insulin repair, 323

insurance crisis, 322

integration, 318

Intelligence Quotient (IQ), 115

interferon, 88, 91, 121

intermediate-density lipoproteins (IDL), 27

intermittent claudication, 288

International Association for Cancer Victors and Friends, 279

International Chiropractors Association, 21, 105, 112

International Food Information Council, 102

International Foundation for Homeopathy, 21

International Journal of Cancer, 266

International Journal of Clinical & Experimental Hypnosis, 10

International Journal of Obesity, 32

International Units (IU), 51, 53

intestinal toxins, 117

Inuit (Greenland), 64

inulin; in echinacea, 90

iodine, 69; deficiency of, 69, 200; sources of, 69

iodized salt, 69

IQ. *See* Intelligence Quotient (IQ)

iris, 243, 247

irisquinone, 274

iron, 25, 69; deficiency of, 26, 41, 61, 70; detoxification and, 70; learning disabilities and, 70; mouth ulcers and, 71; sources of, 70; spirulina and, 81

iron sulfate, 81

iron supplementation, 70

irritable bowel syndrome, 63, 147; biofeedback and, 5; botanical therapies for, 147; calcium deficiency and, 63; colonic therapy for, 147; fiber and, 28; magnesium deficiency and, 65; nutritional therapies for, 147; stress reduction therapies for, 148

iscador, 270

ischemic heart disease (IHD), 54

isoleucine, 29

isometric exercises, 101

Isoptin, 190

Ito, N., 87

IU. *See* International Units (IU)

IVF. *See* in vitro fertilization (IVF)

J

Jahnke, R., 132

JAMA. *See Journal of the American Medical Association*

Janssen, O., 90

317, 319, 322, 323, 324
linoleic acid, 195
lipid peroxides, 138
lipids, 26, 28–29
lipoproteins, 27
lisinopril, 190
Listerine, 236
lithium, 71; algae and, 81; carbonate, 177
lithium ointment, 71
Liu, C., 86
liver; chi energy within, 3; cholesterol and, 27
liver disease, 117
Livingston, Virginia, 271
Livingston Foundation Medical Center, 272, 279
Livingston therapy, 271
London, R. S., 64
London School of Hygiene and Tropical Medicine, 125
Long Beach Press Telegram, 224
Long Island Jewish Medical Center, 209
longevity; exercise and, 109, 302; healthy breakfasts and, 303; shiitake mushrooms and, 91; vitamin C and, 50
Longevity, 27, 125
Louis Harris and Associates, 32
Love, Susan, 200
Love, Medicine & Miracles (Siegel), 10, 14, 263, 272, 277
low birth-weight babies, 216, 219
low-density lipoproteins (LDL), 27, 28; exercise and, 99, 138; ginseng and, 86; heart disease and, 295; spirulina and, 81; vitamin C and, 48
Lown Cardiovascular Center, 286
LSD, 155, 164, 165
Lu, W., 88
Ludvig Boltzmann Institute, Austria, 90
Lukas Klinik, Switzerland, 90
lung cancer, 41
lungs, chi energy within, 3
Lust, Benedict, 11, 12
lymphoma, 264, 269, 271, 272
lysergic acid diethylamide (LSD). *See* LSD
lysine, 29

M

Ma, Q., 183
ma huang (ephedra sinica), 88
macrophage phagocytosis, 90
macrophages, 265
macular degeneration, 248; biofeedback for, 248; nutritional therapies for, 248; surgery for, 249
Macular Degeneration: Major Cause of Central Vision Loss, 248
magnesium, 63, 74, 88, 143; bones and, 312; deficiency of, 64, 293; depression and, 317; sexual health and, 192; sources of, 63; stress and, 133; supplementation, 64
magnesium chelate, 203
magnesium citrate, 121
magnesium supplements, 65
Maharishi Amrit Kalash (MAK), 301
Maharishi Mahesh Yogi, 11, 301
maitake mushrooms (grifola frondosa), 88, 89; for prostate cancer, 269
MAK. *See* Maharishi Amrit Kalash (MAK)
male erectile dysfunction, 190. *See also* impotence
male health problems; benign prostatic hypertrophy, 193–96; impotence, 189–92; premature ejaculation, 193; prostatitis, 196–97
malignant tumors, 264
malnutrition, spirulina treatment for, 81
malocclusions, 236–37
mammogram, 200, 267
manganese, 67, 68, 121; algae and, 81; deficiency of, 71; disease prevention and, 71; epilepsy and, 72; sources of, 71
manganese SOD, 71
manganese supplementation, 72
manic depression; lithium and, 71; serotonin levels and, 176; zinc and, 75
mantra, 10, 11
mao-tung-ching (ilex puibeceus), 138, 292

MAP 30, 83
March of Dimes Birth Defects Foundation, 214
Margolis, Simeon, 306
marijuana, 155, 163
Marinelli, Rick, 194
Mark, Daniel, 291
Marti, James, on the future of alternative medicine, 325–29
Martin, M. F., 31
Martorano, Joseph, 208
Massachusetts Institute of Technology (MIT), 180
massage, 1, 2, 3, 4; deep, 18; depression and, 177; education in China, 17; headaches and, 141, 144; infant, 224; lowering blood pressure and, 290; lymphatic, 254; stress reduction and, 126, 129; treating mental disorder with, 184
mastoiditis, 254
maternal morbidity, and cesarean sections, 222
Maternal Serum Alpha-Fetoprotein test (MSAFP), 214
matricaria chamomilla, 83
maturity-onset diabetes, 67
MaxEPAS, 143
Maximum Life Span (Walford), 301
May, L., 52
Mayo Clinic, 30
Mayo Clinic Health Letter, 141
McGill University (Montreal), 225
McKinlay, John, 189, 190, 191, 192
meat, amino acids in, 29
M. D. Anderson Cancer Center of the University of Texas, 41
Medicaid, 8
Medical College of Pennsylvania, 200
Medical College of Virginia, 180
Medical College of Wisconsin, 132, 206
Medical Herbalism: A Clinical Newsletter for the Herbal Practitioner, 149
Medicare, 8
Medicine, Microbiology and Immunology, 71

throats, 259; on spleen, 121; on throat cankers, 260; on toxic heavy metals, 115; on ulcer treatment, 149; on yeast infections, 210

music therapy, 17

Mutual of Omaha, 13, 282

myelomas, 264

myocardial infarction, 283, 295. *See also* heart attacks

myocardium, 283

myoglobin, 69

myopia, 248–49

mysophobia, 181

N

NACA. *See* National Association of Childbirth Assistants (NACA)

nacardipine, 190

Nagai, T., 83

Nanjing Children's Hospital, 81

Naprosyn, 149

Naproxen, 149

NAS. *See* National Academy of Sciences (NAS)

nasal nicotine solutions, 167

nasal polyps, nutritional therapies for, 256–57

Nathan, Neil, 272

National Academy of Sciences (NAS), 30, 31, 164, 266

National Alliance for the Mentally Ill, 186

National Anorexic Aid Society, Inc., 36

National Association of Anorexia Nervosa and Associated Disorders, 36

National Association of Childbirth Assistants (NACA), 228

National Cancer Center Hospital, Tokyo, 274

National Cancer Institute, 49, 54, 85, 119, 269, 272, 273, 279, 303

National Center for Health Statistics (NCHS), 50, 219, 221, 224

National Center for Homeopathy, 9, 21

National Center for Research Resources, 180

National Center for Sleep Disorders—National Institutes of Health, 179

National Cholesterol Education Program Guidelines (American) Heart Association), *291*

National Chronic Fatigue Syndrome Association, 152

National Clearinghouse for Alcohol and Drug Information, 170

National College of Naturopathic Medicine, 200

National Commission for the Certification of Acupuncturists, 3, 21

National Council on Aging, Family Caregivers Program, 314

National Council on Alcoholism, 170

National Depressive and Manic Depressive Association, 186

National Digestive Disease Information Clearinghouse, 148, 152

National Exercise for Life Institute, 108

National Eye Institute, 250

National Eye Research Foundation, 261

National Foundation for Colitis, 152

National Foundation of Depressive Illness, 186

National Heart, Lung and Blood Institute, 286

National High Blood Pressure Education Program, 135

National High Blood Pressure Information Center, 152

National Institute on Aging, 180, 202, 302

National Institute of Allergy and Infectious Diseases, 198, 212, 241, 261

National Institute of Dental Research, 234, 236, 237, 241

National Institute of Diabetes and Digestive and Kidney Diseases, 147

National Institute of Hygiene (Budapest), 214

National Institute for Occupational Safety and Health (NIOSH), 124

National Institute of Mental Health (NIMH), 135, 173, 174, 175, 181, 182, 183, 186; Eating Disorders Program, 36

National Institute on Aging Information Center, 314

National Institutes of Health, 133, 217, 221

National Mental Health Association, 186

National Osteoporosis Association, 314

National Osteoporosis Foundation, 310

National Research Council, National Academy of Sciences, 36

National Sudden Infant Death Foundation, 228

National Women's Health Network, 212, 228, 241

Natural Healing, 89

Natural Health, 17, 87, 114, 131, 149, 177, 179, 180, 206, 208, 221, 226, 295, 310, 312

Natural Health, Natural Medicine (Weil), 6

natural killer (NK) cells, 265, 274

Natural Products Bureau of Drug Research, 141

Natural Resources Defense Council, 114

Naturopathic Applications of the Botanical Remedies (Mitchell), 83

naturopathic licensing; in Montana, 12; in Oregon, 12

naturopathic medicine, 1, 11, 12; consulting doctors of, *13;* degrees in, *12;* view of disease, *12*

naturopathy, 322, 324

NCHS. *See* National Center for Health Statistics (NCHS)

nearsightedness, 248

neem oil, 254

neodymium-iron-boron magnets, 237

nerve deafness, 251

nervous system, 27
network chiropractors, 6, 318
neural tube defect, 214; babies born with, 213; folic acid and, 46, 214; testing for, 215
neurofibrillary tangles, 305
Neurological Research Laboratory at the Bartholin Institute, Copenhagen, 157
neurotransmitters, 45, 184
Neustaedter, Randall, 255
neutrophils, 90
New Age Journal, 17
New Body, 125, 208
New England Journal of Medicine, 2, 41, 57, 109, 183, 302, 310, 311
New England Research Institute, 189
New York Hospital, Cornell Medical Center, 203
New York Medical College, 252
The New York Times Guide to Personal Health (Brody), 230, 237
New Zealand Medical Journal, 141
Newbold, H., 45
Ni, Maoshing, 245, 247, 308
niacin, 42, 43, 139, 143
niacinamide, 43, 44, 143
Nic-Anon, 170
nicotinamide, 184
nicotinamide adenine dinucleotide, 43
nicotine, 155, 166, 292; for addiction to, 167–68; aerosol, 167; alternative treatment in patches, 167; physiological effects of, 166; sleep quality and, 179
nicotinic acid, 43, 184
Nieman, D., 289
nifedipine, 190
NIMH. *See* National Institute of Mental Health (NIMH)
NIOSH. *See* National Institute for Occupational Safety and Health (NIOSH)
nitrates, 178; headaches and preservatives with, 142
nitrogen dioxide, 116
nitroglycerine, 283, 286, *294*
nitrous dioxide, 166
nitrous oxide, 221

NK. *See* natural killer (NK) cells
non-Hodgkin's lymphomas, 264
nonsteroidal anti-inflammatory drugs (NSAID), 149, 150
nontoxic healing methods, 12
norepinephrine, 17, 175, 177
nose, 243, 256, 257, 260
NSAID. *See* nonsteroidal anti-inflammatory drugs (NSAID)
nucleic acid, 47
nucleoprotein synthesis, 46
Nuprin, 149
nurse-midwives, holistic, 216
nutrition, *218, 322, 325;* aging and, 302–4; disease and deficiency in, 25; guidelines for, 30, *30;* natural, *25;* for optimal health, 13, 19, 31, 35; for pregnant women, 218–19; stress reduction and, 131, 134
Nutrition and Cancer, 50
Nutrition Research Newsletter, 53, 54
Nutrition Today, 33, 35
nutritional supplements, 13
nutritional therapy, for Alzheimer's disease, 308; for cancer, 266, 272; for cataracts, 245; for depression, 177–78; for enlarged prostate, 195; for headaches, 142; for heart disease, 290; for hypertension, 146; for impotence, 191; for macular degeneration, 248; for Meniere's disease (vertigo), 253; for menopause symptoms, 203; for menstrual cramps, 205; for nasal polyps, 257; for osteoporosis, 312; for otitis media, 255; for premenstrual syndrome, 207; for sinusitis, 258; stress reduction and, 134; for tinnitus, 256
nutritional yeast, 47

O

oats, 28
obeline, and smoking cessation, 168

obesity, 32–33, 70
objective response, 269
O'Brien, Jim, 141
obstetricians, holistic, 222
Occupational Safety and Health Administration (OSHA), 124
Office of Alternative Medicine—National Institutes of Health, 10, 21
Office on Smoking and Health, Public Information Branch, 170
Office of Technology Assessment, 272, 276
office toxins, 117
Ohio State University College of Medicine, 201
oil of cloves, 233
olive oil, 28
omega-3 fatty acids, 290
Oncology News, 269
onions, 139
ophediophobia, 181
ophthalmologist, 243
opiates, 156, 164
optic nerve, glaucoma and, 247
Optimal Aging Program—Medical College of Pennsylvania, 110
optimal health; Ayurvedic medicine and, 5; nutrition for, 13, 19
Optometric Extension Program Foundation, Inc., 261
oral cancer, 229
oral contraceptives; nutrient deficiencies and, 43, 46; vaginitis and, 209
oral hygiene, 230–31, 235, 240
Oregon Health Sciences University, 178
Organon of Medicine (Hahnemann), 9
organs, inflammation of, 29
Ornish, Dean, 286, 287, 288, 289, 290, 292, 295; "Reversal Program," 13
Ornstein, R., 74
orthodontic braces, 237
Orthomolecular Nutrition, 71
OSHA. *See* Occupational Safety and Health Administration (OSHA)
osteomalacia, 51, 63

osteopathic medicine, 14–15; for
menstrual cramps, 205
osteopaths, 9, 17, 18
osteoporosis; aging and, 299,
309–10; botanical medicines
for, 310; calcium supple-
ments for, 312; causes of,
310; coping therapies,
310–12; dong quai and, 84;
estrogen replacement and,
203, 288; exercise to prevent, 100, 110, 302, 311–12;
fluoride and, 68; inadequate
calcium and, 62, 224; magnesium and, 64; nutritional
therapies for, 312; phosphorus and, 65; postmenopausal,
310; risks for, 63; vitamin
and mineral therapies for,
312–15
otitis media, 254; Ayurvedic
medicine for, 254; botanical
medicines for, 255; chronic,
254; homeopathic remedies
for, 255; nutritional therapies for, 255; surgery for,
255; treatments of, 254;
types of, 254; vitamins and
minerals, 255
otoliths, 252
otosclerosis, 251, 256
outer ear, 250
ovarian cancer, 6
ovaries, 201, 204
overeating, 33
overexercise, 101
overtraining, 317
ovulation stimulation, 216
oxalic acid, 62
oxidation-reduction reactions, 67
oxygen circulation, and exercise, 99
oxysterols, 295
Ozaki, Y., 84

P

PABA, 118, 121
Pacific yew tree, 6
Paffenbarger, Ralph, Jr., 111, 302
*Pain in Infants, Children, and
Adolescents* (Yee and
Aubuchon), 2
Pakkenberg, Bente, 157

Palmer, Daniel David, 6
panax ginseng. *See* ginseng
panax quinquefolium, 86
panic disorders, 173, 181, 184;
causes of, 181; homeopathic
therapies, 182; psychotherapy for, 182; treatments
for, 181
Panos, Maesimund, 142
pantetheine, 295
pantothenic acid, 42, 88, 133
Pap smear, 266
Papaver somniferum, 164
papaverine injection therapy, 192
paradoxical intention, 182
paranoia, 182
paranoid schizophrenia, 182
parasympathetic cardiac arrhythmia, 5
Parent's Magazine, 215
Parker, G., 142
Parkinson's disease, 56–57
Patanjali, 15
Patient Care, 100, 106, 110
Pauling, Linus, 39, 53; vitamin C
recommendations by, 48, 49
PBS. *See* Public Broadcasting
System (PBS)
PCBs. *See* polychlorinated
biphenyls (PCBs)
PCP, 165
PDAT. *See* pre-senile dementia of
the Alzheimer's type
(PDAT)
PDD. *See* premenstrual dysphoric
disorder (PDD)
pectin, 115
pediatric sickle-cell anemia, 5
pellagra, 43
pelvic cancer, 9
pelvic inflammatory disease, 209
penis, 189
people with disabilities; calisthenics for, 107; exercise for, 98;
swimming and, 105
peptic ulcers, 148, 150
peptides, 17, 29
Perceptual and Motion Skills, 15
*Perfect Health: The Complete
Mind/Body Guide*
(Chopra), 4
perforated ulcer, 149
Peridex, 236
periodontal disease(s); advanced,
236; high copper levels and,

68; screening and recording,
235; selenium and, 73; slowing irreversible, 236
peripheral vision; glaucoma
and, 247
Perlman, David, 184, 235
Pero, Ronald, 7
pessimism; heart disease and, 291
pesticides, 29, 115
Petrov Research Institute of
Oncology, 271
Pettingale, Keith, 273
peyote, 164, 165
pharmaceutical drugs, 6, 79, 155;
advances in, 327
pharynx, 259
phencyclidine hydrochloride. *See*
PCP
phenylalanine, 29
Phenylbutazone, 83
phenytoin, 46
Phillips, S., 85
Phobia Society of America, 186
phobias, 173, 184; causes of, 181;
homeopathic therapies for,
182; hypnosis and, 10; psychotherapy for, 182; simple,
181; social, 181; treatments
for, 181; visualization
and, 15
phosphorus, 65; for healthy teeth,
229; sources of, 65
photoreflective keratotomy, 249
phycocyanin, 81
physical therapists, 15
physically challenged people, athletic competitions and, 109
physicians, holistic, *16,* 19
*Physician's Handbook: The
Livingston-Wheeler Medical
Clinic* (Livingston), 271
phytates, 74
phytoestrogens, 203, 310
piezoelectricity, 311
Ping-Pong, 106
piroxicam, 149
Pizzorno, Joseph, 28, 32, 63, 82,
138, 210, 306, 309; on alcoholism treatments, 159; on
bitter melon, 82; on botanical medicines, 130; on carnitine, 139; on chamomile, 83;
on depression treatments,
176; on detoxifying kidneys,
121; on dong quai, 84; on

and, 10; pregnancy and, 219; stopping, 3, 28, 292
sobriety, 168
Social Readjustment Rating Scale, *127–29*
social supports; cancer and, 272–74; stress reduction and, 132
Society of American Gastrointestinal Endoscopic Surgeons, 279
Sodhi, Virender, 138, 144, 194, 196, 251, 253, 254, 306
sodium, 63, 66, 291; deficiency of, 66; sources of, 66
sodium chloride, 63
solid extracts, 81
sorbitol, 232
Sound, Listening and Learning Center, 261
Southern Illinois School of Medicine, 142
Southern Medical Journal, 252
Southwest College, Arizona, 12
Sowers, Fran, 224
soybeans, 310
Special Olympics, 109
Spencer, J., 252
sphincteric incontinence, 5
Spiegel, David, 10, 14, 15, 273
spina bifida, 213
spinal cord injuries, 5
spinal fractures, 310
spinal manipulation, 6, 7. *See also* chiropractic medicine
spiral relaxation, 132
spirulina, 323; benefits of, 81–82; nutrients in, 81; species of, 81
Spirulina: Nature's Superfood (Morgan and Moorhead), 81
spleen; chi energy within, 3; functions of, 121
spontaneous abortion, 214
Springer, Eileen, 217
squamous-cell carcinoma, 118
squeeze technique, 193
St. John's Wort (hypericum perforatum), 176
standardized extracts, of botanical medicine, 81
Stanford University, 302
Stanford University Hospital, 273
Stanford University Medical Center, 2, 4

Stanford University School of Medicine, 15, 111
starch, 27
starvation diets, 32
state of mind, 318
Steinman, David, 87
Stephan, Peter, 191
Stephan Clinic (London), 191
Stephens, Paul, 233
steroid-dependent asthma, 16
steroids, 247
Still, Andrew Taylor, 14
stillbirth, 214
stirrup, 254
Stoney, Catherine, 291
STP, 164
strabismus, 250
strength training; building of bones and, 311; heart health and, 302
strep throat, 259
streptokinase, 287
stress, 126; biofeedback and, 5, 150; coping with, 125, 129, 134; diet and, 131; disabilities and disorders and, 126; exercise reduces, 100, 131; hormones and, 17; job-related, 125; measuring levels of, 126; potassium and, 66; the Social Readjustment Rating Scale and, *127–29*; therapies to reduce, 125, 134; ulcers and, 150. *See also* relaxation; "relaxation response"
stress incontinence, 202
The Stress Protection Plan (Chaitow), 178
stress reduction; beta-carotene and, 6; exercise hints for, 131; heart disease and, 295; hypertension therapies for, 146; for irritable bowel syndrome, 148; meditation and, 11, 125; social supports and, 132; summary of therapies for, *134*; yoga and, 15, 125, 150, 295
Stress Reduction Clinic—University of Massachusetts, 134
Stress Without Distress (Selye), 126
stroke, 138; as cause of death, 13; preventing, 39

Strome, M., 252
strychnine alkaloids, 191
strychnos nux vomica, 191
subluxations, 6, 7
substantia nigra, 56
sucrose, 26
sudden cardiac death (SCD), 284
Sudden Infant Death Syndrome (SIDS), 226
sugar, 26, 31
sugarless gum, 230, 232
Suharno, D., 42
suicide, 173
sulfur, 67; sources of, 67
sulfur dioxide, 116
sunflower oil, 28
sunglasses, 244, 245
sunlight radiation, 118
Sunnybrook Health Sciences Centre, 253
sunscreen lotions, 118
super foods, 323
superoxide dismutase, 71
supragingival plaque, 235
surfactant, 225
surgery, 267, 268, 273
Swartout, Glen, 244
Sweden; banning of amalgam fillings in, 234; dental implants in, 238
swimming, 102, 103, 105, 109
Sydiskis, R., 82
Syme, Leonard, 132
"Synthetic Antineoplastons and Analogs," 268
Syracuse Cancer Research Institute, 270, 279

T

table salt. *See* sodium chloride
Tagamet, 149
tai chi, 2, 8, 107, 131, 133, 181, 218, 322
tamoxifen, 200
Tanizaki, Y., 16
tannic acids, 230
Tao, 2
taraxacum officinale, 84
Tarotogenesis, Carcinogenesis & Mutagenesis, 87
Tarp, U., 73
tartar, 235
taxol, 6

W

Waite, P., 141
Walford, Roy, 301
Walker, Morton, 194
walking; benefits of, 99, 106;
    brisk, 103, 104, 109; stress
    reduction and, 131;
    water, 110
The Walking Handbook
    (Johnson), 106
Walsh, B., 84
Walsh, William, 184
Wang, G., 274
Warren, Tom, 307–8
water, 25, 26, 35; exercise pro-
    grams, 110; fortified with
    fluoride, 232, 233; toxins in,
    119–20; walkers, 110
Water Piks, 231
wax, ear, 251
Wedeen, R., 115
weight control, 10, 100
weightlifting, progressive, 145
weight-loss programs, 32, 33
Weil, Andrew, 6, 84, 85, 91, 143
Weinhouse, Beth, 257, 258
Weintraub, Michael, 252
Weisman, Thomas, 6, 7, 317,
    319, 322
Weiss, Ed, 317, 320, 321,
    323, 324
Weiss, Gillian, 251
Weiss, Rick, 8
Weizman, Jody, 206
Well Being Journal, 147
Wellness Medicine (Ander-
    son), 76
West, 239
Western Psychiatric Institute and
    Clinic, 178
WHO. *See* World Health
    Organization (WHO)
whole foods, 13
*Wiener Medizinische
    Wochenschrift,* 86
Wikstrom, J., 73
Wilbur, JoEllen, 203
Williams, D., 270
Williams, Gurney, III, 125
withdrawal; from alcohol 156;
    from central nervous system

depressants, 166; from
    cocaine, 162; from drugs,
    156, 330; from nicotine,
    168; from opiates, 164
Wolf, Michele, 98, 265
Wolfe, Honora Lee, 205
women; health guidelines for, 201
Woodside, D. B., 35
worker's compensation, 8
World Health Organization
    (WHO), 3, 6, 30, 55
World Journal of Surgery, 5
*World Medicine: The EastWest
    Guide to Healing Your Body*
    (Monte), 15
Wray, D., 71
Wurtman, Richard, 180

X

X-ray therapy, 267
X-rays, 219
xanthine oxidase, 290
xerophthalmia, 41
xin shen ling (XSL), 183
XJL, 159
XSL. *See* xin shen ling (XSL)
xylitol, 232

Y

Yale University School of
    Medicine, 132
yams; Mexican, 6; wild, 203, 310
Yau, Terrence, 54
yeast infections, 201, 202; aci-
    dophilus and, 209; botanical
    medicines for, 210; homeo-
    pathic medicines for, 210;
    preventing, 209; symptoms
    of, 208; treatments for, 209;
    vitamin and mineral thera-
    pies for, 210
yin and yang, 2
Yo San University of Traditional
    Chinese Medicine, 245, 308
Yoder, Barbara, 162, 167
yoga, 14–15, 19, 181; cancer
    treatment and, 4; headaches
    and, 143; for heart disease

reversal, 1, 295; high blood
    pressure and, 290; pregnan-
    cy and, 218; relaxation
    responses through, 129, 133;
    relaxation responses
    through, 134; "Reversal
    Program" and, 13
yogis, 15
Your Health, 141, 142, 143, 159,
    180, 206, 208, 237, 246,
    255, 270
*Your Nature, Your Health—
    Chinese Herbs in
    Constitutional Therapy*
    (Dharmananda), 192, 193
"yo-yo cycle," 161
Yuan, Chung San, 138, 292

Z

Zestril, 190
zhuling polysaccharide, 274
Zimmerman, David, 193,
    208, 236
*Zimmerman's Guide to
    Nonprescription Drugs*
    (Zimmerman), 39, 193,
    209, 233
zinc, 67, 73, 88; adrenal glands
    and, 133; AIDS and, 74;
    alcoholism treatments and,
    158; in algae, 81; benefits
    of, *75;* cancer and, 266; for
    cataracts, 246; deficiency of,
    61, 74, 301; depression and,
    179; diabetes and, 74; head
    injuries and, 74; HIV and,
    74; immune system disease
    and, 75; liver and, 121;
    lymph detoxification and,
    122; premenstrual syndrome
    and, 75; prostate disorders
    and, 195; rheumatoid arthri-
    tis and, 75; sex drive and,
    191; sources of, 74; for
    ulcers, 150
zinc sulfate, 248
zinc supplementation, 75
zoophobia, 181